Medical Terminology Basics

Medical Terminology Basics

PROGRAMMED INSTRUCTION

Y. H. Hui, PhD

Science Technology System

JONES AND BARTLETT PUBLISHERS

Sudbury, Massachusetts

BOSTON   TORONTO   LONDON   SINGAPORE

World Headquarters

Jones and Bartlett Publishers
40 Tall Pine Drive
Sudbury, MA 01776
978-443-5000
info@jbpub.com
www.jbpub.com

Jones and Bartlett Publishers
Canada
6339 Ormindale Way
Mississauga, Ontario L5V 1J2
Canada

Jones and Bartlett Publishers
International
Barb House, Barb Mews
London W6 7PA
United Kingdom

Jones and Bartlett's books and products are available through most bookstores and online booksellers. To contact Jones and Bartlett Publishers directly, call 800-832-0034, fax 978-443-8000, or visit our website, www.jbpub.com.

Substantial discounts on bulk quantities of Jones and Bartlett's publications are available to corporations, professional associations, and other qualified organizations. For details and specific discount information, contact the special sales department at Jones and Bartlett via the above contact information or send an email to specialsales@jbpub.com.

The author, editor, and publisher have made every effort to provide accurate information. However, they are not responsible for errors, omissions, or for any outcomes related to the use of the contents of this book and take no responsibility for the use of the products and procedures described. Treatments and side effects described in this book may not be applicable to all people; likewise, some people may require a dose or experience a side effect that is not described herein. Drugs and medical devices are discussed that may have limited availability controlled by the Food and Drug Administration (FDA) for use only in a research study or clinical trial. Research, clinical practice, and government regulations often change the accepted standard in this field. When consideration is being given to use of any drug in the clinical setting, the health care provider or reader is responsible for determining FDA status of the drug, reading the package insert, and reviewing prescribing information for the most up-to-date recommendations on dose, precautions, and contraindications, and determining the appropriate usage for the product. This is especially important in the case of drugs that are new or seldom used.

Production Credits

Publisher: David Cella
Acquisitions Editor: Kristine Jones
Associate Editor: Maro Gartside
Production Manager: Julie Champagne Bolduc
Production Assistant: Jessica Steele Newfell
Marketing Manager: Grace Richards
Manufacturing and Inventory Control Supervisor: Amy Bacus
Interior Design and Composition: Publishers' Design and Production Services
Cover Design: Kristin E. Parker
Cover Image: © Madartists/Dreamstime.com
Printing and Binding: Malloy, Inc.
Cover Printing: Malloy, Inc.

Library of Congress Cataloging-in-Publication Data

Hui, Y. H. (Yiu H.)
    Medical terminology basics : programmed instruction / Y. H. Hui.
            p. cm.
    Includes bibliographical references and index.
    ISBN 978-0-7637-6618-4 (pbk. : alk. paper)
    1. Medicine—Terminology—Programmed instruction.   I. Title.
    R123.H85 2010
    610.1'4—dc22
        2009019780

6048

Printed in the United States of America

14   13   12   11   10   10 9 8 7 6 5 4 3 2

Contents

Preface

Academic books on medical terminology began to appear in the United States in the late 1950s and early 1960s. At that time, most authors were professors teaching medical terminology courses to college students in a health field. Many of us respect their creativity, dedication, and decision to publish college textbooks in this relatively new discipline in the United States. They received little guidance from other textbooks on medical terminology and relied more on personal experience gained from clinical settings and teaching in a health field.

Over the last 50 years, medical terminology has evolved into a required course for most careers in the allied health fields, such as nursing, physical therapy, and clinical laboratory service. With millions of students enrolled in medical terminology courses, the number of available college textbooks has risen into the hundreds, including both print and electronic media.

The traditional and basic design of the contents of a medical terminology book varies according to the extent of coverage, course units, didactic approaches, student competency, and many other considerations. The contents in *Medical Terminology Basics: Programmed Instruction* are based on a didactic approach using programmed instruction and are designed to achieve these goals:

1. Successful learning of the basics of medical terminology by repetitive processes

2. Obligatory, but minimal, supervision by an instructor

3. Flexibility for both instructors and students: supervision, self-regulated progress, and time portioned for a step-by-step teaching and learning approach

4. Fulfillment of academic requirements for a course on the basics of medical terminology

The introduction of this book provides further details about these four goals. There are only a few medical terminology books that use programmed instruction because its acceptance as a classroom text is dependent on two important academic considerations: 1) curriculum requirements and 2) the unique profile or needs of students. You, as instructors and students, will determine if this book has fulfilled your expectations in teaching and learning objectives.

With the advance of the Internet, *Medical Terminology Basics: Programmed Instruction* makes full use of the resource powers of the electronic medium to accomplish the goals of the printed product. Supplements are available for students and instructors, including interactive websites and downloadable resources. Visit http://healthprofessions.jbpub.com/medtermbasics/preview for more information about the extensive online supplements available with this text.

I hope that this book and the accompanying electronic resources will serve all of your needs. I welcome comments on the general and specific approaches of this book and its websites as well as reports of any errors.

—Y.H. Hui

Acknowledgments

I am grateful to one special colleague, among others, for the completion of *Medical Terminology Basics: Programmed Instruction*—my long-time partner in writing and publishing, Peggy Stanfield. In 1993, we completed a 900-page manuscript on programmed instruction in medical terminology. For reasons beyond our control, the project was never published. In 2001, she gave me permission to *select*, *use*, *revise*, and *update* parts of the manuscript in order to prepare a smaller book on medical terminology using the same didactic approaches. It took nearly 10 years for me to complete this new project. Without her assistance—and blessing—it is unlikely that *Medical Terminology Basics: Programmed Instruction* would have been published.

We all know how hard it is to prepare the manuscript for a technical book. Actually, the production of both a book and its accompanying websites poses equal difficulty, though the challenges are of a different type. Many people were involved in the production of this book and its websites. I have been fortunate to have a number of committed people from Jones and Bartlett lend their support and expertise to the finished product. You are the best judge of the quality of their work.

Introduction: A Guide to Using This Book

Pronunciations

For many of us, pronouncing a medical word is difficult. In learning medical terminology, the process is easier if we learn to pronounce the words at the same time we learn their meanings. Traditionally, the pronunciation of any word in the English language is governed by phonetics, rules, and symbols, as outlined in reliable dictionaries for various disciplines. Unfortunately, each reference source carries its own set of symbols to represent various sounds as determined by the author or the publisher in any discipline, medical or otherwise. This is especially true when a source uses symbols of various origins, such as Greek, Latin, mathematical, chemical, and so on. The macron (ā) and breve (ă) diacritical marks are very common. Authors, editors, and publishers of medical terminology are very careful in choosing their pronunciation symbols when the intended users of a book are undergraduate students, especially freshmen or sophomores. Depending on the target audience, books on medical terminology implement one of the following pronunciation systems:

1. Traditional phonetics in the English language with rules and symbols

2. Traditional phonetics in the English language with rules and no symbols

3. Applicable phonetics using simple rules only

4. A combination of the above approaches

This book uses Option 2 with selected application of Option 4. In general, pronunciation is indicated by a simple phonetic spelling with no *diacritical* markings, as indicated below.

1. The primary accent is indicated by an underline, e.g., cerebellum (seh′-reh-<u>bel</u>-um).

2. The secondary accent is indicated by (′), e.g., cerebellum (seh′-reh-<u>bel</u>-um).

3. When an unmarked vowel ends a syllable, it is long, e.g., immune (i-mun′).

4. When a syllable ends with a consonant, its unmarked vowel is short, e.g., cranial (<u>kra</u>-ne-al).

To give you a frame of reference, the following list shows how diacritical markings or symbols can be used in addition to the four simple phonetic rules above to indicate the pronunciation of a medical term.

1. A *long* vowel sound is indicated by a macron (ˉ), as in the examples below:
   a   urease (u̱-re-ās); abate (ah-bāt)
   e   lead (lēd); scabies (ska̱-bēz)
   i   askaracide (as-ka̱r-ah-sīd); bile (bīl)
   o   ohms (ōmz); hormone (ho̱r-mōn)
   u   ampule (a̱m-pūl); femur (fe̱-mūr)
   oo   oophoron (oo-fōr-on)

2. A *short* vowel that *is* the syllable or that *ends* the syllable is indicated by a breve (˘):
   a   apophysis (ă-po̱f-i-sis)
   e   edema (ĕ-dē̱m-ah); effusion (ĕ-fū̱s-ion)
   i   immunity (ĭ-mŭ̱n-i-te′); oxidation (oks′-sĭ-da̱-shun)
   o   otic (ŏ-tic); official (ŏ-fi̱sh-al)
   u   avoirdupois (av-er-dû-poiz)
   oo   book (bŏ̱ok)

Coverage and Goals

How much information is covered in any college medical terminology book depends on many factors, such as:

1. Whether the book is intended to be used as reference or as an undergraduate text

2. Competency of targeted users

3. Length of the college course

4. Depth and breadth of information

5. Didactic approaches

   Medical Terminology Basics: Programmed Instruction is designed for an introductory course on basic medical terminology and for students and instructors who prefer a book with some flexibility in the teaching and learning process. It is not intended to be comprehensive.

   This book features a repetitive learning process, which means that each medical term and its components are repeated at least twice (and sometimes more) in each chapter. The number of terms that can be included in this book is consequently limited by such an approach. The aspects of basic physiology and anatomy are explained when applicable to a particular medical term, but it is expected that the student will rely on other resources for more detail. The medical terms related to the most common body systems are presented, since it is impossible and impractical to cover all aspects of the human body systems.

   The basic goals of this book are:

1. The student will learn the most basic medical terms in order to form a foundation for education or training in an allied health field.

2. The student will achieve this goal in the shortest or minimum possible time required by the educational curriculum and course credits.

3. The student can achieve this goal in or outside a classroom, assuming proper supervision is exercised.

Student Activities

Beginning with Chapter 3, students learn medical terms in *Medical Terminology Basics: Programmed Instruction* by using three basic approaches:

1. The first part of each chapter provides programmed instructions. If students complete this part as directed, they will learn the basic medical terms covered in the chapter.

2. The second part of each chapter provides a Progress Check that reinforces the terms the student learned in the first part of the chapter.

3. The websites accompanying this book are another source of student activities. Visit http://healthprofessions.jbpub.com/medtermbasics/preview for details.

Supplemental Tools

Each chapter profiles two boxes of supplemental information. As these supplemental tools are not discussed within the blocks, the boxes will not be cited or referred to in the text.

Students taking this course are either enrolled in a college health program or interested in doing so. One box in each chapter provides a short description of several careers in the health professions. The goal of these boxes is to assist students in making educated decisions about their future career ambitions.

The second box in each chapter provides a short list of abbreviations that are important in the medical field. The abbreviations are tested in the Progress Check for each chapter. The best way for students to learn medical abbreviations is, of course, in a clinical setting; students will have a chance to do so when they work in the medical field.

Premises

The students should be aware of the following premises when using this or any other medical terminology college textbook:

1. *Terms coverage.* There are hundreds of thousands of medical terms in the health field, as illustrated by available dictionaries, some of which contain as many as 5000 printed pages. Frequently, some terms are present in some texts but not in others.

2. *Word parts.* The technique in each book is to teach students the basic components of each medical term so they will know how to develop medical terms from such components. This presents two challenges. First, many medical terms cannot be developed because they do not comply with the rules governing word components. Second, some medical terms do not have components; they are simply medical terms by themselves and cannot be built from standard components taught in available textbooks.

3. *Pronunciations.* Most textbooks try to be consistent when they present the phonetic spellings of medical terms. No two books use the same system of phonetic spelling.

Students can best obtain clarifications from their instructors. Using Internet search engines is currently the preferred method of learning and ascertaining more details about specific medical terms.

Learning and Teaching Resources on the Website

This book has a website that provides additional learning and teaching resources for students and instructors. Visit http://healthprofessions.jbpub.com/medtermbasics/ preview for more information.

The Fundamentals of Personalized Instruction Programs

Using the Blocks

BLOCK	DATA AND ANSWERS	DESCRIPTIONS AND QUESTIONS
1-1		A personalized instructional program (PIP) is designed to help you learn subject matter with minimal supervision from your instructor. One such program uses a block, which is usually one or more lines of words containing one or more blanks (_____). The blank is in the right column. Write your answer in this blank and then compare your answer with the correct answer, given in the left column.
	PIP block	You have just learned the definition of ___PIP___, and an example of one such program is a ___block___. Compare your answers with the answers provided.
1-2	feedback	One benefit of using a PIP is feedback. By checking the answer, you provide yourself with ___feedback___. Look at the answer now.
1-3	instant	Another benefit of a PIP is instant feedback. When you check the answer, the feedback is ___instant___. Look at the answer now.
1-4	pace	A PIP gives you the opportunity to learn at your own ___pace___. Check the answer now.
1-5	homework	Some instructors assign sections of a PIP as homework to supplement lectures or another required textbook. If so, the assignment becomes ___homework___ like any other reading assignment. Check the answer now.

3

BLOCK	DATA AND ANSWERS	DESCRIPTIONS AND QUESTIONS
1-6	test answer	Other instructors assign sections of a PIP as a test for some classroom lectures. To treat this assignment as a _test_ , you must cover the _answer_ column. Check the answer now.
1-7	check	To use PIP properly and efficiently, you will need to use some basic guides. One guide is checking the answer. Always _check_ the answer after you have filled in a blank space.
1-8	correct	Another guide is to make sure that you correct your wrong answer. If you check the answer and it is different from yours, you must _correct_ it.
1-9	go back do not skip	Another important guide is to never skip any block as you proceed. It is essential that you do not skip any block because each block builds upon the previous one. You can always go back to previous blocks to review. In a PIP you can _go back_ to check some previous blocks, but please _do not skip_ any block by jumping ahead.
1-10	personalized instructional program usually one or more lines of words containing one or more blanks	A PIP is a _personized instructional program_. A block is _usually one or more lines of words containing one or more blanks_
1-11	check correct	Always _check_ the answer after you have filled in the blank space(s). Always _correct_ your answer if it is wrong.

BLOCK	DATA AND ANSWERS	DESCRIPTIONS AND QUESTIONS
1-12	instant feedback pace	By checking the answer, you receive ___instant feedback___ on the correctness of your answer. A PIP permits you to learn subject matter at your own ___pace___.
1-13	medical terminology health	What is medical terminology? Every health field has its own vocabulary. All health professionals have a basic understanding of medical words, although to a different extent. For example, a dental hygienist knows fewer medical terms than a dentist does, but they both have the same basic background training in or understanding of medical terminology. That is why you are required to take a course in ___medical___ ___terminology___: because you are planning a career in the ___health___ field.
1-14	terms	How will you learn medical terminology? Now that you are familiar with the procedures and mechanics involved in using a PIP, you will be introduced to the scientific discipline of medical terminology. This is the study of medical terms, words, vocabulary, glossaries, descriptions, and names. For convenience, we will call all of these "terms." Medical terminology is the study of medical ___terms___.
1-15	communicate	By acquiring a basic knowledge of the components of medical terms, all health professionals can communicate with one another. The objective of learning medical terminology is to make sure that all individuals in the health care field can ___communicate___ with one another when medical terms are involved.

BLOCK	DATA AND ANSWERS	DESCRIPTIONS AND QUESTIONS
1-16		You will learn a specific number of medical terms by using the PIP system in one of three ways designed by your instructor.
		In one method, the instructor assigns the students to study certain blocks in one class meeting. During the next meeting, the instructor gives a test on those blocks. This simple
	blocks	arrangement requires you to study certain _blocks_ and
	test	take a _test_.
1-17		In a second approach, the instructor requires students to study specific lectures and then assigns blocks as homework to prepare for the next class, discussion, or quiz. That is,
	lectures	the students must study the _lectures_ and the
	assigned blocks	_assigned_ _blocks_.
1-18		In a third approach, the instructor lectures from one textbook and gives home assignments from this book. The student
	both (or	is expected to learn the material in _both_ _or_
	two)	_two_ books on medical terminology.
1-19		The remaining units in this book will help you to master medical terminology in two stages. During the first stage you will learn the basics of using word components or parts to understand and build medical terms.
	two	In the PIP system, there are _two_ stages in learning
	build	medical terminology. The first stage teaches you to _build_
	terms, components	medical _terms_ from word _components_
	parts	or _parts_.

BLOCK	DATA AND ANSWERS	DESCRIPTIONS AND QUESTIONS
1-20		The second stage is to apply the knowledge acquired in the first stage to build medical terms for specific body organs, functions, clinical conditions, and disorders.
	medical terms	First, you learn how to build _medical_ _terms_
	components, parts	from word _components_ or _parts_.
	medical terms	Then, you will use the same approach to build _medical_ _terms_ from word
	components, parts	_components_ or _parts_ for specific body
	organs, functions, clinical	_organs_, _functions_, _clinical_
	conditions, disorders	_conditions_, and _disorders_.
1-21		The next unit provides you with eight keys to building medical terms using their components or parts.
	eight	That is, using the _eight_ keys, you will learn how to put
	components	together the appropriate word _components_
	parts, medical	or _parts_ to build all types of _medical_
	terms	_terms_.

Eight Keys to Building Medical Terms

BLOCK	DATA AND ANSWERS	DESCRIPTIONS AND QUESTIONS
2-1	words	Words in the English language, including medical terms, are made up of component parts. By systematically combining these component parts, we can construct _____ in any scientific discipline, especially the medical field. Refer to **Table 2.1** (which contains the word roots, combining forms, prefixes, and suffixes relevant to the medical field).
2-2	word root, root word	Every word has a root, sometimes also known as a base or a stem. We also can call it a word root, word base, or word stem. Some textbooks use the term "word root," some use "root word," and some use these terms interchangeably—which is what this book does. Thus, the fundamental component of a word is known as the _____ _____ or _____ _____.
2-3	terms eight keys	This book provides eight keys to building medical terms from word roots. Note that, although this book uses eight keys, you may see other books that give eight, nine, or ten keys. Ask your instructor for guidance when comparing different systems. You will be learning how to build medical _____ by using _____ _____.

TABLE 2.1   Word Components in this Chapter

WORD ROOTS	COMBINING FORMS	PREFIXES
ache	angi/o	a-
bile	bil/i	an-
cholecyst	cardi/o	anti-
cusis	cerebr/o	brady-
cyan	cor/e	de-
derma	enter/o	dis-
dermat	erythr/o	dys-
endometr	gastr/o	eu-
erythr	hem/o	ex-
feca	lapar/o	hemi-
fore	laryng/o	hemo-
gall	lymph/o	hyper-
gastr	melan/o	mal-
genesis	myc/o	pan-
head	nat/a	quadri-
infect	nephr/o	**SUFFIXES**
lapar	neur/o	-al
muc	oncy/o	-algia
neur	oste/o	-cytes
nutrition	ot/o	-ectasis
ophthalm	pelv/i	-emia
pareun	psych/o	-gram
phobia	rachi/o	-ia
presby	rhin/o	-itis
skin	stomat/o	-logist
spinal	trache/o	-logy
stenosis		-lysis
stomat		-metry
stone		-osis
tension		-ous
therapy		-pathy
toxin		-phoria
zoo		-plegia
		-pnea
		-porosis
		-scopy
		-tion
		-tocia
		-us

BLOCK	DATA AND ANSWERS	DESCRIPTIONS AND QUESTIONS
2-4		Medical terms derive from English, French, German, Spanish, Greek, Italian, Latin, and many other languages. The eight keys described here are applicable to the majority of the medical terms used in this country by a variety of health professionals. Of course, there are exceptions to every key. Consider the following. First, different medical dictionaries may provide different definitions, pronunciations, and/or word parts for the same medical term. Second, one instructor's interpretation of a medical term (meaning, pronunciation, and/or word parts) may differ from that of another instructor. Consult your instructor if you come across such variations.

BOX 2.1

Allied Health Professions

Medicine: cardiovascular technologists and technicians, nuclear medicine technologists, surgical technologists, medical assistants

Dentistry: dental hygienists, dental assistants

Nursing: registered nurses, licensed practical nurses, licensed vocational nurses

Pharmacy: pharmacy technicians, pharmacy aides

Dietetics: dietitians, dietetic technicians, dietetic assistants

Optometry: dispensing opticians

Emergency Medical Services: emergency medical technicians and paramedics

Imaging Modalities: radiologic technologists and technicians, radiation therapists

Respiratory Care: respiratory therapists

Physical Therapy: physical therapists, physical therapists assistants and aides

Veterinary Medicine: veterinary technologists and technicians, animal care and service workers

Miscellaneous: clinical laboratory (medical) technologists and technicians; medical, dental, and ophthalmic laboratory technicians; nursing, psychiatric, and home health aides; medical assistants

Source: P. S. Stanfield, N. Cross, Y. H. Hui, eds. *Introduction to the Health Professions*, 5th ed. (Sudbury, MA: Jones & Bartlett, 2009).

BLOCK	DATA AND ANSWERS	DESCRIPTIONS AND QUESTIONS
2-5		A word root has many characteristics including but not limited to the following: 1. It is usually derived from Greek or Latin. 2. It is the foundation upon which other components of a word are attached. 3. It can be a noun, an adjective, and so on. 4. It can occur as a simple group of letters derived from the first part of a complete word, such as a noun or an adjective. This is more common than other forms. 5. Although a word root in a medical term usually refers to a part of the body, it is not always so. All forms of word roots will be represented throughout this book. Another word component is a prefix. *pre-* means before; prefixes go before the word root.
	term prefix, root	Thus, one way to build a medical _____ is by combining a _____ with a word _____.

BOX 2.2 **Abbreviations**	
q	every
qd	once a day
qod	every other day
Q ____ h	every _____ other hour
bid	twice a day
tid	three times a day
qid	four times a day
hs	at bedtime (hour of sleep)
ac	before meals
pc	after meals
prn	when needed
ad lib	as desired
stat	immediately

BLOCK	DATA AND ANSWERS	DESCRIPTIONS AND QUESTIONS
2-6		**Key 1:** A prefix and a word root can be combined to form a medical term.
	prefix, root	When a _____ joins a word _____, it complies
	1, term	with Key __ to form a medical _____.
2-7		There are many prefixes.
	hypertension (hahy'-per-ten-shun')	For example, hypertension means high blood pressure.
		hyper- is a prefix meaning above or more than normal.
		"tension" is a word root meaning force. In medicine, tension refers to blood pressure.
2-8	prefix, higher, above, more than normal	*hyper-* is a _____ meaning _____, _____, or _____ _____ _____.
	word root	"tension" is a _____ _____ and refers to
	blood pressure	_____ _____.
	high blood pressure	Hypertension is _____ _____ _____.
2-9	malnutrition (mal-nu'-tri-shun)	Malnutrition means bad nutrition.
		mal- is a prefix meaning bad.
		"nutrition" is a word root meaning nourishing, nourishment, food, etc.
2-10	bad	The prefix *mal-* means _____.
	malnutrition	The medical term for bad nutrition is _____.
2-11	agenesis (ey-jen-uh-sis)	Agenesis means without development.
		a- is a prefix meaning without.
		"genesis" is a word root meaning generation (development).

BLOCK	DATA AND ANSWERS	DESCRIPTIONS AND QUESTIONS
2-12	prefix, without root generation, development	*a-* is a _____ meaning _____. "genesis" is a word _____ meaning _____ or _____.
2-13	antitoxin (an'-ti-<u>tok</u>-sin')	Antitoxin means against a toxic substance. *anti-* is a prefix meaning against. "toxin" is a word root meaning a toxic substance.
2-14	disinfect (dis'-in-<u>fekt</u>)	Disinfect means to free of infection. *dis-* is a prefix meaning to free of, separate from, or undo. "infect" is a word root meaning to contaminate with a harmful agent.
2-15	prefix, against root, a toxic substance	*anti-* is a _____ meaning _____. "toxin" is a word _____ meaning ___ _____ _____.
2-16	prefix, to free of separate from, undo root, to contaminate with a harmful agent	*dis-* is a _____ meaning _____ _____ _____, _____ _____, or _____. "infect" is a word _____ meaning _____ _____ _____ __ _____ _____.
2-17	against a toxic substance to free of infection	Antitoxin means _____ ___ _____ _____. Disinfect means _____ _____ _____ _____.
2-18		Another type of word component is a suffix. A suffix is placed at the end of a word root. We can combine a word root with a suffix to form a medical term.

BLOCK	DATA AND ANSWERS	DESCRIPTIONS AND QUESTIONS
2-19		**Key 2:** A word root and a suffix can be combined to form a medical term.
	root, suffix 2, term	When a word _____ joins a _____, it complies with Key __ to form a medical _____.
2-20	dermatitis (derm'-ah-<u>ti</u>-tis)	Dermatitis means inflammation of the skin. "dermat" is a word root meaning the skin. -*itis* is a suffix meaning inflammation.
	suffix, inflammation	-*itis* is a _____ meaning _____.
	root, the skin	"dermat" is a word _____ meaning _____ _____.
2-21		In medicine, when -*itis* is added to a medical word component describing a body part or organ, it means the latter is inflamed.
	terms root, part, organ, -*itis*	Many medical _____ can be built by combining a word _____ referring to a body _____ or _____ with the suffix _____.
2-22	gastritis (ga'-<u>strahy</u>-tis	Gastritis is inflammation of the stomach.
	endometritis (en-doh'-mi-<u>trahy</u>-tis)	Endometritis is inflammation of the lining of the uterus.
	cholecystitis (koh'-luh-si'-<u>stahy</u>-tis)	Cholecystitis is inflammation of the gallbladder.
2-23		"gastr" is a word root meaning the stomach. "endometr" is a word root meaning the lining of the uterus. "cholecyst" is a word root meaning the gallbladder. -*itis* is a suffix meaning inflammation.

BLOCK	DATA AND ANSWERS	DESCRIPTIONS AND QUESTIONS
2-24	inflammation of the stomach, "gastr" Endometritis "endometr" Cholecystitis "cholecyst" gallbladder -*itis*, inflammation	Gastritis is _____ _____ _____ _____, and its word root is _____. _____ is inflammation of the lining of the uterus, and its word root is _____. _____ is inflammation of the gallbladder. The word root is _____, meaning _____. The suffix is _____, meaning _____.
2-25	cyanosis (sahy'-uh-<u>noh</u>-sis)	Cyanosis is the condition of being blue or a disease of blueness. Thus, it also means blueness of the skin. "cyan" is a word root meaning blue. -*osis* is a suffix meaning the condition of.
2-26	word root, blue -*osis* the condition of blueness, blueness of the skin	"cyan" is a _____ _____ meaning _____. _____ is a suffix meaning the condition of. Cyanosis is _____ _____ _____ _____ or _____ _____ _____ _____.
2-27	mucus (myoo-<u>kuhs</u>)	Mucus is a thick, slippery fluid produced by the membranes lining certain organs, such as the nose, mouth, throat, and vagina. Mucus is the Latin word for a semi-fluid, slimy discharge. It is a singular noun with the following word components: "muc" is a word root referring to slippery fluid. -*us* is a suffix indicating a singular noun.
2-28	mucous (myoo-<u>kuhs</u>)	Mucous means pertaining to mucus or is an adjective for mucus. -*ous* is a suffix meaning pertaining to.

BLOCK	DATA AND ANSWERS	DESCRIPTIONS AND QUESTIONS
2-29	a thick, slippery fluid produced by the membranes lining certain organs, such as the nose, mouth, throat, and vagina, Mucus is the Latin word for a semi-fluid slimy discharge	Mucus is __ _____, _____ _____ _____ ____ _____ _____ _____ _____ _____, _____ _____ _____ _____, _____, _____, _____. _____ _____ _____ _____ _____ __ _____, _____ _____.
2-30	suffix, a singular noun	-us is a _____ indicating __ _____ _____.
	suffix, pertaining to	-ous is a _____ meaning _____ _____.
2-31	pertaining to mucus adjective	Mucous means _____ _____ _____ and is an _____ for mucus.
2-32		*Key 3:* A prefix and a suffix can be combined to form a medical term.
	prefix, suffix 3, term	When a _____ joins a _____, it complies with Key __ to form a medical _____.
2-33	dystocia (dis'-<u>to</u>-zee-ah)	Dystocia means difficult labor.
		dys- is a prefix meaning difficult.
		-tocia is a suffix meaning labor (childbirth).
2-34	euphoria (u'-<u>for</u>-e-ah)	Euphoria is the state of well-being.
		eu- is a prefix meaning good or well-being.
		-phoria is a suffix meaning bearing, the state of.

BLOCK	DATA AND ANSWERS	DESCRIPTIONS AND QUESTIONS
2-35	prefix, difficult	*dys-* is a _____ meaning _____.
	-tocia	_____ is a suffix meaning labor.
	eu-	_____ is a prefix meaning well-being.
	suffix, state of	*-phoria* is a _____ meaning _____ _____.
2-36	difficult labor	Dystocia is _____ _____.
	the state of well-being	Euphoria is _____ _____ _____ _____.
2-37	anemia (ah'-<u>ne</u>-me-ah)	Anemia means no, not, or without blood. In medicine, it refers to reduced red blood cells.
		An- is a prefix meaning no, not, or without.
		-emia is a suffix meaning condition of blood.
2-38	quadriplegia (quad'-ri-<u>ple</u>-jah)	Quadriplegia is paralysis of all four extremities.
		quadri- is a prefix meaning four.
		-plegia is a suffix meaning paralysis.
2-39	Anemia	_____ means no, not, or without blood.
	an-, -emia	The prefix is _____, and the suffix is _____.
	Quadriplegia	_____ is paralysis of all four extremities.
	quadri-, -plegia	The prefix is _____ and the suffix is _____.
2-40	no, not, without blood	Anemia means _____, _____, or _____ _____.
	reduced red blood cells	In medicine, anemia means _____ _____ _____ _____.
	paralysis of all four extremities	Quadriplegia is _____ _____ _____ _____ _____.

BLOCK	DATA AND ANSWERS	DESCRIPTIONS AND QUESTIONS
2-41	bradypnea (brad'-ip-<u>ne</u>-ah)	Bradypnea is slow breathing. *brady-* is a prefix meaning slow. *-pnea* is a suffix meaning breathing.
2-42	polyphagia (pau'-li-<u>fa</u>-je'-ah)	Polyphagia is excessive eating. *poly-* is a prefix meaning many or excessive. *-phagia* is a suffix meaning eating.
2-43	Bradypnea *brady-* *-pnea*	_____ is slow breathing. _____ is a prefix meaning slow. _____ is a suffix meaning breathing.
2-44	Polyphagia *poly-*, prefix suffix, eating	_____ is excessive eating. _____ is a _____ meaning many or excessive. *-phagia* is a _____ meaning _____.
2-45	 term root, root	We can combine a word root with another word root to form a medical term. One way to build a medical _____ is by combining one word _____ with another word _____.
2-46	 root root, 4 term	**Key 4:** One word root can be combined with another word root to form a medical term. When one word _____ joins with another word _____, it complies with Key __ to form a medical _____.
2-47		A compound word is formed when we join one word with another word. When we join two word roots, we may be joining two words, thus forming a compound word.

BLOCK	DATA AND ANSWERS	DESCRIPTIONS AND QUESTIONS
2-48	root root, compound	When one word _____ is combined with another word _____, a _____ word may be formed. Three examples are headache, gallstone, and foreskin, all common medical terms familiar to most of us.
2-49	headache (hed-ache)	A headache refers to pain in the head. "head" is a word root. "ache" is a word root. In this case, the combination can be considered a simple word or a compound word.
2-50	gallstone (gall-s-tone)	Gallstone is a stone in the gallbladder. "gall" is a word root meaning gallbladder. "stone" is a word root meaning stone.
2-51	foreskin (for-s-kin)	Foreskin is the retractable fold of skin in the front part of the penis. "fore" is a word root meaning front. "skin" is a word root meaning skin.
2-52	zoophobia (zoh'-uh-foh-bee-uh)	Zoophobia is fear of animals. "zoo" is a word root meaning zoo. "phobia" is a word root meaning fear or afraid of. (Note that "phobia" can be a word root or a suffix.)
2-53	the fear of or the condition of being afraid of animals	Zoophobia is _____ _____ _____ _____ _____ _____ _____ _____ _____ _____ _____.
2-54	presbycusis (prez'-bi-kyu-sas)	Presbycusis is a hearing problem due to old age. "presby" is a word root meaning old age. "cusis" is a word root meaning hearing problem.

BLOCK	DATA AND ANSWERS	DESCRIPTIONS AND QUESTIONS
2-55	Presbycusis	_____ is a hearing problem due to old age.
	"presby"	The first word root is _____, meaning old age.
	"cusis"	The second word root is _____, meaning hearing problem.
2-56		Some medical terms are built by combining three components: a prefix, a word root, and a suffix, in that order.
	prefix, root	That is, if you combine a _____, a word _____, and
	suffix, term	a _____, a medical _____ is formed.
2-57		**Key 5:** One prefix and one word root can be combined with a suffix to form a medical term.
	prefix, root, suffix	When a _____, a word _____, and a _____
	5	are combined in that order, it complies with Key __ to form a
	term	medical _____.
2-58	hemigastrectomy (hem′-i-ga-<u>strek</u>-to-me)	Hemigastrectomy is removal of half of the stomach.
2-59		*hemi-* is a prefix meaning half.
		"gastr" is a word root meaning stomach.
		-ectomy is a suffix meaning removal.
	5	This method of building the medical term for hemigastrectomy complies with Key __.
2-60	panencephalitis (pan′-en-sefa′-<u>li</u>- tis)	Panencephalitis is inflammation of the entire brain.
		pan- is a prefix meaning entire.
		"encephal" is a word root meaning the brain.
		-itis is a suffix meaning inflammation.

BLOCK	DATA AND ANSWERS	DESCRIPTIONS AND QUESTIONS
2-61	prefix, entire "encephal," word root suffix, inflammation	*pan-* is a _____ meaning _____. _____ is a _____ _____ meaning brain. *-itis* is a _____ meaning _____.
2-62	prefix, half word root stomach suffix, removal	*hemi-* is a _____ meaning _____. *gastr-* is a _____ _____ meaning _____. *-ectomy* is a _____ meaning _____.
2-63	Panencephalitis Hemigastrectomy 5	_____ is inflammation of the entire brain. _____ is removal of half of the stomach. Both medical terms are built by combining a prefix, a word root, and a suffix. This method of building a medical term complies with Key __.
2-64	defecation (de′-fi-<u>ka</u>-shun)	Defecation is the process of excreting human feces. *de-* is a prefix meaning to come down. "feca" is a word root meaning feces. *-tion* is a suffix meaning process.
2-65	hyperalbuminemia (hi′-per-al-byoo′-mih-<u>nee</u>-mee-ah)	Hyperalbuminemia is an excess of specific protein substances in the blood. *hyper-* is a prefix meaning over, excessive. "albumin" is a word root referring to specific protein substances in the blood. *-emia* is a suffix meaning blood.

BLOCK	DATA AND ANSWERS	DESCRIPTIONS AND QUESTIONS
2-66	*de-* word root, feces *-tion* the process of excreting human feces	_____ is a prefix meaning to come down. "feca" is a _____ _____ meaning _____. _____ is a suffix meaning process. Defecation is _____ _____ ____ _____ _____ _____.
2-67	*hyper-*, prefix word root specific protein substances in blood *-emia* Hyperalbuminemia	_____ is a _____ meaning over, excessive. "albumin" is a _____ _____ meaning _____ _____ _____ ___ _____. _____ is a suffix meaning blood. _____ is an excess of specific protein substances in the blood.
2-68	exophthalmia (ek'-sof-thal-me-ah)	Exophthalmia is protrusion of the eyeballs due to a hormonal disorder. *ex-* is a prefix meaning outward, away from (e.g., away from the face or protrusion). "ophthalm" is a word root referring to the eyes or eyeballs. *-ia* is a suffix meaning condition.
2-69	dyspareunia (dis'-puh-roo-nee-uh)	Dyspareunia is difficult, painful mating or sexual intercourse. *dys-* is a prefix meaning difficult or painful. "pareun" is a word root meaning mating or intercourse. *-ia* is a suffix meaning condition.

BLOCK	DATA AND ANSWERS	DESCRIPTIONS AND QUESTIONS
2-70	*ex-* "ophthalm" *-ia* Exophthalmia	_____ is a prefix meaning outward, away from (e.g., away from the face or protrusion). _____ is a word root referring to the eyes or eyeballs. _____ is a suffix meaning condition. _____ is protrusion of the eyeballs due to a hormonal disorder.
2-71	difficult, painful mating or sexual intercourse prefix, difficult painful word root mating, intercourse suffix, condition	Dyspareunia is _____, _____ _____ _____ _____ _____. *dys-* is a _____ meaning _____ or _____. *pareun-* is a _____ _____ meaning _____ or _____. *-ia* is a _____ meaning _____.
2-72		There is another word component that we have not yet discussed: the combining form. A combining form is a word root to which a final vowel (usually the letter "o") is added. In this book, we represent the combining form by a word root, a slash (/), and a vowel, e.g., word root/vowel.
	combining form word root, slash vowel word root/vowel	Thus, a _____ _____ is a combination of a _____ _____, a _____, and a _____. The connection between the two components is represented as _____ _____ throughout this book.

BLOCK	DATA AND ANSWERS	DESCRIPTIONS AND QUESTIONS
2-73		*Key 6:* A suffix can be joined to a combining form to create a medical term.
	term	Thus, one way to build a medical _____ is by
	combining form	combining one _____ _____ with a
	suffix, 6	_____. This is Key __.
2-74	neurologist (nyoo'-<u>rol</u>-uh-jist)	A neurologist is a physician who specializes in the nervous system.
		"neur" is a word root meaning nerve.
		"neur/o" is the combining form.
		-*logist* is a suffix meaning one who specializes.
		Thus, this medical term has two components: a combining form ("neur/o") and a suffix (-*logist*).
2-75	word root, nerve	"neur" is a _____ _____ meaning _____.
	combining form	"neur/o" is the _____ _____ of "neur."
	suffix, one who specializes	-*logist* is a _____ meaning _____ _____ _____.
	a physician specializing in the	A neurologist is __ _____ _____ ___ _____ _____ _____.
	nervous system	
	combining form	When a _____ _____ is added to
	suffix, 6	a _____, it complies with Key __ to form a medical
	term	_____.
2-76	erythrocytes (i-<u>rith</u>-ruh-sahyt')	Erythrocytes means red cells. In medicine and biology these are the red blood cells.
		"erythr" is a word root meaning red.
		"erythr/o" is the combining form.
		-*cytes* is a suffix meaning cell.

BLOCK	DATA AND ANSWERS	DESCRIPTIONS AND QUESTIONS
2-77	combining form red suffix, cells red cells the red blood cells	"erythr/o" is a _____ _____ meaning _____. -*cytes* is a _____ meaning _____. Erythrocytes means _____ _____. In medicine and biology it refers to _____ _____ _____ _____.
2-78	laparoscopy (<u>lap</u>-er-uh-skoh'-pee)	Laparoscopy is use of a scope to penetrate the abdomen wall to study the abdominal cavity. "lapar" is a word root meaning abdominal wall. "lapar/o" is the combining form. -*scopy* is a suffix referring to testing or examining with a scope.
2-79	nephropathy (nuh'-fro-<u>puh</u>-thee)	Nephropathy is disease of the kidney. "nephr/o" is the combining form. -*pathy* is a suffix meaning disease, disorder, or pathological condition.
2-80	"lapar/o" suffix, testing examining with a scope	_____ is a combining form meaning abdominal wall. -*scopy* is a _____ meaning _____ or _____ _____ __ _____.
2-81	combining form kidney -*pathy*	"nephr/o" is a _____ _____ meaning _____. _____ is a suffix meaning disease, disorder, or pathological condition.
2-82	Laparoscopy disease of the kidney	_____ is using a scope to penetrate the abdomen wall to study the abdominal cavity. Nephropathy is _____ _____ _____ _____.

BLOCK	DATA AND ANSWERS	DESCRIPTIONS AND QUESTIONS
2-83	cardiology (<u>kahr</u>-dee-ol'-uh-jee)	Cardiology is the study of the heart. "cardi/o" is a combining form meaning the heart. *-logy* is a suffix meaning the study of.
2-84	osteoporosis (os'-tee-oh-puh-<u>roh</u>-sis)	Osteoporosis is the condition of pores or holes in the bone. "oste/o" is a combining form meaning bones. *-porosis* is a suffix meaning holes or pores.
2-85	"cardi/o" suffix, the study of	_____ is a combining form meaning the heart. *-logy* is a _____ meaning _____ _____ ____.
2-86	combining form bones *-porosis*	"oste/o" is a _____ _____ meaning _____. _____ is a suffix meaning holes or pores.
2-87	the study of the heart Osteoporosis	Cardiology is _____ _____ ____ _____ _____. _____ is the condition of pores or holes in the bone.
2-88		**Key 7:** A combining form can be joined to a word root to create a medical term.
	combining form word root, term 7	That is, if you join a _____ _____ with a _____ _____, a medical _____ is formed. This complies with Key __.
2-89	melanoderma (mel'-lan-uh-<u>dur</u>-ma)	Melanoderma is discoloration of the skin. "melan/o" is a combining form meaning black. "derma" is the word root for skin. Thus, this medical term has two components: a combining form ("melan/o") and a word root ("derma").

BLOCK	DATA AND ANSWERS	DESCRIPTIONS AND QUESTIONS
2-90	hemophobia (he′-mo-<u>foh</u>-bee-uh)	Hemophobia is fear of blood. "hem/o" is a combining form meaning blood. "phobia" is a root word meaning fear or condition of being afraid of.
2-91	combining form black "derma"	"melan/o" is a _____ _____ meaning _____. _____ is a word root meaning skin.
2-92	"hem/o" root word, fear being afraid of	_____ is a combining form meaning blood. "phobia" is a _____ _____ meaning _____ or _____ _____ _____.
2-93	discoloration of the skin Hemophobia	Melanoderma is _____ _____ _____ _____. _____ is fear of blood.
2-94	psychotherapy (sahy′-<u>koh</u>-ther-uh-pee)	Psychotherapy means treatment of the mind or soul. "psych/o" is a combining form meaning mind or soul. "therapy" is a root word meaning treatment.
2-95	tracheostenosis (trey′-kee-oh-ste-<u>no</u>-sis)	Tracheostenosis is narrowing or constriction of the windpipe. "trache/o" is a combining form meaning windpipe. "stenosis" is a root word meaning narrowing or constriction.
2-96	cerebrospinal (ser′-eh-broh-<u>spy</u>-nal)	Cerebrospinal means (space flowing) through the brain and spinal cord. "cerebr/o" is a combining form meaning brain. "spinal" is a root word meaning spine.
2-97	"psych/o" root word treatment	_____ is a combining form meaning mind or soul. "therapy" is a _____ _____ meaning _____.

BLOCK	DATA AND ANSWERS	DESCRIPTIONS AND QUESTIONS
2-98	combining form windpipe "stenosis"	"trache/o" is a _____ _____ meaning _____. _____ is a root word meaning narrowing or constriction.
2-99	"cerebr/o" root word spine	_____ is a combining form meaning brain. "spinal" is a _____ _____ referring to the _____.
2-100	(space flowing) through the brain and spinal cord treatment of the mind or soul narrowing or constriction of the windpipe	Cerebrospinal means _____ _____ _____ _____ _____ _____ _____ _____. Psychotherapy means _____ _____ _____ _____ _____ _____. Tracheostenosis is _____ _____ _____ _____ _____ _____.
2-101		Keys 6 and 7 have not explored the complexity of the combining form. Key 8 addresses the many variations of the definitions used in these two keys. **Key 8:** There are variations of the basic combining forms in building medical terms. Variation 1: Applications and functions of the vowels. Variation 2: Keeping or deleting a vowel when two vowels would be adjacent in a medical term. Variation 3: Keeping or deleting a vowel when more than one combining form is present.
2-102		Variation 1: Applications and functions of the vowels. The vowel in a combining form can be any of the following: a, e, i, o, and u.

BLOCK	DATA AND ANSWERS	DESCRIPTIONS AND QUESTIONS
2-103	word root, vowel, a, e i, o, u	Thus, a combining form is made up of a _____ _____, slash, and a _____, which can be ___, ___, _, ___, or ___.
2-104		The vowel in a combining form serves two important purposes: 1. To link two components of a medical term 2. To facilitate pronunciation
2-105	To link two components of a medical term To facilitate pronunciation	The vowel in a combining form has two uses: 1. _____ _____ _____ _____ _____ __ _____ _____ 2. _____ _____ _____
2-106		Of the five vowels: "o" is most common. "i" is found in some combining forms. "e" is found in several combining forms. "a" is rare but appears in a limited number of combining forms. "u" is seldom found in combining forms.
2-107	"o", "u"	You have seen several combination forms with the vowel "o" under Keys 6 and 7. The most common vowel used to create a combining form is ___. The most uncommon vowel used is ___. The following gives one more example of a medical term with the vowel "o."

BLOCK	DATA AND ANSWERS	DESCRIPTIONS AND QUESTIONS
2-108	gynecology (gigh'-neh-<u>kol</u>-oh-jee)	Gynecology means study of women. In medicine and biology, it means the branch of medicine that studies diseases and disorders of the female reproductive system. "gynec/o" is a combining form meaning women. -*logy* is a suffix meaning the study of.
2-109	biliary (<u>bil</u>-ee-er'-ee)	The vowel "i" is used in some combining forms. "biliary" means pertaining to the bile. Bile is a bitter, alkaline, brownish-yellow or greenish-yellow fluid that is secreted by the liver and stored in the gallbladder. Bile also is called gall. "bil/i" is a combining form meaning bile. -*ary* is a suffix meaning pertaining to.
2-110	pelvimetry (pel'-<u>vim</u>-i-tree)	Pelvimetry is the process of measuring the pelvis. "pelv/i" is a combining form meaning pelvis. -*metry* is a suffix meaning the process of measuring.
2-111	"bil/i" suffix, pertaining to	_____ is a combining form meaning bile. -*ary* is a _____ meaning _____ ____.
2-112	"pelv/i" -*metry*	_____ is a combining form meaning pelvis. _____ is a suffix meaning the process of measuring.

BLOCK	DATA AND ANSWERS	DESCRIPTIONS AND QUESTIONS
2-113	the process of measuring the pelvis	Pelvimetry is _____ _____ _____ _____ _____ _____.
	a bitter, alkaline brownish-yellow or greenish-yellow fluid that is secreted by the liver and stored in the gallbladder	Bile is __ _____, _____, _____ _____ _____ _____ _____ __ _____ ____ ____ _____ _____ _____ ___ _____ _____.
	gall	Bile also is called _____.
	pertaining to the bile	Biliary means _____ _____ _____ _____.
2-114	corectasis (kor′-ek-ta-sis)	The vowel "e" is found in some combination forms.
		Corectasis is dilation of the pupil.
		"cor/e" is a combining form meaning pupil.
		-ectasis is a suffix meaning dilation.
		Note that one "e" is deleted when the two word parts are combined. This facilitates pronunciation. See later blocks for more details.
2-115	natal (na-tal)	Although uncommon, the vowel "a" is occasionally used in combination forms.
		Natal means pertaining to birth.
		"nat/a" is the combining form.
		-al is a suffix meaning pertaining to.
		Note that one "a" is deleted when the two word parts are combined. This facilitates pronunciation. See later blocks in this chapter for more details.

BLOCK	DATA AND ANSWERS	DESCRIPTIONS AND QUESTIONS
2-116	"cor/e" -ectasis	_____ is a combining form meaning pupil. _____ is a suffix meaning dilation.
2-117	combining form birth -al	"nat/a" is a _____ _____ meaning _____. _____ is a suffix meaning pertaining to.
2-118	"natal" corectasis	_____ means pertaining to birth. _____ is dilation of the pupil.
2-119		Variation 2: Keeping or deleting a vowel when two vowels would be adjacent in a medical term. Sometimes the vowel "o" is not included in the medical term itself after the combining form is joined to a suffix (Key 6). The next few blocks give examples.
2-120	stomatitis (<u>sto</u>-mah-ti'-tis)	Stomatitis is inflammation of the mouth. "stomat/o" is a combining form meaning the mouth. -itis is a suffix meaning inflammation. When two vowels would be adjacent in a medical term, the one belonging to the combining form is usually deleted. This facilitates pronunciation of the medical term.
2-121	rachialgia (ray'-kee-<u>al</u>-jia)	Rachialgia is pain in the spine. "rachi/o" is a combining form meaning spine. -algia is a suffix meaning pain. When two vowels would be adjacent in a medical term, the one belonging to the combining form is usually deleted. The one not deleted is usually attached to a word part with a consonant. This facilitates pronunciation of the medical term.

BLOCK	DATA AND ANSWERS	DESCRIPTIONS AND QUESTIONS
2-122	"stomat/o" suffix, inflammation	_____ is a combining form meaning the mouth. -*itis* is a _____ meaning _____.
2-123	combining form spine suffix, pain	"rachi/o" is a _____ _____ meaning _____. -*algia* is a _____ meaning _____.
2-124	inflammation of the mouth Rachialgia	Stomatitis is _____ ____ _____ _____. _____ is pain in the spine.
2-125	gastroenterologist (gas-troh-en-tuh-rol'-uh-jist)	Variation 3: Keeping or deleting a vowel when more than one combining form is present. Some medical terms contain two or more combining forms. A gastroenterologist is a physician who specializes in the study of the stomach and intestine. "gastr/o" is a combining form meaning stomach. "enter/o" is a combining form meaning intestine. -*logist* is a suffix meaning one specializing in. Note that both vowels are kept. This facilitates pronunciation. Also, no two vowels are adjacent.
2-126	otorhinolaryngology (oh'-toh-rahy-noh'-lar-ing-gol-uh-jee)	Otorhinolaryngology is the study of the ear, nose, and throat. "ot/o" is a combining form meaning ear. "rhin/o" is a combining form meaning nose. "laryng/o" is a combining form meaning throat or larynx. -*logy* is a suffix meaning study of. Note that all three vowels are kept. This facilitates pronunciation. Also, no two vowels are adjacent.

BLOCK	DATA AND ANSWERS	DESCRIPTIONS AND QUESTIONS
2-127	stomach	"gastr/o" is a combining form meaning _____.
	intestine	"enter/o" is a combining form meaning _____.
	-logist	_____ is a suffix meaning one specializing in.
2-128	"ot/o"	_____ is a combining form meaning ear.
	"rhin/o"	_____ is a combining form meaning nose.
	"laryng/o"	_____ is a combining form meaning throat or larynx.
	-logy	_____ is a suffix meaning the study of.
2-129	Otorhinolaryngology	_____ is the study of the ear, nose, and throat.
	gastroenterologist	A _____ is a physician specializing in the study of the stomach and intestine.
2-130	lymphangiogram (lim'-fan-jee-o-gram)	A lymphangiogram is a picture or record of lymph and blood vessels. This is usually made by taking an x-ray after injecting dye or a similar chemical compound into a blood vessel.
		"lymph/o" is a combining form meaning lymph.
		"angi/o" is a combining form meaning blood.
		-gram is a suffix meaning picture or record.
		Note that the first "o" is dropped because it precedes another vowel, "a."
2-131	onychomycosis (on'-ik-o-mi-ko-sis)	Onychomycosis is a fungal infection of the nails.
		"oncy/o" is a combining form meaning nail.
		"myc/o" is a combining form meaning fungus.
		-osis is a suffix meaning abnormal condition.
		Note that one "o" is deleted because two vowels are adjacent.

BLOCK	DATA AND ANSWERS	DESCRIPTIONS AND QUESTIONS
2-132	-*gram*	_____ is a suffix meaning picture or record.
	"angi/o"	_____ is a combining form meaning blood.
	"lymph/o"	_____ is a combining form meaning lymph.
2-133	fungus	"myc/o" is a combining form meaning _____.
	condition	-*osis* is a suffix meaning _____.
	nails	"oncy/o" is a combining form meaning _____.
2-134	picture or record of lymph and blood vessels	A lymphangiogram is a _____ _____ _____ _____ _____ _____ _____ _____.
	Onychomycosis	_____ is the abnormal condition of fungal infection of the nails.
2-135		The basic rule is to drop one vowel when two vowels are placed side by side. Ease of pronunciation is always a consideration.
		However, there are exemptions to this rule in keeping or deleting a vowel. Your instructor will explain when this occurs.
2-136		Let us now review the eight keys to building medical terms.
	term	Key 1 states that a medical _____ can be built by
	prefix, root	combining a _____ with a word _____.
2-137	term	Key 2 states that a medical _____ can be built by
	root, suffix	combining a word _____ with a _____.
2-138	term	Key 3 states that a medical _____ can be built by
	prefix, suffix	combining a _____ with a _____.
2-139	term	Key 4 states that a medical _____ can be built by
	root, root	combining a word _____ with a word _____.
2-140	term	Key 5 states that a medical _____ can be built by
	prefix, root	combining a _____, a word _____, and a
	suffix	_____.

BLOCK	DATA AND ANSWERS	DESCRIPTIONS AND QUESTIONS
2-141	term combining form, suffix	Key 6 states that a medical _____ can be built by adding a _____ _____ to a _____.
2-142	term combining form, word root	Key 7 states that a medical _____ can be built by adding a _____ _____ to a _____ _____.
2-143	there are variations of the basic combining forms in developing medical terms	Key 8 states that _____ _____ _____ _____ _____ _____ _____ _____ _____ _____ _____ _____.
2-144		Although the eight keys provide basic rules for developing medical terms, there are many exceptions to each key. We encourage you to make use of printed and electronic resources and the expertise of your instructors to clarify these exceptions.
2-145	head, body, legs, muscle, hair, eyes, ears, and so on. (If you have named others, please use the Internet or other resources to confirm their accuracy.)	The next stage of your training is to learn to build medical terms for the human body systems by using the principles of the eight keys. All of us are familiar with our bodies. Examples of parts of the human body are: _____ _____ _____ _____ _____ _____ _____ _____ _____. (Name as many as you can.) Some, but not all, body systems are covered in the remaining chapters of this book.

Progress Check

A. Multiple Choice

1. A word root meaning red is:
   a. erythr
   b. ache
   c. neur
   d. phobia

2. A word root meaning development is:
   a. cusis
   b. muc
   c. genesis
   d. phobia

3. A combining form meaning blood is:
   a. cardi/o
   b. bil/i
   c. neur/o
   d. angi/o

4. A combining form meaning the ear is:
   a. oste/o
   b. ot/o
   c. oncy/o
   d. orth/o

5. A prefix meaning to come down is:
   a. de-
   b. dis-
   c. eu-
   d. an-

6. A prefix meaning half is:
   a. hemi-
   b. quadri-
   c. peri-
   d. brady-

7. A suffix meaning pain is:
   a. -cyte
   b. -ia
   c. -algia
   d. -logy

8. A suffix meaning breakdown is:
   a. -itis
   b. -lysis
   c. -al
   d. -gram

B. Definitions and Word Components

	TERM	DEFINITION	PREFIX	WORD ROOT	VOWEL	WORD ROOT	VOWEL	SUFFIX
1.	antitoxin							
2.	biliary							
3.	disinfect							
4.	endometritis							
5.	mucous							
6.	quadriplegia							
7.	zoophobia							
8.	hemophobia							
9.	cerebrospinal							
10.	natal							

C. Medical Terms and Their Definitions

	TERM	DEFINITION
1.		condition of fungal infection of the nails
2.	corectasis	
3.		incision into the spine
4.	pelvimetry	
5.		treatment of the mind or soul
6.	tracheostenosis	
7.		discoloration of the skin
8.	nephropathy	
9.		use of a scope to penetrate the abdomen wall to study the abdominal cavity
10.	albumin	
11.		condition of protrusion of the eyeballs due to a hormonal disorder
12.	dyspareunia	
13.		removal of half of the stomach
14.	presbycusis	
15.		inflammation of the entire brain
16.	hemolysis	
17.		slow breathing
18.	dystocia	
19.		state of well-being
20.	cholecystitis	

D. Abbreviations

	ABBREVIATION	MEANING
1.	q	
2.	qd	
3.	qod	
4.	Q ___ h	
5.	bid	
6.	tid	
7.	qid	
8.	hs	
9.	ac	
10.	pc	
11.	prn	
12.	ad lib	
13.	stat	

PART

II

Programmed Instruction for Medical Terminology Related to Body Systems

Whole-Body Terminology

BLOCK	DATA AND ANSWERS	DESCRIPTION AND QUESTIONS
3-1		The structural units of the body are: cell, tissue, organ, and system.
		The smallest structural unit of the human body is the cell. A cell is made up of a substance called protoplasm surrounded by a cell membrane. The protoplasm is divided into two parts: cytoplasm (large) and nucleoplasm (small). The small unit of nucleoplasm is surrounded by another membrane and is called a nucleus.
	cell (sel) protoplasm (pro-to-plazm), cell membrane (sel mem-bran), cytoplasm (si'-to-plazm), nucleoplasm (nu'-kle-o-plazm), nucleus (nu'-kle-us), chromosomes (kro-ma-som), mitosis (mi'-to-sis)	Chromosomes are scattered throughout the nucleus. Each cell performs special functions necessary to maintain its life. Cells multiply or reproduce by dividing. This process is called mitosis.
		See **Figure 3.1** and **Table 3.1** (which contains the word roots, combining forms, prefixes, and suffixes relevant to this subject).

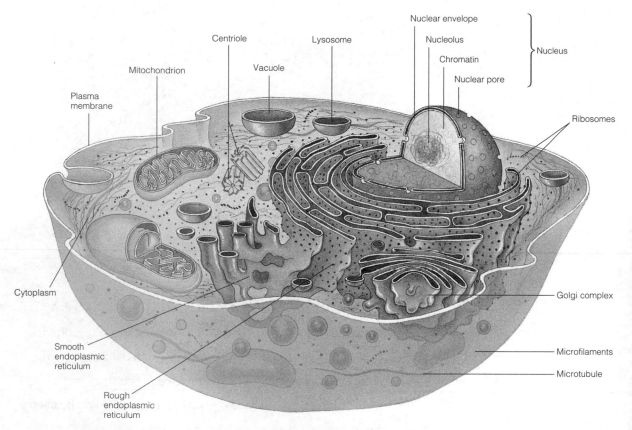

FIGURE 3.1   Structure of the general eukaryotic cell

TABLE 3.1   Word Components in this Chapter

WORD ROOTS	COMBINING FORMS	PREFIXES
cardi	cardi/o	endo-
chondri	chondri/o	epi-
crani	chrom/o	hypo-
crin	crani/o	mito-
epitheli	crin/o	proto-
gastr	cyt/o	SUFFIXES
ili	gastr/o	-ac
inguin	ili/o	-al
lumb	inguin/o	-ant
lymph	intestin/o	-ar
muscul	lumb/o	-atic
nerv	lymph/o	-crine
nucle	mit/o	-ic
peritone	muscul/o	-osis

TABLE 3.1   Word Components in this Chapter (continued)

WORD ROOTS	COMBINING FORMS	SUFFIXES
plasm	nerv/o	-ous
pleur	nucle/o	-some
quadr	peritone/o	-us
skelet	pleur/o	
spin	prot/o	
theli	quadr/o	
thor	skelet/o	
thorac	spin/o	
umbilic	thorac/o	
vascul	umbilic/o	
	vascul/o	

BLOCK	DATA AND ANSWERS	DESCRIPTION AND QUESTIONS
3-2		The original meaning of the word "protoplasm" is first something molded or first created thing. Now, biologists define it as the gelatinous fluid in living tissue. At present, it also is considered a word root. However, the medical components of protoplasm are as follows: "prot/o" is a combining form meaning first or to create. *proto-* is also a prefix. "plasm" is a word root meaning molded, created, or formed.
3-3	combining form first, to create *proto-* word root molded, created, formed	"prot/o" is a __Combining__ __Form__ meaning __first__ or to __create__. "prot/o" can also be a prefix: __proto__ "plasm" is a __word__ __root__ meaning __molded__, __created__, or __formed__.

BLOCK	DATA AND ANSWERS	DESCRIPTION AND QUESTIONS
3-4		A nucleus is a spherical round body within a cell and is made up of protoplasm, called nucleoplasm, which contains genes or chromosomes. The nucleus is surrounded by a thin nuclear membrane and the cytoplasm (the large remaining part of the protoplasm).
		"nucleus" is a word root meaning a central body or unit.
		"nucle" is a word root meaning a nucleus.
		"nucle/o" is the combining form.
		-us is a suffix that indicates a singular noun.
3-5		"nucleus" is a word root meaning a central body or unit.
	"nucle"	_nucle_ is a word root meaning nucleus.
	"nucle/o"	_nucle/o_ is a combining form meaning nucleus.
	-us	_us_ is a suffix that indicates a singular noun.
3-6		"cytoplasm" is a root word meaning the gelatinous fluid outside the nucleus.
		"nucleoplasm" is a root word meaning the gelatinous fluid inside the nucleus.
		"cyt/o" is a combining form meaning cell, container, or receptacle.
		"nucle/o" is a combining form meaning nucleus.
3-7	Cytoplasm	_cytoplasm_ is gelatinous fluid outside the nucleus.
	Nucleoplasm	_nucleoplasm_ is gelatinous fluid inside the nucleus.

BLOCK	DATA AND ANSWERS	DESCRIPTION AND QUESTIONS
3-8	a combining form cell, container receptacle a combining form nucleus	"cyt/o" is a _Combining form_ meaning _cell_, _container_, or _receptacle_. "nucle/o" is a _combining form_ meaning _nucleus_.
3-9		Chromosomes are special threadlike substances in the nucleus that contain the genetic makeup of humans and exhibit a special color when treated with a certain dye. "chrom/o" is a combining form meaning color. -somes is a suffix referring to a specified or special body.
3-10	combining form, color -somes Chromosomes are special threadlike substances in a special body that contain the genetic makeup of humans and exhibit a special color when treated with a certain dye	"chrom/o" is a _combining_ _form_ meaning _Color_. _-Somes_ is a suffix meaning a specified or special body. Define chromosomes, accounting for both the root word "chrom/o" and the suffix -somes: _Chromosomes are special_ _threadlike substances in a_ _special body that contain_ _the genetic makeup of_ _humans and exhibit a_ _special color when_ _treated with a certain dye_.
3-11		Mitosis is a condition of threading (literally, "the threads [genetic materials] are multiplying"). In biology, mitosis is the process in which chromosomes are duplicated to reproduce life. "mit/o" is a combining form meaning threads. mito- also is a prefix. -osis is a suffix meaning condition or process.

BLOCK	DATA AND ANSWERS	DESCRIPTION AND QUESTIONS
3-12	"mit/o"	_mit/o_ is a combining form meaning threads.
	mito-	_mito_ is also a prefix meaning threads.
	suffix, condition	_-osis_ is a _suffix_ meaning _condition_ or
	process	_process_.
3-13	a substance making up the cell	Protoplasm is _a substance making up the cell_.
	protoplasm making up the nucleus	Nucleoplasm is _protoplasm making up the nucleus_.
	protoplasm outside the nucleus	Cytoplasm is _protoplasm outside the nucleus_.
3-14		The next few blocks review what we have learned about cells and other basic structures of the human body.
3-15	smallest	A cell is the _smallest_ structural unit of the human body.
3-16	membrane	A cell has a skin or wall called a _membrane_.
	in, out	A cell can screen substances trying to move _in_ or _out_ of the cell.
	cells	A tissue is a group of _cells_ with a special
	function	_function_ in the body.
3-17		A cell is made up of a substance called
	protoplasm	_protoplasm_.
	nucleus	A cell contains a small body called a _nucleus_.
	round	Structurally, the small body is _round_ or
	spheroid	_spheroid_.
		The small body contains human genetic materials called
	genes, chromosomes	_genes_ or _chromosomes_.
		The protoplasm inside the nucleus is called
	nucleoplasm	_nucleoplasm_.

BLOCK	DATA AND ANSWERS	DESCRIPTION AND QUESTIONS
3-18	to maintain its life, to reproduce	The special functions of a cell are _to maintain its life_ and _to reproduce_.
3-19	special threadlike substances in a body that contain the genetic makeup of humans and exhibit a special color when treated with a certain dye	Chromosomes are _special threadlike substances in a body that contain the genetic makeup of humans and exhibit a special color when treated with a certain dye_.
3-20	mitosis	The process in which cells multiply or reproduce by dividing is called _mitosis_.
3-21	tissue (tish-oo)	Recall the components of a cell: nucleus, protoplasm, nucleoplasm, genes (chromosomes), cytoplasm, and cell membrane. Some cells form a group because they have special responsibilities or functions in the body. Collectively, they are called tissue. A group of tissues in turn form a structure called an organ. For example, many cells combine to form a tissue that can perform certain functions of the liver. A group of such tissues join to form the liver, an organ.

BLOCK	DATA AND ANSWERS	DESCRIPTION AND QUESTIONS
3-22	epithelial tissue (ep'-i-the-le-al tish-oo)	There are many tissues in the body. They include epithelial tissue, connective tissue, muscle tissue, and nerve tissue.
		Epithelial tissue refers to the skin and lining surfaces. The skin has three main functions: protection, absorption, and secretion.
	connective tissue (ko'-nek-tiv tish-oo)	A connective tissue is one of the fibrous tissues of the body. Connective tissues serve a binding function for special parts of the body (e.g., bones and tendons).
	muscle tissue (mus-el tish-oo)	A muscle tissue is a tissue that contracts or relaxes (e.g., that in the arm and heart).
	nerve tissue (nerv tish-oo)	A nerve tissue is a collection of nerve fibers that conduct electrical impulses that control and coordinate body activities.
3-23	epithelium (ep-ih-thee-lee-um)	The epithelium is the outside layer of cells.
		epi- is a prefix meaning upon, on, outside, or top.
		"thelium" is a word root meaning nipple, holes, or apertures.
		Accordingly, epithelium refers to a layer of cells outside holes and apertures—in this case, skin.
		"epitheli" is a root word meaning skin.
		-al is a suffix meaning pertaining to.

BLOCK	DATA AND ANSWERS	DESCRIPTION AND QUESTIONS
3-24	the skin and lining surfaces	The epithelial tissue refers to _the_ _skin_ _and_ _lining_ _surfaces_.
	protection absorption, secretion	The skin has three main functions: _protection_, _absorption_, and _secretion_.
	prefix, upon, on outside, top	*epi-* is a _prefix_ meaning _upon_, _on_, _outside_, or _top_.
	root, nipple holes, apertures	"thelium" is a word _root_ meaning _nipple_, _holes_, or _apertures_.
	"epitheli," root	_epitheli_ is a word _root_ meaning skin.
	-al	_al_ is a suffix meaning pertaining to.
3-25	the fibrous tissues of the body	Connective tissue refers to _the_ _fibrous_ _tissues_ _of_ _the_ _body_.
	to bind some parts of the body (e.g., bones and tendons)	The function of connective tissue is _to_ _bind_ _some_ _parts_ _of_ _the_ _body_ _(e.g.,_ _bones_ _and_ _tendons)_.
3-26	a tissue that contracts or relaxes	Muscle tissue is _a_ _tissue_ _that_ _contracts_ or _releases_.
	nerve fibers that conduct electrical impulses that control and coordinate body activities	Nerve tissue is _nerve_ _fibers that_ _conduct_ _electrical_ _impulses_ _that_ _control_ _and_ _coordinate_ _body_ _activities_.

BLOCK	DATA AND ANSWERS	DESCRIPTION AND QUESTIONS
3-27	organ (<u>or</u>-gan)	A group of tissues that combine to perform special functions in the body is called an organ (e.g., heart, lungs, liver).
	system (<u>sis</u>-tem)	A set of body organs that work together for a common purpose is called a system. There are many systems in the body.
		Body systems include the skin and related parts, muscle and bones, heart and circulation, digestion and metabolism, respiration, nerves, urinary and reproductive functions, hormones, and the senses (e.g., sight, hearing, smell). The body has nine such systems, and we will study each of them in detail in this book. First, let us study the functions and medical parts of each system.
3-28	integumentary system (in-<u>teg</u>'-u-men-<u>ter</u>-e sis-tem)	The integumentary system consists of the skin and accessory organs such as nail, hair, and oil and sweat glands. In Latin, "integument" means covering.
	the skin and accessory organs such as nail, hair, and oil and sweat glands	The integumentary system consists of __the skin and accessory organs such as nails, hair, and oil and sweat glands__.
	covering	In Latin, the word "integument" means __covering__.
3-29	musculoskeletal system (mus-ku'-lo-<u>skel</u>-e-tal sis-tem)	The musculoskeletal system consists of the skeleton and muscles of the body.
		"muscul" is a root word meaning muscle.
		"muscul/o" is a combining form meaning muscle.
		"skelet" is a root word meaning skeleton, bones of the body.
		"skelet/o" is the combining form.
		-al is a suffix meaning pertaining to.

BLOCK	DATA AND ANSWERS	DESCRIPTION AND QUESTIONS
3-30	combining form muscle	"muscul/o" is a <u>Combining</u> <u>form</u> meaning <u>muscle</u>.
	combining form skeleton, bones of the body	"skelet/o" is a <u>Combining</u> <u>form</u> meaning <u>skeleton</u>, <u>bones</u> <u>of</u> <u>the</u> <u>body</u>.
	suffix, pertaining to	-al is a <u>Suffix</u> meaning <u>pertaing</u> <u>to</u>.
	the muscle and skeleton of the body	"Musculoskeletal" refers to <u>the</u> <u>muscle</u> <u>and</u> <u>skeleton</u> <u>of</u> <u>the</u> <u>body</u>
3-31	cardiovascular system (kar′-de-o-<u>vas</u>-ku-lar sis-tem)	The cardiovascular system consists of the heart, blood vessels, and the circulating blood.
		"cardi" is a root word meaning heart.
		"cardi/o" is the combining form.
		"vascular" is a word root referring to vessels that carry body fluids like blood and lymph.
		"vascul" is a word root referring to vessels that carry certain body fluids such as blood and lymph.
		"vascul/o" is the combining form.
		-ar is a suffix meaning pertaining to.
3-32	combining form heart	"cardi/o" is a <u>Combining</u> <u>form</u> meaning <u>heart</u>.
	"vascul/o"	<u>vasvulo</u> is a combining form referring to vessels that carry body fluids like blood and lymph.
	suffix, pertaining to	-ar is a <u>Suffix</u> meaning <u>pertaining</u> <u>to</u>.
	the	The cardiovascular system consists of <u>the</u>
	heart, blood vessels circulating blood	<u>heart</u>, <u>blood</u> <u>vessels</u>, and <u>circulating</u> <u>blood</u>.

BLOCK	DATA AND ANSWERS	DESCRIPTION AND QUESTIONS
3-33		One component of the blood is its fluid or lymph fluid.
	lymph (limf) lymphatic vessels (lim-<u>fat</u>-ik <u>ves</u>-selz)	Lymph fluid comes from the blood. It filters into the spaces between the cells and returns to the blood via lymphatic vessels. For example, the spleen is the largest lymphatic organ of the body. This network of fluid, blood, vessels, organs, and
	lymphatic system (lim-<u>fat</u>-ik <u>sis</u>-tem)	transport dynamics is the lymphatic system.
		The lymphatic system is usually considered part of the circulatory or cardiovascular system.
3-34		"lymph" is a root word meaning lymph.
		"lymph/o" is a combining form meaning lymph.
		-*atic* is a suffix meaning pertaining to.
3-35	lymph lymph fluid lymphatic	The fluid formed in tissues spaces is called _____ or _____ _____, which is transported throughout the body by a network of _____ vessels.
3-36	"lymph"	_____ is a root word meaning lymph.
	"lymph/o"	_____ is the combining form.
	-*atic*	_____ is a suffix meaning pertaining to.
3-37	gastrointestinal system (gas'-tro-in-<u>tes</u>-ti-nal sis-tem)	The gastrointestinal system refers to the mouth, salivary glands, esophagus, stomach, intestines, rectum, and the accessory organs the liver, gallbladder, and pancreas.
		"gastr/o" is a combining form meaning stomach.
		"intestin/o" is a combining form meaning intestine.
		-*al* is a suffix meaning pertaining to.

BOX 3.1
Allied Health Professions

Dietitians and Dietetic Technicians

Dietitians are professionals trained in applying the principles of nutrition to food selection and meal preparation. They help prevent and treat illnesses by promoting healthy eating habits, scientifically evaluating clients' diets, and suggesting diet modifications. They counsel individuals and groups; set up and supervise food service systems for institutions such as schools, hospitals, and prisons; promote sound eating habits through education; and conduct research. Major areas of specialization include clinical, management, community, business and industry, and consultant dietetics. Dietitians also work as educators and researchers.

A dietetic technician, registered (DTR), works as a member of the food service, management, and health care team, independently or in consultation with a registered dietitian. The dietetic technician supervises support staff, monitors cost-control procedures, interprets and implements quality assurance procedures, counsels individuals or small groups, screens patients/clients for nutritional status, and develops nutrition care plans. The dietetic technician helps to supervise food production and service; plans menus; tests new products for use in the facility; and selects, schedules, and conducts orientation programs for personnel. The technician may also be involved in selecting personnel and providing on-the-job training. The dietetic technician obtains, evaluates, and uses dietary histories to plan nutritional care for patients. Using this information, the technician guides families and individuals in selecting food, preparing it, and planning menus based on nutritional needs. The dietetic technician has an active part in calculating nutrient intakes and dietary patterns.

A great resource is the American Dietetic Association at www.eatright.org.

Source: P. S. Stanfield, N. Cross, Y. H. Hui, eds. *Introduction to the Health Professions*, 5th ed. (Sudbury, MA: Jones & Bartlett, 2009).

BLOCK	DATA AND ANSWERS	DESCRIPTION AND QUESTIONS
3-38	combining form stomach	"gastr/o" is a _____ _____ meaning _____.
	combining form intestine	"intestin/o" is a _____ _____ meaning _____.
	suffix, pertaining to	-*al* is a _____ meaning _____ ____.
3-39	the	The gastrointestinal system includes: _____
	mouth, salivary glands	_____, _____ _____,
	esophagus, stomach	_____, _____,
	intestines, rectum, and	_____, _____, _____
	the accessory organs	_____ _____ _____
	liver, gallbladder, and	_____, _____, _____
	pancreas	_____.

BLOCK	DATA AND ANSWERS	DESCRIPTION AND QUESTIONS
3-40	respiratory system (res-pir-ah-<u>to</u>-re <u>sis</u>-tem)	The respiratory system is responsible for taking in oxygen and removing carbon dioxide. It involves the nose, pharynx, larynx, trachea, bronchi, and lungs. The route or passageway from the nose and through a series of "tubes" or "organs" to the lungs is called the respiratory tract.
	oxygen carbon dioxide	The respiratory system takes in _____ and releases _____ _____.
	nose pharynx, larynx, trachea bronchi, lungs	The respiratory system includes: _____, _____, _____, _____, _____, and _____.
3-41	genitourinary system (jen'-i-<u>to</u>-u-rih-ner'e <u>sis</u>-tem)	The genitourinary system is responsible for body sexual functions and the disposal of liquid body waste (urine). The system consists of the reproductive and urinary organs. The urinary organs are the kidneys, ureters, bladder, and urethra. The reproductive organs are the gonads and various external genitalia and internal parts.
3-42	sexual, waste disposal	The genitourinary system is responsible for two types of functions: _____ and _____ _____.
	the kidneys ureters, bladder urethra	The urinary organs are _____ _____, _____, _____, and _____.
	the gonads and various external genitalia and internal parts	The sex organs are _____ _____ _____ _____ _____ _____ _____ _____ _____.

BLOCK	DATA AND ANSWERS	DESCRIPTION AND QUESTIONS
3-43	endocrine system (<u>en</u>-do-krin sis-tem)	Endocrine means internal secretion. The endocrine system refers to the glands that make hormones and release them into the circulatory system. *endo-* is a prefix meaning internal, innermost, or within. "crine" is a word root meaning secrete. *-crine* also is a suffix.
3-44	prefix, internal suffix, secrete internal secretion the glands that make hormones and release them into the circulatory system	*endo-* is a _____ meaning _____. *-crine* is a _____ meaning _____. "endocrine" means _____ _____. The endocrine system refers to _____ _____ _____ _____ _____ _____ _____ _____ _____ _____ _____ _____.
3-45	nervous system (<u>ner</u>-vus sis-tem)	The nervous system comprises the brain, spinal cord, and nerves. "nerve" is a word root meaning nerve. "nerv/o" is the combining form. *-ous* is a suffix meaning pertaining to.
3-46	"nerv/o" suffix, pertaining to the brain the spinal cord, nerves	_____ is a combining form meaning nerve. *-ous* is a _____ meaning _____ ____. The nervous system is made up of _____ _____, _____ _____ _____, and _____.

BLOCK	DATA AND ANSWERS	DESCRIPTION AND QUESTIONS
3-47		The last body system is the sensory system or system of the senses (eyes, ears, and nose). We are all familiar with our senses of sight, hearing, and smell. The senses of touch and taste will not be discussed in this book.
3-48		The body has two main groups of cavities, those facing the front (ventral) and those facing the back (dorsal) of the body. Each of these cavities is further divided into smaller cavities that contain specific organs. **Figure 3.2** depicts the dorsal and ventral body cavities.
3-49	pleural (<u>plu</u>-ral) pleurae (<u>plu</u>-ray) thoracic (tho-<u>rass</u>-ic)	The pleural cavity is the body cavity that surrounds the lungs. This cavity is lined by double folded membranes known as pleurae. The thoracic or chest cavity contains: 1. The hearts, lungs, and supporting structures 2. Other structures associated with hormonal, nervous, and digestive systems

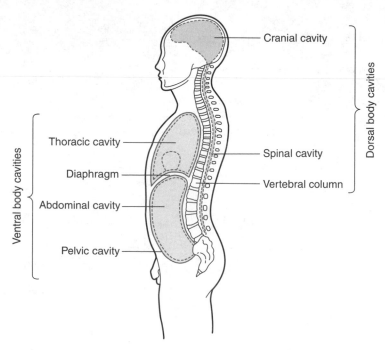

FIGURE 3.2   Sagittal section of the body, showing the dorsal and ventral body cavities

BLOCK	DATA AND ANSWERS	DESCRIPTION AND QUESTIONS
3-50		"pleur" is a root word referring to the pleural cavity or the membranes lining the lungs. "pleur/o" is the combining form. -al is a suffix meaning pertaining to. "thorac" and "thor" are both root words meaning chest. "thorac/o" is the combining form. -ic is a suffix meaning pertaining to. "thoracic" is an adjective describing the chest.
3-51	"pleur" "pleur/o" suffix, pertaining to	_____ is a root word meaning the pleural cavity or the membranes lining the lungs. _____ is the combining form. -al is a _____ meaning _____ ____.
3-52	"thorac," "thor" "thorac/o" suffix, pertaining to	_____ and _____ are both root words meaning chest. _____ is a combining form meaning chest. -ic is a _____ meaning _____ ____.
3-53	the body cavity that surrounds the lungs	The pleural cavity is _____ _____ _____ _____ _____ _____ _____.
3-54	peritoneal cavity (per'-i-to-<u>ne</u>-al <u>kav</u>-i-te)	The peritoneal cavity contains the stomach, intestines, liver, gallbladder, pancreas, spleen, reproductive organs, and urinary bladder. This space also is known as the abdominopelvic cavity. Although there is no physical partition, we can also refer to the abdominal cavity and the pelvic cavity. "peritone" is a word root meaning a membrane covering the entire abdominal wall. "peritone/o" is the combining form. -al is a suffix meaning pertaining to.

BLOCK	DATA AND ANSWERS	DESCRIPTION AND QUESTIONS
3-55	a membrane covering the entire abdominal wall	"peritone" is a word root meaning __ _____ _____ _____ _____ _____ _____.
	combining form a membrane covering the entire abdominal wall	"peritone/o" is a _____ _____ meaning __ _____ _____ _____ _____ _____ _____.
	-al	_____ is a suffix meaning pertaining to.
3-56	the stomach, intestines, liver gallbladder, pancreas spleen, reproductive organs, urinary bladder	The peritoneal cavity refers to the space containing _____ _____, _____, _____, _____, _____, _____, _____ _____, and _____ _____.
	abdominopelvic cavity	This entire space is also known as the _____ _____.
	the abdominal cavity, the pelvic cavity	We may divide this space further into _____ _____ _____ and _____ _____ _____ (though there is no physical barrier between them).
3-57	diaphragm (<u>di</u>-ah-fram)	The diaphragm is a dome-shaped muscle separating the abdominal and thoracic cavities.
3-58	a dome-shaped muscle separating the abdominal and thoracic cavities	The diaphragm is __ _____ _____ _____ _____ _____ _____ _____ _____.

BLOCK	DATA AND ANSWERS	DESCRIPTION AND QUESTIONS
3-59		Let us now look at the cavities at the back (dorsal) of the body.
	cranial cavity (kra-ne-al <u>kav</u>-i-te)	The cranial cavity is the space enclosed by skull bones, containing the brain.
	spinal cavity (<u>spi</u>-nal <u>kav</u>-i-te)	The spinal cavity inside the spinal column is the space containing the spinal cord.
		"crani" is a word root meaning skull.
		"crani/o" is the combining form.
		"spine" is a word root meaning spine.
		"spin/o" is the combining form.
		-al is a suffix meaning pertaining to.
3-60	"crani"	_____ is a word root meaning skull.
	"crani/o"	_____ is a combining form meaning skull.
	"spine"	_____ is a word root meaning spine.
	"spin/o"	_____ is a combining form meaning spine.
	-al	_____ is a suffix meaning pertaining to.
3-61	brain	The cranial cavity contains the _____.
3-62	spinal cord	The spinal cavity contains the _____ _____.
3-63	mediastinum (me'-de-ah-<u>sti</u>-num)	The mediastinum is the mass of tissues and organs separating the two lobes of the lungs and separating the sternum in front and the vertebral column behind. The mediastinum includes: the heart, its large and small vessels, and all respiratory branches leading to the lungs from the nose.

BLOCK	DATA AND ANSWERS	DESCRIPTION AND QUESTIONS
3-64		A human's body parts can be studied from many angles, or more appropriately, from many planes. Body planes are imaginary lines that divide the body in anatomic diagrams. See **Figure 3.3**.
	sagittal (<u>saj</u>-i-tal), frontal (<u>frun</u>-tal), coronal (ko-<u>ro</u>-nal), transverse (trans-<u>vers</u>)	There are three major body planes: sagittal, frontal (or coronal), and transverse.
		A sagittal plane divides the body into right and left portions. The portions may or may not be equal. When it runs through the midline, it is called a mid-sagittal plane. If so, then the right and left portion are equal. Otherwise, it is called a para-sagittal plane.
		A frontal or coronal plane divides the body into anterior and posterior sections (front and back).
		A transverse plane divides the body into superior and inferior sections (top and bottom).

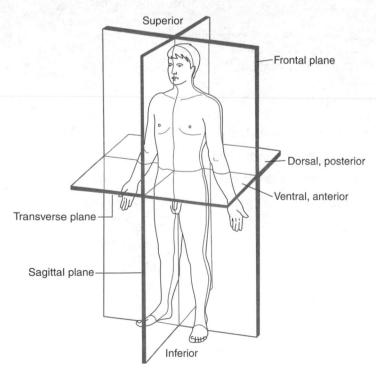

FIGURE 3.3 Body planes and directions

BLOCK	DATA AND ANSWERS	DESCRIPTION AND QUESTIONS
3-65	a plane that divides the body into right and left portions the portions may or may not be equal	A sagittal plane is ___ _____ _____ _____ _____ _____ _____ _____ _____ _____ _____; _____ _____ _____ _____ _____ _____ ____ _____.
3-66	a plane that divides the body into anterior and posterior sections (front and back)	A frontal or coronal plane is ___ _____ _____ _____ _____ _____ _____ _____ _____ _____ _____ _____ _____ _____.
3-67	a plane that divides the body into superior and inferior sections (top and bottom)	A transverse plane is ___ _____ _____ _____ _____ _____ _____ _____ _____ _____ _____ _____ _____ _____.
3-68	quadrant (<u>kwo</u>-d-rant)	Patients will often point to one area of the abdomen and complain that "this part hurts." However, clinicians and support personnel need to be very explicit in their communications, both oral and written, when describing pain symptoms. To do so, anatomists and clinicians divide the abdomen surface into four general areas called quadrants. See **Figure 3.4**. These imaginary divisions use the belly button (umbilicus or navel) as a reference point. The four quadrants are separated by a vertical and a horizontal line through the navel. As a result, as seen in Figure 3.4, we have: the right upper quadrant (RUQ); left upper quadrant (LUQ); right lower quadrant (RLQ); and left lower quadrant (LLQ).

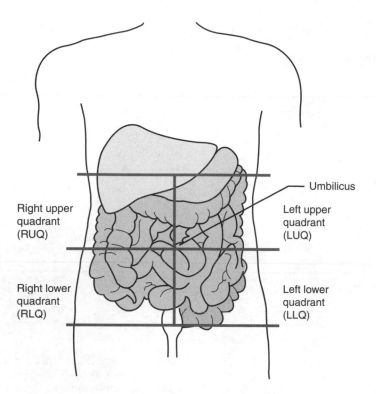

FIGURE 3.4 Abdominal quadrants

BLOCK	DATA AND ANSWERS	DESCRIPTION AND QUESTIONS
3-69		"quarter" is a root word meaning one of four.
		"quadrant" is another word root meaning quarter or one of four.
		"quadr" is a word root meaning quadrant.
		"quadr/o" is the combining form.
		-*ant* is a suffix meaning the "thing of which" (in this case, "four of which").

BLOCK	DATA AND ANSWERS	DESCRIPTION AND QUESTIONS
3-70	"quadrant"	In addition to "quarter," _____ is another root word meaning one of four.
	"quadr"	_____ is a word root meaning one of four.
	"quadr/o"	_____ is the combining form.
	-ant	_____ is a suffix meaning the "thing of which."
3-71		To be even more specific in identifying different parts of the abdomen, clinicians further divide the area into nine regions.
		Some textbooks call them Region 1, 2, 3, and so on. Others simply describe them without using numbers. We follow the second approach. Consult **Figure 3.5** when studying the next few blocks for the nine regions.

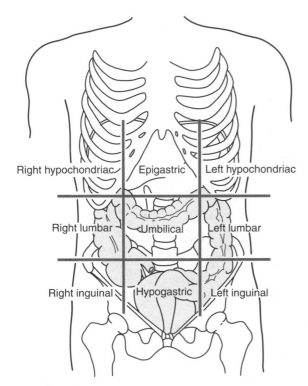

FIGURE 3.5   Abdominal regions

BLOCK	DATA AND ANSWERS	DESCRIPTION AND QUESTIONS
3-72	hypochondriac (hi-poh'-<u>koh</u>-dree-ak)	The right hypochondriac region is located in the upper-right area of the abdomen, covering the right lobe of the liver and the gallbladder.
		The left hypochondriac region is located in the upper-left area of the abdomen, covering a small portion of the stomach and a portion of the large intestine.
		"hypochondrium" is a noun meaning abdomen.
		"hypochrondriac" is an adjective describing the abdomen.
		hypo- is a prefix meaning below or under.
		"chondri" is a word root meaning cartridge. It also means lump or groats depending on the medical usage.
		"chondri/o" is the combining form.
		-ac is a suffix meaning pertaining to.
3-73	prefix, below under	*hypo-* is a _____ meaning _____ or _____.
	word root cartridge, lump, groats	"chondri" is a _____ _____ meaning _____, _____, or _____.
	"chondri/o"	_____ is the combining form of "chondri."
	-ac	_____ is a suffix meaning pertaining to.
3-74	epigastric (ep-ih-<u>gas</u>-trik) region	The epigastric region is located between the right and left hypochondriac regions, beneath the cartilage of the lower ribs. It covers parts of the right and left lobes of the liver and a major portion of the stomach.
		epi- is a prefix meaning over, upon, or above.
		"gastr" is a root word meaning stomach.
		"gastr/o" is the combining form.
		-ic is a suffix meaning pertaining to.

BLOCK	DATA AND ANSWERS	DESCRIPTION AND QUESTIONS
3-75	the right lobe of the liver and the gallbladder	The right hypochondriac region covers _____ _____ _____ _____ _____ _____ _____ _____ _____.
3-76	a small portion of the stomach and a portion of the large intestine	The left hypochondriac region covers ___ _____ _____ _____ _____ _____ _____ __ _____ _____ _____ _____ _____.
3-77	the right and left lobes of the liver and a major portion of the stomach	The epigastric region covers _____ _____ _____ _____ _____ _____ _____ _____ _____ __ _____ _____ _____ _____ _____.
3-78	abdomen	Hypochondrium refers to the _____.
3-79	Hypochondriac	_____ is an adjective meaning abdomen.
3-80	in the upper-right area of the abdomen covering the right lobe of the liver and the gallbladder	The right hypochondriac region is located ____ _____ _____ _____ _____ _____ _____ _____ _____ _____ _____ ____ _____ _____ _____ _____ _____.
3-81	in the upper-left area of the abdomen covering a small portion of the stomach and a portion of the large intestine	The left hypochondriac region is located ____ _____ _____ _____ _____ _____ _____ _____ __ _____ _____ _____ _____ _____ _____ _____ __ _____ _____ _____ _____ _____.
3-82	prefix, over, upon

combining form stomach

-ic | *epi-* is a _____ meaning _____ or _____.

"gastr/o" is a _____ _____ meaning _____.

_____ is a suffix meaning pertaining to. |

BLOCK	DATA AND ANSWERS	DESCRIPTION AND QUESTIONS
3-83	Located between the right and left hypochondriac regions beneath the cartilage of the lower ribs, it covers parts of the right and left lobes of the liver and a major portion of the stomach	Define the epigastric region: _____ _____ _____ _____ _____ _____ _____ _____, _____ _____ _____ ____ _____ _____ _____; ___ _____ _____ _____ _____ _____ _____ _____ _____ _____ _____ _____ _____ ___ _____ _____ _____ _____ _____
3-84		The right lumbar region is located in the middle-right area of the abdomen covering portions of the large and small intestines. The left lumbar region is located in the middle-left area of the abdomen, covering portions of the small intestine and a part of the colon. Lumbar means loins. "lumb" is a word root meaning loins. "lumb/o" is the combining form. -ar is a suffix meaning pertaining to.
3-85		The umbilical region is located in the middle area of the abdomen, between the right and left lumbar regions and directly underneath the epigastric region. This region includes portions of the small intestine and a portion of the transverse colon. "umbilicus" is a root word meaning navel. "umbilic" is a root word meaning navel. "umbilic/o is the combining form. -al is a suffix meaning pertaining to.

BLOCK	DATA AND ANSWERS	DESCRIPTION AND QUESTIONS
3-86	portions of the large and small intestines	The right lumbar region covers the following organs: _____ ____ _____ _____ _____ _____ _____.
	portions of the small intestine and a part of the colon	The left lumbar region covers the following organs: _____ ____ _____ _____ _____ _____ __ _____ ____ _____ _____.
3-87	"lumb" "lumb/o" -_ar_	_____ is a word root meaning loins. _____ is the combining form. _____ is a suffix meaning pertaining to.
3-88	navel "umbilic/o" suffix, pertaining to	"umbilic" is a root word meaning _____. _____ is the combining form. -_al_ is a _____ meaning _____ _____.
3-89	portions of the small intestine and a portion of the transverse colon	The umbilical region includes the following organs: _____ ____ _____ _____ _____ _____ __ _____ _____ _____ _____ _____.
3-90	in the middle-right area of the abdomen covering portions of the large and small intestines	The right lumbar region is located ____ _____ _____ _____ _____ _____ _____ _____ _____ ____ ____ _____ _____ _____ _____.
3-91	in the middle-left area of the abdomen covering portions of the small intestine and a part of the colon	The left lumbar region is located ____ _____ _____ _____ _____ _____ _____ _____ _____ ____ _____ _____ _____ __ _____ ____ _____ _____.

BLOCK	DATA AND ANSWERS	DESCRIPTION AND QUESTIONS
3-92	in the middle area of the abdomen between the right and left lumbar regions and directly underneath the epigastric region, this region includes portions of the small intestine and a portion of the transverse colon	The umbilical region is located ____ _____ _____ _____ _____ _____ _____, _____ _____ _____ _____ _____ _____ _____ _____ _____ _____ _____ _____ _____; _____ _____ _____ _____ _____ _____ _____ _____ _____ ___ _____ _____ _____ _____ _____.
3-93	right inguinal (ing'-gwi-nal), iliac (ill'-ee-ac) region	The right inguinal (iliac) region is located in the lower-right area of the abdomen, under the right lumbar region. It covers portions of the small intestine and the cecum.
3-94		The left inguinal (iliac) region is located in the lower-left area of the abdomen, under the left lumbar region. It covers portions of the colon and the small intestine.
3-95		"inguin" is a word root meaning groin. "inguin/o" is the combining form. -al is a suffix meaning pertaining to.
3-96	ilium (ill-ee-um)	"ilium" is a word root referring to the largest of the three hip bones. "ili" is a word root referring to the largest of the three hip bones. "ili/o" is the combining form. -ac is a suffix meaning pertaining to.
3-97	left inguinal (iliac) region	The _____ _____ _____ _____ covers portions of the colon and the small intestine.

BLOCK	DATA AND ANSWERS	DESCRIPTION AND QUESTIONS
3-98	right inguinal (iliac) region	The _____ _____ _____ _____ covers portions of the small intestine and the cecum.
3-99	combining form groin -al	"inguin/o" is a _____ _____ meaning _____. A suffix for the word root of "inguin" is _____.
3-100	"ilium" or "ili" "ili/o" -ac	_____ or ____ is a word root referring to the largest of the three hip bones. _____ is a combining form referring to the largest of the three hip bones. _____ is a suffix meaning pertaining to.
3-101	word root groin word root, the largest of the three hip bones	"inguinal" is a _____ _____ meaning _____. "ilium" is a _____ _____ referring to _____ _____ ____ _____ _____ _____ _____.
3-102	portions of the colon and the small intestine	The left inguinal (iliac) region covers _____ ____ _____ _____ _____ _____ _____ _____.
3-103	portions of the small intestine and the cecum	The right inguinal (iliac) region covers _____ ____ _____ _____ _____ _____ _____ _____.
3-104		The hypogastric region is located in the lower-middle area of the abdomen, under the umbilical region. It comprises the urinary bladder, portions of the small intestine, and the appendix.

BLOCK	DATA AND ANSWERS	DESCRIPTION AND QUESTIONS
3-105		Hypogastric means under or below the stomach.
		hypo- is a prefix meaning under.
		"gastr" is a root word meaning stomach.
		"gastr/o" is the combining form.
		-ic is a suffix meaning pertaining to.
3-106	under or below the stomach	Hypogastric means _____ _____ _____ _____ _____.
	the urinary bladder, portions of the small intestine, the appendix	The hypogastric region covers _____ _____ _____, _____ _____ _____ _____ _____, and _____ _____.
3-107	*hypo-*	_____ is a prefix meaning under.
	root word stomach	"gastr" is a _____ _____ meaning _____.
	combining form stomach	"gastr/o" is a _____ _____ meaning _____.
	-ic	_____ is a suffix meaning pertaining to.

BLOCK	DATA AND ANSWERS	DESCRIPTION AND QUESTIONS
3-108	Located in the lower-right area of the abdomen, under the right lumbar region, covering portions of the small intestine and the cecum	Define the right inguinal (iliac) region: _____ ___ _____ _____ _____ _____ _____ _____, _____ _____ _____ _____ _____, _____ _____ ____ _____ _____ _____ _____ _____ _____
	Located in the lower-left area of the abdomen, under the left lumbar region, covering portions of the colon and the small intestine	Define the left inguinal (iliac) region: _____ ____ _____ _____ _____ _____ _____ _____, _____ _____ _____ _____ _____, _____ _____ _____ _____ _____ _____ _____ _____
	Located in the lower-middle area of the abdomen, under the umbilical region, the urinary bladder, portions of the small intestine, the appendix	Define the hypogastric region: _____ ____ ____ _____ _____ ____ _____ _____, _____ _____ _____ _____; _____ _____ _____, _____ ____ _____ _____ _____, and _____ _____
3-109		In this chapter, you have learned whole-body terminology affecting: cells, organs, tissues, planes, regions, and quadrants. The remaining chapters cover each of the nine body systems and medical terms associated with them. The next chapter concentrates on the skin system.

BOX 3.2 Abbreviations	
CAD	coronary heart disease
CLL	chronic lymphatic leukemia
COPD	chronic obstructive pulmonary disorder
FEF	forced expiratory flow
ID	intradermal
KUB	kidney, ureter, bladder
MCH	mean corpuscular hemoglobin
MS	multiple sclerosis
RE	right eye
REM	rapid eye movement
SLE	systemic lupus erythematosus
TKR	total knee replacement
TSH	thyroid stimulating hormone
UGI	upper gastrointestinal

Progress Check

A. Multiple Choice

1. A word root meaning secrete is:
   a. nucle
   b. peritone
   c. crine
   d. epitheli

2. A word root meaning groin is:
   a. chondri
   b. plasm
   c. thor
   d. inguin

3. A word root meaning vessel is:
   a. lymph
   b. vascul
   c. muscul
   d. nerve

4. A combining form meaning heart is:
   a. cardi/o
   b. chondri/o
   c. gastr/o
   d. lymph/o

5. A combining form meaning threads or threading is:
   a. lymph/o
   b. gastr/o
   c. mit/o
   d. nerv/o

6. A combining form meaning membranes lining the lungs:
   a. lymph/o
   b. pleur/o
   c. spin/o
   d. quadr/o

7. A combining form meaning hip bone is:
   a. ili/o
   b. inguin/o
   c. chondri/o
   d. cyt/o

8. A prefix meaning inside, within, and internal is:
   a. electro-
   b. hypo-
   c. exo-
   d. endo-

9. A prefix meaning over, upon, or above is:
   a. epi-
   b. ambi-
   c. circum-
   d. dia-

10. A suffix meaning pertaining to is:
    a. -atic
    b. -crine
    c. -us
    d. -dome

11. A suffix identifying a noun as singular is:
    a. -al
    b. -us
    c. -ic
    d. -ton

12. A suffix meaning container or receptacle is:

    a. -ic

    b. -osis

    c. -ant

    d. -some

B. Matching

1. nucleus	**a.** membrane lining the abdominal wall
2. epithelium	**b.** fluid
3. peritoneal	**c.** groin
4. crine	**d.** hip bone
5. hypochondrium	**e.** mid-abdominal segment of body
6. inguinal	**f.** membranes, lung
7. ilium	**g.** secrete
8. lumbar	**h.** skin
9. pleural	**i.** spheroid round body
10. lymph	**j.** upper region of abdomen below ribs

C. Medical Terms and Their Definitions

	TERM	DEFINITION
1.	connective tissue	
2.		dome-shaped muscle separating the abdominal and thoracic cavities
3.	epigastric region	
4.		consists of the skin and accessory organs, such as nail, hair, and oil and sweat glands; in Latin, integument means covering
5.	mediastinum	
6.		space containing the stomach, intestines, liver, gallbladder, pancreas, spleen, reproductive organs, and urinary bladder
7.	sagittal plane	
8.		group of cells combined to form a structure that has a special responsibility or function in the body
9.	transverse plane	
10.		root word meaning navel

D. Abbreviations

	ABBREVIATION	MEANING
1.	CAD	
2.	CLL	
3.	COPD	
4.	FEF	
5.	ID	
6.	KUB	
7.	MCH	
8.	MS	
9.	RE	
10.	REM	
11.	SLE	
12.	TKR	
13.	TSH	
14.	UGI	

The Integumentary System

BLOCK	DATA AND ANSWERS	DESCRIPTIONS AND ANSWERS
4-1	epithelium (ep'-ih-<u>thee</u>-lee-um) integument (in-teg-u-ment)	Epithelium is the tissue that covers the internal and external surfaces of the body. The external covering of the body is the skin (integument). The integumentary system is composed of the skin and its accessory organs: hair, nails, sweat, and sebaceous glands. This system is the largest organ of the body. See **Figure 4.1** and **Table 4.1** (which contains the word roots, combining forms, prefixes, and suffixes relevant to this subject).
4-2	skin integument integumentary integumentary	The external covering of the body is the _____ or _____. The _____ system is composed of the skin and its accessory organs. The skin, or _____, system is the largest organ of the body.
4-3	 hair, nails sweat, sebaceous glands	The accessory organs of the skin are: hair, nails, sweat, and sebaceous glands. The accessory organs of the skin are: _____, _____, _____, and _____ _____.

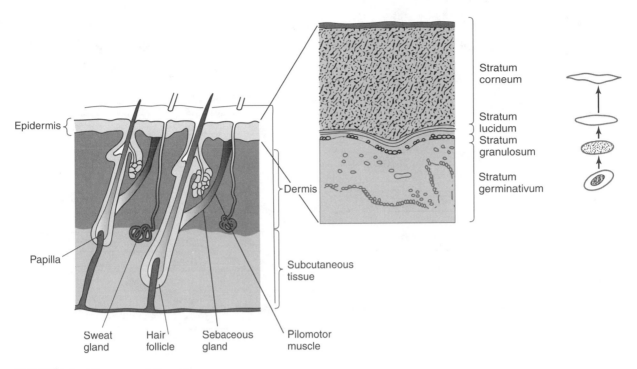

FIGURE 4.1 Diagram of the skin

TABLE 4.1 Word Components in this Chapter

WORD ROOTS	COMBINING FORMS	PREFIXES
abrasion	aut/o	auto-
aut	cap/o	cryo-
cap	corpor/o	dys-
coni	crur/o	electro-
corpor	cry/o	epi-
crur	crypt/o	hetero-
cry	cutane/o	hyper-
crypt	derm/o	intra-
cutane	dermat/o	sub-
cyte	desiccat/o	SUFFIXES
derma	echar/o	-al
dermal	electr/o	-cyte
dermat	fibr/o	-ectomy
desiccat	heter/o	-elastica
echar	kerat/o	-ion

TABLE 4.1 Word Components in this Chapter (continued)

WORD ROOTS	COMBINING FORMS	SUFFIXES
electr	melan/o	-is
epiderm	onych/o	-itis
epitheli	ped/o	-logist
fibr	rhytid/o	-logy
genic	seb/o	-malacia
heter	ungu/o	-oma
kerat	xer/o	-osis
melan		-ous
onych		-phagia
pachy		-plasty
ped		-rrhea
pigmentosum		-therapy
rhytid		-tome
seb		-tomy
senile		
surgery		
therapy		
tinea		
ungu		
unguium		
xer		

BLOCK	DATA AND ANSWERS	DESCRIPTIONS AND ANSWERS
4-4	epidermis (ep'-ih-der-mis), dermis (<u>der</u>-mis)	The skin has two layers: epidermis and the dermis. *epi-* is a prefix meaning upon. "dermis" is a root word meaning skin. The epidermis is the top layer of the skin, and it is composed of four layers called strata. The dermis is the second layer under the epidermis. It has two parts, an upper and lower layer. Dermis is the basic medical word or word root for skin from which several word roots have developed. Thus, the major word roots for skin include, but are not limited to, "dermis," "derm," "derma," "dermal," and "dermat." However, their usage in many medical texts is not uniform. Although they also are used throughout this book, the most common and uniform medical components for skin are two combining forms, "derm/o" and "dermat/o." To complicate the matter, "cutane" is another word root for skin and its combining form is "cutane/o."
4-5	 epidermis dermis	The skin has two layers. The top layer is the _____. The bottom layer is the _____. The skin has several word roots and two combining forms.
4-6	"dermis", "derm" "derma", "dermal", "dermat" "derm/o" "dermat/o" word root "cutane/o"	The word roots are _____, _____, _____, _____, and _____. The combining forms are _____ and _____. "cutane" is a _____ _____ meaning skin. The combining form is _____.

BLOCK	DATA AND ANSWERS	DESCRIPTIONS AND ANSWERS
4-7	dermatology (der'-mah-<u>tol</u>-o-je)	Dermatology is the study of the skin. "dermat/o" is a combining form meaning skin. -*logy* is a suffix meaning the study of.
4-8	the study of the skin skin the study of	Dermatology is _____ _____ ____ _____ _____. "dermat/o" means _____. -*logy* means _____ _____ ____.
4-9	dermatologist (der'-mah-<u>tol</u>-o-jist)	A dermatologist is a physician who specializes in the treatment of skin diseases. "dermat/o" is a combining form meaning skin. -*logist* is a suffix meaning one who specializes in the study of.
4-10	combining form skin suffix, one who specializes in the study of a physician who specializes in skin diseases	"dermat/o" is a _____ _____ meaning _____. -*logist* is a _____ meaning _____ _____ _____ ___ _____ _____ ____. A dermatologist is __ _____ _____ _____ ___ _____ _____.
4-11	dermatotome (der-mah-<u>to</u>-tom)	A dermatotome is an instrument that cuts the skin. "dermat/o" is a combining form meaning skin. -*tome* is a suffix meaning instrument for cutting.
4-12	combining form skin suffix, an instrument to cut an instrument that cuts the skin	"dermat/o" is a _____ _____ meaning _____. -*tome* is a _____ meaning _____ _____ ____ _____. A dermatotome is _____ _____ _____ _____ _____ _____.

BLOCK	DATA AND ANSWERS	DESCRIPTIONS AND ANSWERS
4-13	dermatitis (der′-mah-<u>ti</u>-tis)	Inflammation of the skin is called dermatitis. "dermat" is a word root meaning skin. -*itis* is a suffix meaning inflammation.
4-14	word root, skin suffix inflammation inflammation of the skin	"dermat" is a _____ _____ meaning _____. -*itis* is a _____ meaning _____. Dermatitis is _____ _____ _____ _____.
4-15	seborrheic dermatitis (seb-<u>o</u>-re-ik der′-mah-<u>ti</u>-tis)	Seborrheic dermatitis is an inflammation of the skin with an oily appearance (yellowish, greasy scaling). "seb/o" is a combining form meaning oil. -*rrhea* is a noun suffix meaning discharge. -*rrheic* is an adjective suffix meaning discharging. "dermat/o" is a combining form meaning skin. -*itis* is a suffix meaning inflammation.
4-16	"seb/o" -*rrhea* "dermat/o" -*itis*	_____ is a combining form meaning oil. _____ is a suffix meaning discharge. _____ is a combining form meaning skin. _____ is a suffix meaning inflammation.
4-17	seborrheic dermatitis	_____ _____ is an inflammation of the skin with an oily appearance.
4-18	dermatotherapy (der-mat′-o-<u>ther</u>-ah-pe)	Dermatotherapy is treatment of the skin. "dermat/o" is a combining form meaning skin. -*therapy* is a suffix meaning treatment. (Note that therapy also can be a noun and a word root.)

BLOCK	DATA AND ANSWERS	DESCRIPTIONS AND ANSWERS
4-19	"dermat/o" *-therapy* Dermatotherapy	_____ is a combining form meaning skin. _____ is a suffix meaning treatment. _____ is the treatment of the skin.
4-20	dermatofibroma (der-mat'-o-fi-<u>bro</u>-mah)	A dermatofibroma is a fibrous tumor of the skin. "dermat/o" is a combining form meaning skin. "fibr" is a root word meaning fiber. *-oma* is a suffix meaning tumor.
4-21	"dermat/o" "fibr" *-oma* dermatofibroma	_____ is a combining form meaning skin. _____ is a root word meaning fiber. _____ is a suffix meaning tumor. A _____ is a fibrous tumor of the skin.
4-22	dermatoconiosis (der-mat-<u>o</u>-ko'-ne-<u>o</u>-sis)	People are sometimes sensitive to dust in the air. Dermatoconiosis is an abnormal condition of the skin caused by dust, usually in the workplace. "dermat/o" is a combining form meaning skin. "coni" is a root word meaning dust. *-osis* is a suffix meaning condition.
4-23	"dermat/o" "coni" *-osis* Dermatoconiosis	_____ is a combining form meaning skin. _____ is a root word meaning dust. _____ is a suffix meaning condition. _____ is an abnormal condition of the skin caused by dust.

BLOCK	DATA AND ANSWERS	DESCRIPTIONS AND ANSWERS
4-24	epidermal (ep'-ih-<u>der</u>-mal)	So far, we have studied the derivative "derma" as the beginning of a medical term. This word root can also be used in the middle of a medical term. Epidermal means pertaining to something on top of the skin. *epi-* is a prefix meaning upon. "derm" is a word root meaning skin. *-al* is a suffix meaning pertaining to.
4-25	prefix, upon word root, skin suffix, pertaining to Epidermal	*epi-* is a _____ meaning _____. "derm" is a _____ _____ meaning _____. *-al* is a _____ meaning _____ _____. _____ means pertaining to something on top of the skin.
4-26	xeroderma pigmentosum (ze-ro-<u>der</u>-mah pig'-men-<u>to</u>-sum)	The word root "derma" also can be used at the end of a medical term. Xeroderma pigmentosum is a fatal disorder in which skin is dry and pigmented, with brown spots and ulcers (Kaposi's disease). "xer/o" is a combining form meaning dry. "derma" is a root word meaning skin. Pigmentosum is a medical word meaning pigmented condition.
4-27	"xer/o" "derma" Pigmentosum Xeroderma pigmentosum	_____ is a combining form meaning dry. _____ is a root word meaning skin. _____ is a medical word meaning pigmented condition. _____ _____ is a fatal disorder in which skin is dry and pigmented, with brown spots and ulcers (Kaposi's disease).

BLOCK	DATA AND ANSWERS	DESCRIPTIONS AND ANSWERS
4-28	keratoderma (keh-rat'-o-der-mah)	Keratoderma means horny skin texture. "kerat/o" is a combining form meaning horny substance. "derma" is a root word meaning skin.
4-29	"kerat/o"	_____ is a combining form meaning horny substance.
	"derma"	_____ is a root word meaning skin.
	keratoderma	Horny skin texture is called _____.
4-30	pachyderma (pak'-ih-der-mah)	Pachyderma is abnormal thickening of the skin. "pachy" is a word root meaning abnormal thickening. "derma" is a word root meaning skin.
4-31	word root abnormal thickening	"pachy" is a _____ _____ meaning _____ _____.
	word root, skin	"derma" is a _____ _____ meaning _____.
	abnormal thickening of the skin	Pachyderma is _____ _____ ____ _____ _____.
4-32	epithelium (ep'-ih-thee-lee-um)	Epithelium is the tissue (made of cells) that covers the internal and external surfaces of the body. The adjective for epithelium is epithelial.
	intraepidermal epithelioma (in-trah-ep'-ih-der-mal ep'-ih-the-le-o-mah)	Intraepidermal epithelioma is a tumor of the skin consisting mainly of epithelial cells. *intra-* is a prefix meaning within. "epidermal" is a root word meaning epidermis. "epitheli" is a root word meaning epithelium. *-oma* is a suffix meaning tumor.

BLOCK	DATA AND ANSWERS	DESCRIPTIONS AND ANSWERS
4-33	prefix, within	*intra-* is a _____ meaning _____.
	root word epidermis	"epidermal" is a _____ _____ meaning _____.
	root word epithelium	"epitheli" is a _____ _____ meaning _____.
	suffix, tumor	*-oma* is a _____ meaning _____.
4-34	a tumor of the skin consisting mainly of epithelial cells	Intraepidermal epithelioma is __ _____ ____ _____ _____ _____ _____ ____ _____ _____.
4-35	keratin (keh-rat′-<u>in</u>)	Keratin is a chemical component of the skin (epidermis), hair, nails, and teeth. All of these body parts sometimes have horny tissues. "kerat" is a word root. "kerat/o" is a combining form. Some patients may develop a skin condition in which the cells become hardened and horny, resembling the nails, though not as hard. Because of this resemblance, the word component "kerat" is used in any clinical circumstances referring to the skin instead of the nails. The next few blocks explore the use of the component "kerat" to characterize skin hardening.
4-36	keratogenic (keh-rat′-o-<u>jen</u>-ik)	Keratogenic means originating in horny tissue. "kerat/o" is a combining form meaning horny. "genic" is a root word meaning originating in.
4-37	"kerat/o"	_____ is a combining form meaning horny.
	"genic"	_____ is a root word meaning originating in.
	Keratogenic	_____ means originating in horny tissue.

BOX 4.1
Allied Health Professions

Dental Hygienists and Dental Assistants

Dental hygienists clean teeth and provide other preventive dental care; they also teach patients how to practice good oral hygiene. Hygienists examine patients' teeth and gums, recording the presence of diseases or abnormalities. They remove calculus, stains, and plaque from teeth; take and develop dental x-rays; and apply cavity-preventive agents such as fluorides and pit and fissure sealants. In some states, hygienists administer local anesthetics and anesthetic gas; place and carve filling materials, temporary fillings, and periodontal dressings; remove sutures; and smooth and polish metal restorations.

Dental assistants perform a variety of patient care, office, and laboratory duties. They work at chairside as dentists examine and treat patients. They make patients as comfortable as possible in the dental chair, prepare them for treatment, and obtain dental records. Assistants hand instruments and materials to dentists, and keep patients' mouths dry and clear by using suction or other devices. They also sterilize and disinfect instruments and equipment, prepare tray setups for dental procedures, and instruct patients on postoperative and general oral health care.

Some dental assistants prepare materials for making impressions and restorations, expose radiographs, and process dental x-ray film as directed by the dentist. State law determines which clinical tasks a dental assistant may perform, but in most states they may remove sutures, apply anesthetic and cavity-preventive agents to the teeth and oral tissue, remove excess cement used in the filling process, and place rubber dams on the teeth to isolate them for individual treatment.

Those with laboratory duties make casts of the teeth and mouth from impressions taken by dentists, clean and polish removable appliances, and make temporary crowns. Dental assistants with office duties arrange and confirm appointments, receive patients, keep treatment records, send bills, receive payments, and order dental supplies and materials. Dental assistants should not be confused with dental hygienists, who are licensed to perform a wider variety of clinical tasks.

The following are some resources for further information:

- American Dental Hygienists Association, Division of Education, www.adha.org

- Dental Assisting National Board, www.danb.org

- American Dental Assistants Association, www.dentalassistant.org

- National Association of Dental Assistants, www.ndaonline.org

Source: P.S. Stanfield, N. Cross, Y. H. Hui, eds. *Introduction to the Health Professions*, 5th ed. (Sudbury, MA: Jones & Bartlett, 2009).

BLOCK	DATA AND ANSWERS	DESCRIPTIONS AND ANSWERS
4-38	keratosis (keh′-rah-<u>to</u>-sis) "kerat/o" -*osis* Keratosis	Keratosis is a horny skin growth. "kerat/o" is a combining form meaning horny skin. -*osis* is a suffix meaning condition. _____ is a combining form meaning horny skin. _____ is a suffix meaning condition. _____ is a condition of a horny growth of the skin.
4-39	dyskeratosis (dis-keh′-rah-to-sis)	Dyskeratosis is faulty development of the epidermis in which it has abnormal, premature, or imperfect keratin formation (keratinization). *dys-* is a prefix meaning bad or faulty. "kerat/o" is a combining form meaning keratin. -*osis* is a suffix meaning condition.
4-40	prefix, bad, faulty combining form keratin suffix, condition	*dys-* is a _____ meaning _____ or _____. "kerat/o" is a _____ _____ meaning _____. -*osis* is a _____ meaning _____.
4-41	the faulty development of epidermis with abnormal, premature, or imperfect keratin formation	Dyskeratosis is _____ _____ _____ ____ _____ _____ _____, _____, ____ _____ _____ _____.
4-42	keratosis pilaris (keh′-rah-to-sis pih-lah-ris)	Keratosis pilaris is a condition in which hard elevations form around hair follicles. Keratosis is a horny or hardening skin condition. Pilaris refers to hair follicles.

BLOCK	DATA AND ANSWERS	DESCRIPTIONS AND ANSWERS
4-43	combining form keratin	"kerat/o" is a _____ _____ meaning _____.
	suffix, condition	-*osis* is a _____ meaning _____.
	a horny or hardening skin condition	Keratosis is ___ _____ _____ _____ _____ _____.
	hair follicle	Pilaris means _____ _____.
4-44	hard elevations formed around hair follicles	Keratosis pilaris refers to _____ _____ _____ _____ _____ _____.
4-45		The next few blocks explore another part of the skin: finger- and toenails.
	tinea unguium (<u>tin</u>-e-ah ung-<u>gwe</u>-um)	Tinea unguium is a fungal infection of the fingernails. It is commonly called ringworm.
		Tinea is a fungal infection that can affect many different parts of the body.
		"ungu" and "unguium" are root words meaning fingernails.
		"ungu/o" is a combining form meaning nail.
4-46	a fungal infection	Tinea is ___ _____ _____.
	root word fingernails	"unguium" is a _____ _____ meaning _____.
	a fungal infection of the fingernails	Tinea unguium is ___ _____ _____ _____ _____ _____.

BLOCK	DATA AND ANSWERS	DESCRIPTIONS AND ANSWERS
4-47	onychocryptosis (on'-ih-ko-krip-<u>to</u>-sis)	Onychocryptosis is the condition of having hidden (or ingrown) nails (toe). "onych/o" is a combining form meaning nail. "crypt" is a root word meaning hidden (or ingrown). "crypt/o" is a combining form meaning crypt. -osis is a suffix meaning condition.
4-48	"onych/o" "crypt" -osis	_____ is a combining form meaning nail. _____ is a root word meaning hidden (or ingrown). _____ is a suffix meaning condition.
4-49	onychocryptosis	The medical term for ingrown toenails is _____.
4-50	onychophagia (on'-ih-kofa-je-ah) Onychophagia	Onychophagia is biting of fingernails. "onych/o" is a combining form meaning nail. -phagia is a suffix meaning eating. _____ is nail biting.
4-51	"onych/o" -phagia	_____ is a combining form meaning nail. _____ is a suffix meaning eating.
4-52	onychitis (on'-ih-<u>ki</u>-tis)	Review: "onych/o" is a combining form meaning nail. -itis is a suffix meaning inflammation. Build a medical term (with pronunciation) meaning inflammation of the nail: _____ _____
4-53	"onych/o" -itis	_____ is a combining form meaning nail. _____ is a suffix meaning inflammation.

BLOCK	DATA AND ANSWERS	DESCRIPTIONS AND ANSWERS
4-54		Review:
		"onchy/o" is a combining form meaning nail.
		-malacia is a suffix meaning softening.
		Build a medical term meaning softening of the nails:
	onychomalacia	_____
	(on'-ih-<u>ko</u>-mal-a-se-ah)	_____
4-55	"onych/o"	_____ is a combining form meaning nail.
	-malacia	_____ is a suffix meaning softening.
4-56		*-ectomy* is a suffix meaning cut off, remove surgically or excise.
	Onychectomy	_____ refers to excision of a nail.
4-57	"onych/o"	_____ is a combining form meaning nail.
	-ectomy	_____ is a suffix meaning cut off, remove surgically, or excise.
4-58		In the remaining blocks in this chapter, we will study other clinical conditions of the skin such as color, treatment, cancer, and surgery.
	melanin (mel-<u>ah</u>-nin)	Some cells form melanin, a necessary color pigment (dark or black) in the skin. These cells are called melanocytes.
	melanocyte (mel-ah-<u>no</u>-sit)	"melan/o" is a combining form meaning dark or black.
		"cyte" is a root word meaning cell.
		-cyte is also a suffix.
4-59	"melan/o"	_____ is a combining form meaning dark or black.
	"cyte"	_____ is a root word meaning cell.
	melanocyte	A _____ is a cell that forms melanin.

BLOCK	DATA AND ANSWERS	DESCRIPTIONS AND ANSWERS
4-60		*sub-* is a prefix meaning under or beneath.
		"cutane" is a root word meaning skin.
		-ous is a suffix meaning pertaining to.
	subcutaneous (sub′-ku-<u>ta</u>-ne-us)	Subcutaneous means under the skin. (For example, in clinical medicine, a subcutaneous injection is injected under the skin.)
4-61	prefix, under	*sub-* is a _____ meaning _____.
	word root, skin	"cutane" is a _____ _____ meaning _____.
	suffix, pertaining to	*-ous* is a _____ meaning _____ _____.
4-62	under the skin	"Subcutaneous" means _____ _____ _____.
		An injection just beneath the skin is
	subcutaneous	_____.
4-63	cutis hyperelastica (ku-<u>tis</u> hi′-per-el-as-<u>tih</u>-kah)	Cutis hyperelastica is excess elasticity of the skin or loose skin.
		"cutis" is a root word meaning skin.
		hyper- is a prefix meaning excess or too much.
		-elastica is a suffix meaning elastic.
4-64	"cutis"	_____ is a root word meaning skin.
4-65	prefix, excess, too much	*hyper-* is a _____ meaning _____ or _____ _____.
	suffix, elastic	*-elastica* is a _____ meaning _____.
4-66	Cutis hyperelastica	_____ _____ is looseness, or excess elasticity, of the skin.

BLOCK	DATA AND ANSWERS	DESCRIPTIONS AND ANSWERS
4-67	autodermatoplasty (au-to-der-mat-o-<u>plas</u>-te)	Autodermatoplasty is plastic repair using a patient's own skin for the skin graft. "aut/o" is a combining form meaning self. *auto-* is also a prefix. "dermat/o" is a combining form meaning skin. *-plasty* is a suffix meaning plastic repair.
4-68	combining form self	"aut/o" is a _____ _____ meaning _____.
	combining form skin	"dermat/o" is a _____ _____ meaning _____.
	suffix, plastic repair	*-plasty* is a _____ meaning _____ _____.
4-69	plastic repair using a patient's own skin for the skin graft	Autodermatoplasty is _____ _____ _____ __ _____ _____ _____ _____ _____ _____ _____.
4-70	heterodermatoplasty (het'-eh-ro-der-mat-o-<u>plas</u>-te)	Heterodermatoplasty means plastic repair using skin from a donor for a skin graft. "heter/o" is a combining form meaning other, other than usual, different, or not the same. *hetero-* also is a prefix. "dermat/o" is a combining form meaning skin. *-plasty* is a suffix meaning plastic repair.

BLOCK	DATA AND ANSWERS	DESCRIPTIONS AND ANSWERS
4-71	combining form other, other than usual not the same	"heter/o" is a _____ _____ meaning _____, _____ _____ _____, or _____ _____ _____.
	prefix, other other than usual, not the same	*hetero-* is a _____ meaning _____, _____ _____ _____, or _____ _____ _____.
	combining form skin	"dermat/o" is a _____ _____ meaning _____.
	suffix, plastic repair	*-plasty* is a _____ meaning _____ _____.
4-72	plastic repair using skin from a donor for the skin graft	Heterodermatoplasty is _____ _____ _____ _____ _____ __ _____ _____ _____ _____ _____.
4-73	rhytidectomy (rit'-ih-<u>dek</u>-to-me)	Rhytidectomy is the process of surgically removing wrinkles. "rhytid" is a word root meaning wrinkles. "rhytid/o" is a combining form meaning wrinkles. *-ectomy* is a suffix meaning cut off, removing surgically, or excising.
4-74	"rhytid" *-ectomy*	_____ is a word root meaning wrinkles. _____ is a suffix meaning excision.
4-75	Rhytidectomy	_____ is the excision of wrinkles.
4-76	rhytidoplasty (rit-id-o-<u>plas</u>-te)	Rhytidoplasty is the plastic repair of wrinkles. "rhytid/o" is a combining form meaning wrinkles. *-plasty* is a suffix meaning plastic repair.
4-77	"rhytid/o" *-plasty*	_____ is a combining form meaning wrinkles. _____ is a suffix meaning plastic repair.

BLOCK	DATA AND ANSWERS	DESCRIPTIONS AND ANSWERS
4-78	Rhytidoplasty	_____ is the plastic repair of wrinkles.
4-79	tinea (<u>tin</u>-ee-ah)	The next few blocks discuss ringworm infection of the skin. Recall that "tinea" is a word root for ringworm, which causes chronic fungal infection of the skin.
4-80	capitis (cap-<u>ih</u>-tis)	Tinea capitis is ringworm infection of the scalp. "capit/o" is a combining form meaning head. *-is* is a suffix indicating the ending of a noun.
4-81	tinca corporis (cor'-<u>poh</u>-ris)	Tinea corporis is a ringworm infection of the non-hairy skin of the body. "corpor/o" is a combining form meaning body.
4-82	tinea cruris (<u>kroo</u>-ris)	Tinea cruris, commonly known as jock itch, is a ringworm infection of the groin. "crur/o" is a combining form meaning leg or thigh.
4-83	tinea pedis (<u>ped</u>-is)	Tinea pedis, commonly known as athlete's foot, is a ringworm infection of the foot. "ped/o" is a combining form meaning foot.
4-84	suffix, the ending of a noun combining form head combining form leg, thigh combining form foot combining form body	*-is* is a _____ indicating _____ _____ ____ __ _____. "capit/o" is a _____ _____ meaning _____. "crur/o" is a _____ _____ meaning _____ or _____. "ped/o" is a _____ _____ meaning _____. "corpor/o" is a _____ _____ meaning _____.

BLOCK	DATA AND ANSWERS	DESCRIPTIONS AND ANSWERS
4-85	a ringworm infection of the scalp	Tinea capitis is ___ _____ _____ _____ _____ _____.
	a ringworm infection of the non-hairy skin of the body	Tinea corporis is ___ _____ _____ _____ _____ _____ _____ _____ _____ _____.
	a ringworm infection of the groin	Tinea cruris is ___ _____ _____ _____ _____ _____.
	a ringworm infection of the foot	Tinea pedis is ___ _____ _____ _____ _____ _____.
4-86		The next few blocks study some surgical procedures associated with the skin.
	cryosurgery (cry-oh-<u>ser</u>-jer-ee)	Cryosurgery uses liquid nitrogen to freeze the skin to treat certain skin cancers.
		"cry/o" is a combining form meaning use of liquid nitrogen to freeze.
		cryo- is a prefix meaning use of liquid nitrogen to freeze.
		"surgery" is a root word meaning surgery.
4-87	"cry/o"	_____ is a combining form meaning use of liquid nitrogen to freeze.
	cryo-	_____ is a prefix meaning use of liquid nitrogen to freeze.
	the use of liquid nitrogen to freeze the skin to treat certain skin cancers	Cryosurgery is _____ _____ _____ _____ _____ _____ _____ _____ _____ _____ _____ _____ _____ _____.

BLOCK	DATA AND ANSWERS	DESCRIPTIONS AND ANSWERS
4-88	electrodesiccation (ee-lek'-troh-<u>des</u>-ih-kay'-shun)	Electrodesiccation is a technique using an electrical spark to dry (destroy) tissue for the removal of skin lesions. "electr/o" is a combining form meaning electricity. *electro-* also is a prefix. "desiccat" is a root word meaning drying. "desiccat/o" is the combining form. *-ion* is a suffix meaning a process or action.
4-89	combining form electricity prefix, electricity "desiccat" "desiccat/o" *-ion* Electrodesiccation	"electr/o" is a _____ _____ meaning _____. *electro-* is a _____ meaning _____. _____ is a root word meaning drying. _____ is a combining form meaning drying. _____ is a suffix meaning a process or action. _____ is the technique of using an electrical spark to dry (destroy) tissue to remove skin lesions.
4-90	dermabrasion (derm'-ah-<u>bray</u>-shun)	Dermabrasion is the removal of the epidermis and a portion of the dermis with sandpaper or brushes in order to eliminate superficial scars or unwanted tattoos. "derm/o" is a combining form meaning skin. "abrasion" is a root word meaning scraping with a hard object.

BLOCK	DATA AND ANSWERS	DESCRIPTIONS AND ANSWERS
4-91	the removal of the epidermis and a portion of the dermis with sandpaper or brushes in order to eliminate superficial scars or unwanted tattoos	Dermabrasion is _____ _____ ____ _____ _____ _____ __ _____ ____ ____ _____ _____ _____ ____ _____ ___ _____ ____ _____ _____ _____ ____ _____ _____.
	scraping with a hard object	Abrasion is _____ _____ __ _____ _____.
4-92	escharotomy (es-kar-<u>ot</u>-oh-mee)	Escharotomy is a surgical incision made in the dead tissue resulting from a severe burn. "eschar" is a root word meaning scab or dry crust. "eschar/o" is the combining form. -tomy is a suffix meaning a surgical incision.
4-93	"eschar" suffix, a surgical incision a surgical incision made in the dead tissue resulting from a severe burn	_____ is a root word meaning scab or dry crust. -tomy is a _____ meaning __ _____ _____. Escharotomy is __ _____ _____ _____ ___ _____ _____ _____ _____ _____ __ _____ _____.

BOX 4.2 Abbreviations	
Bx, bx	biopsy
Decub.	decubitus (ulcer), bedsore
EAHF	eczema, asthma, and hay fever
FS	frozen section
ID	incision and drainage
SC	subcutaneous
SLE	systemic lupus erythematosus
Ung.	ointment
UV	ultraviolet (light)
XP, XDP	xeroderma pigmentosum

Progress Check

A. Multiple Choice

1. A word root meaning leg or thigh is:
   a. derma
   b. crur
   c. fibr
   d. pachy

2. A word root meaning wrinkle is:
   a. rhytid
   b. perine
   c. arthr
   d. orch

3. A word root meaning self is:
   a. sial
   b. pleur
   c. rach
   d. aut

4. A word root meaning hornlike is:
   a. kary
   b. noct
   c. kerat
   d. cheil

5. A combining form meaning foot is:
   a. ped/o
   b. cephal/o
   c. fibul/o
   d. episi/o

6. A combining form meaning cold is
   a. melan/o
   b. col/o

   c. cry/o
   d. xer/o

7. A combining form meaning scab or dry crust is:
   a. seb/o
   b. ungu/o
   c. bil/o
   d. eschar/o

8. A combining form meaning nail is:
   a. narc/o
   b. onych/o
   c. onc/o
   d. crur/o

9. A prefix meaning on top is:
   a. epi-
   b. trans-
   c. sym-
   d. intra-

10. A suffix meaning an instrument for cutting is:
   a. -osis
   b. -phagia
   c. -tome
   d. -tomy

11. A suffix meaning pertaining to is:
   a. -ist
   b. -phagia
   c. -ous
   d. -rrhea

12. A suffix meaning softening is:
   a. -malacia

    b. -megaly

    c. -mastoid

    d. -iasis

13. A suffix meaning tumor is:

    a. -tropia

    b. -opsia

    c. -philia

    d. -oma

B.   Building Medical Terms

Use the following word components to build medical terms matching the definitions given. Some answers may have two words.

abrasion	desiccat	*-ion*
coni	desiccat/o	-oma
coni/o	elastica	onych
crypt	electr	onych/o
crypt/o	electr/o	-osis
cutis	epi-	pedis
derm	eschar	-plasty
derm/o	eschar/o	rhytid
dermat	fibr	rhytid/o
dermat/o	fibr/o	tinea
dermis	hyper-	-tomy

1. technique using an electrical spark to dry (destroy) tissue for the removal of skin lesions

2. fibrous tumor of the skin

3. abnormal condition of the skin caused by dust

4. condition of having hidden (or ingrown) nails (toe)

5. surgical incision made in the dead tissue resulting from a severe burn

6. removal of the epidermis and a portion of the dermis with sandpaper or brushes in order to eliminate superficial scars or unwanted tattoos

7. plastic repair of wrinkles

8. excess elasticity of the skin or loose skin

9. ringworm infection of the foot, commonly known as athlete's foot

10. top layer of the skin

C.   Definitions and Word Components

	TERM	DEFINITION	PREFIX	WORD ROOT	VOWEL	WORD ROOT	VOWEL	SUFFIX
1.	dyskeratosis							
2.	onychophagia							
3.	subcutaneous							

	TERM	DEFINITION	PREFIX	WORD ROOT	VOWEL	WORD ROOT	VOWEL	SUFFIX
4.	autodermatoplasty							
5.	heterodermatoplasty							
6.	keratosis							
7.	intraepidermal							
8.	hyperelastica							
9.	dermatoplasty							
10.	melanocytes							

D. Abbreviations

	ABBREVIATION	MEANING
1.	Bx, bx	
2.	Decub.	
3.	EAHF	
4.	FS	
5.	ID	

	ABBREVIATION	MEANING
6.	SC	
7.	SLE	
8.	Ung.	
9.	UV	
10.	XP, XDP	

The Gastrointestinal System

BLOCK	DATA AND ANSWERS	DESCRIPTIONS AND QUESTIONS
5-1		The gastrointestinal (GI) system, sometimes referred to as the digestive system or alimentary canal, is a continuous tube beginning with the mouth and ending at the anus. The accessory organs are the liver, gallbladder, and pancreas.
		Figures 5.1 through 5.6 provide anatomical diagrams of the GI system. Refer to them frequently for clarification (this applies to most blocks), as studying several figures together gives a better perspective than just looking at one figure because all of the figures are related.
		Table 5.1 gives the word roots, combining forms, prefixes, and suffixes pertaining to the GI tract.
5-2	stomatitis (<u>sto</u>-mah-ti′-tis)	Stomatitis is inflammation of the mouth.
	stomatalgia (<u>sto</u>-mah-tal′-je-ah)	Stomatalgia is pain in the mouth.
	stomatodynia (<u>sto</u>-mat-o-din′-e-ah)	Stomatodynia is another term for pain in the mouth.
	stomatorraphy (<u>sto</u>-mat-or-ah′-fe)	Stomatorraphy is suture of the mouth.

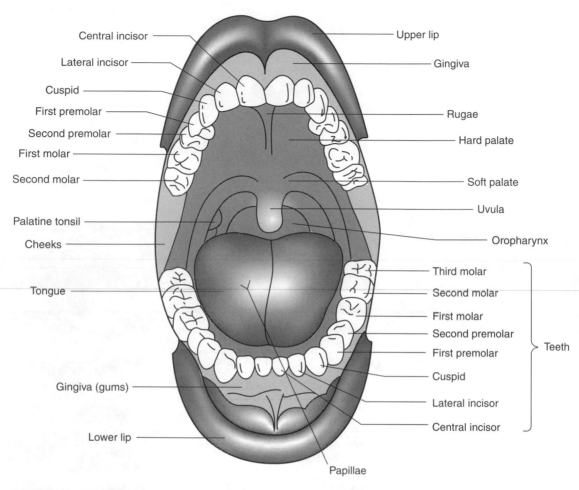

FIGURE 5.1   Oral cavity

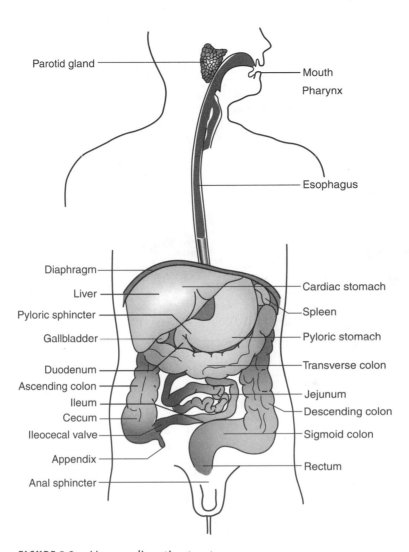

FIGURE 5.2   Human digestive tract

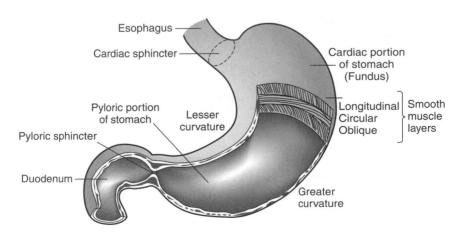

FIGURE 5.3   External and internal anatomy of the stomach

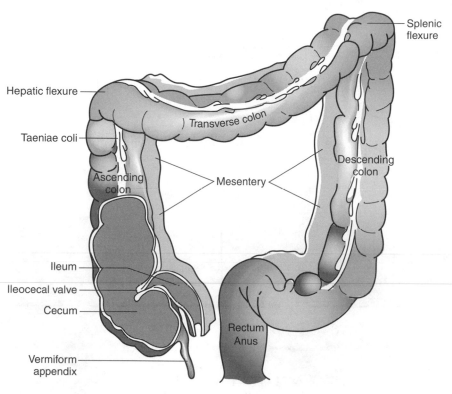

FIGURE 5.4   Large intestine

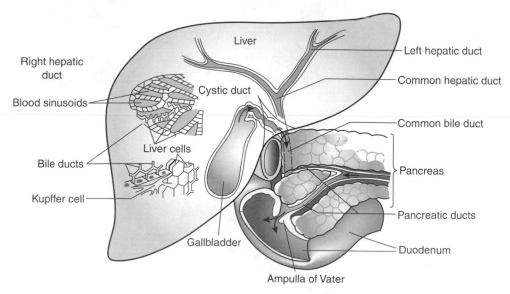

FIGURE 5.5   Liver and its interrelationship with the gallbladder, pancreas, and duodenum

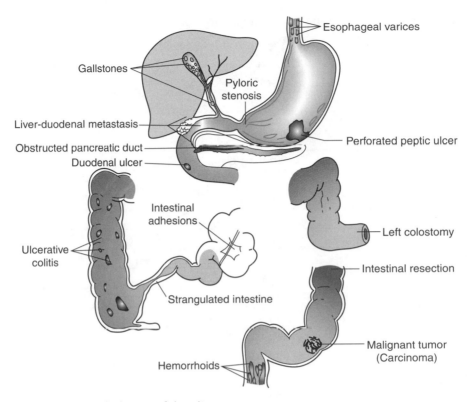

FIGURE 5.6 Pathologies of the alimentary tract

TABLE 5.1 Word Components in this Chapter

WORD ROOTS	COMBINING FORMS	PREFIXES
anal	abdomin/o	a-
anus	an/o	brady-
append	ang/i	hyper-
bili	append/o	hypo-
bucca	bil/i	mal-
cec	cec/o	post-
cheil	cecoile/o	prosth-
chol	cheil/o	sub-
chole	chol/e	**SUFFIXES**
cholecyst	cholangi/o	-al
cholia	cholecyst/o	-algia
colon	choledoch/o	-ary
cyst	cholester/o	-cele
dent	cirrh/o	-centesis
duoden	col/o	-cyst

TABLE 5.1   Word Components in this Chapter (continued)

WORD ROOTS	COMBINING FORMS	SUFFIXES
enter	colon/o	-dontia
esophag	cyst/o	-dynia
gastr	dent/o	-ectomy
gingiv	duoden/o	-emia
gloss	enter/o	-ia
hemorrhoid	esophag/o	-ic
hepat	gastr/o	-ist
ile	gastroenter/o	-itis
jejun	gingiv/o	-logy
jejunum	gloss/o	-malacia
lingu	hemorrhoid/o	-megaly
olig	hepat/o	-oma
palat	ile/o	-osis
pancreat	jejun/o	-tomy
peritone	lingu/o	-pathy
peritoneal	odont/o	-pepsia
pharyng	olig/o	-pexy
pharynx	palat/o	-phagia
proc	pancreat/o	-plasty
procto	peritone/o	-plegia
rect	pharyn/o	-prandial
scope	pharyng/o	-ptosis
sial	proct/o	-rrhaphy
sigmoid	rect/o	-scope
sten	sial/o	-stormy
sterol	sigmoid/o	-tomy
stoma	sten/o	
stomato	stomat/o	
stomy	uvul/a	
uvula		

BLOCK	DATA AND ANSWERS	DESCRIPTIONS AND QUESTIONS
5-3		"stomat/o" is a combining form meaning the mouth.
		-itis is a suffix meaning inflammation.
		-algia is a suffix meaning pain.
		-dynia is another suffix meaning pain.
		-rraphy is a suffix meaning suture.
5-4	inflammation of the mouth	Stomatitis is ___inflammation___ _of_ _the_ ___mouth___.
	pain in the mouth	Stomatalgia is ___pain___ _in_ _the_ ___mouth___.
	pain in the mouth	Stomatodynia is ___pain___ _in_ _the_ ___mouth___.
	suture of the mouth	Stomatorraphy is ___stuture___ _of_ _the_ ___mouth___.
5-5	"stomat/o"	___stomat/o___ is a combining form meaning the mouth.
	-itis	___itis___ is a suffix meaning inflammation.
	-algia	___algia___ is a suffix meaning pain.
	-dynia	___dynia___ is a suffix meaning pain.
	-rraphy	___rraphy___ is a suffix meaning suture.
5-6		Recall that the combining form for mouth is "stomat/o."
		-pathy is a suffix used to indicate a disease state.
	stomatopathy (sto'-mah-to-<u>path</u>-e)	Build a medical term (with pronunciation) meaning any disease of the mouth: ___stomatopathy___ ___(sto - mah-to - path - e)___
5-7	any disease of the mouth	Stomatopathy refers to ___any___ ___disease___ ___in___ ___the___ ___mouth___.

BLOCK	DATA AND ANSWERS	DESCRIPTIONS AND QUESTIONS
5-8	stomatoplasty (sto'-mah-to-plas-te)	*-plasty* is a suffix meaning surgical repair (plastic surgery). Build a medical term meaning surgical repair of the mouth: *stomatoplasty (sto'-mah-to-plas-te)*
5-9	palatoplasty (pal-at-o-plas-te)	"palat/o" is a combining form meaning palate, which is the roof of the mouth. Build a medical term meaning surgical repair of the palate: *palatoplasty*
5-10	gingivectomy (jin-jiv-ek-to-me)	Gingivectomy is surgical removal of gum tissue. "gingiv/o" is a combining form meaning gum. *-ectomy* is a suffix meaning excision.
5-11	a combining form gum a suffix, excision	"gingiv/o" is *a combining form* meaning *gum*. *-ectomy* is *a suffix* meaning *excision*.
5-12	Gingivectomy	*gingivectomy* is surgical removal of gum tissue.
5-13	gingivitis (jin-jiv-i-tis)	*-itis* is a suffix meaning inflammation. Build a medical term meaning inflammation of the gums: *gingivitis*
5-14		There are glands in the mouth that secrete saliva. These glands collectively are called the salivary glands. "sial" is a word root meaning salivary glands. "sial/o" is the combining form.

BLOCK	DATA AND ANSWERS	DESCRIPTIONS AND QUESTIONS
5-15	word root salivary glands suffix inflammation inflammation of· salivary glands	"sial" is a ___word___ ___root___ meaning ___Salivary___ ___glands___. -itis is a ___Suffix___ meaning ___inflammation___. Sialitis refers to ___inflammation___ ___of___ ___Salivary___ ___glands___.
5-16	sialolith (si-al-<u>o</u>-lith)	Sialolith means salivary stone. "sial/o" is a combining form meaning salivary. "lith" is a root word or a suffix (-lith) meaning stone.
5-17	Sialolith "sial/o" "lith"	___Sialolith___ means salivary stone. ___Sialo___ is a combining form meaning salivary. ___lith___ is a root word meaning stone.
5-18	dysphagia (dis-<u>fa</u>-je-ah)	Dysphagia is difficulty in swallowing or eating. dys- is a prefix meaning difficult. -phagia is a suffix meaning swallowing or eating.
5-19	difficulty in swallowing or eating prefix, difficult suffix swallowing, eating	Dysphagia is ___difficulty___ ___in___ ___swallowing___ ___or___ ___eating___. dys- is a ___prefix___ meaning ___difficult___. -phagia is a ___Suffix___ meaning ___swallowing___ or ___eating___.
5-20	 teeth	"dent/o" is a combining form meaning teeth. -ist is a suffix referring to one who specializes in. A dentist is a specialist in ___teeth___.

BLOCK	DATA AND ANSWERS	DESCRIPTIONS AND QUESTIONS
5-21		"odont/o" is another combining form meaning teeth.
		-itis is a suffix meaning inflammation.
	Odontitis	_odontitis_ refers to inflammation of the teeth.
5-22	malocclusion (mal'-ok-<u>klu</u>-zhun)	Malocclusion means poorly aligned teeth.
		mal- is a prefix meaning poor, bad, or difficult.
		Occlusion, as used in dentistry, means alignment. (The literal meaning of occlusion is blockage. In this case, when the teeth fit, the mouth is blocked from the outside.)
5-23	malocclusion	A person with poorly aligned teeth is said to have a _malocclusion_.
	mal-	_mal_ is a prefix that means poor, bad, or difficult.
	Occlusion	_occlusion_, as used in dentistry, means alignment.
5-24		"dent/o" is a combination form meaning teeth.
		-algia is a suffix meaning pain.
		Build a medical term meaning toothache:
	dentalgia (den-<u>tal</u>-je-ah)	_dentalgia_ .
5-25	odontalgia (o-don-<u>tal</u>-je-ah)	Odontalgia is another term for toothache.
		"odont/o" is a combining form meaning teeth.
		-algia is a suffix meaning pain.
5-26	Odontalgia	_odontalgia_ is another term for toothache.
	"odont/o"	_odont/o_ is a combining form meaning teeth.
	-algia	_algia_ is a suffix meaning pain.

BLOCK	DATA AND ANSWERS	DESCRIPTIONS AND QUESTIONS
5-27	prosthodontics (pros-tho-<u>don</u>-tiks)	Prosthodontics refers to adding teeth or replacing some or all of the teeth. "prosth/o" is a combining form meaning add or replace. "odont/o" is a combining form meaning teeth. -ics is a suffix meaning pertaining to or the condition of.
5-28	combining form add, replace combining form teeth suffix, pertaining to the condition of	"prosth/o" is a _____ _____ meaning _____ or _____. "odont/o" is a _____ _____ meaning _____. -ics is a _____ meaning _____ _____ or _____ _____ _____.
5-29	adding teeth or replacement of some or all of the teeth	Prosthodontics is _____ _____ _____ _____ _____ _____ _____ _____ _____ _____ _____ _____.
5-30	oligodontia (ol'-i-go-<u>don</u>-te-ah)	Oligodontia is the condition of having fewer than the normal number of teeth. "olig/o" is a combining form meaning few or scanty. "odont/o" is a combining form meaning teeth. -ia is a suffix meaning condition or pertaining to.
5-31	"olig/o" "odont/o" -ia oligodontia	_____ is a combining form meaning few. _____ is a combining form meaning teeth. _____ is a suffix meaning the condition of or pertaining to. In dentistry, the condition of having fewer than the normal number of teeth is _____.

BLOCK	DATA AND ANSWERS	DESCRIPTIONS AND QUESTIONS
5-32		"gloss/o" is a combining form meaning tongue. -*algia* is a suffix meaning pain. -*dynia* is another suffix meaning pain. -*itis* is a suffix meaning inflammation.
5-33	glossalgia (glos-<u>al</u>-je-a<u>h</u>) <u>glos</u>sodynia (glos-o-<u>de</u>-ne-ah)	Build two terms meaning pain in the tongue: 1. _____ _____ 2. _____ _____
5-34	glossitis (glos-<u>i</u>-tis)	Build a term meaning inflammation of the tongue: _____ _____
5-35	sublingual (sub-<u>ling</u>-wal)	Sublingual means under the tongue. *sub-* is a prefix meaning beneath. "lingu/o" is a combining form meaning tongue. -*al* is a suffix meaning pertaining to.
5-36	*sub-* "lingu/o" -*al* Sublingual	_____ is a prefix meaning beneath. _____ a combining form meaning tongue. _____ is a suffix meaning pertaining to. _____ means under the tongue.
5-37		Recall that "gloss/o" is a combining form for tongue. -*rrhaphy* is a suffix meaning suture. -*oma* is a suffix meaning tumor. -*tomy* is a suffix meaning incision in.

BLOCK	DATA AND ANSWERS	DESCRIPTIONS AND QUESTIONS
5-38		Build medical terms meaning:
	glossorrhaphy (glos-o-<u>raf</u>-e)	suture of the tongue: _____ _____
	glossoma (glos-<u>o</u>-mah)	tumor of the tongue: _____ _____
	glossotomy (glos-<u>ot</u>-o-me)	incision in the tongue: _____ _____
5-39	suture of the tongue	Glossorrhaphy is _____ _____ _____ _____.
	tumor of the tongue	Glossoma is _____ _____ _____ _____.
5-40	"gloss/o"	A combining form meaning tongue is _____.
	-*itis*	A suffix meaning inflammation is _____.
	"glossitis"	Inflammation of the tongue is _____.
5-41		-*pathy* is a suffix meaning disease.
		Build a medical term meaning disease of the tongue:
	glossopathy (glos-<u>op</u>-ath-e)	_____ _____
5-42		-*plegia* is a suffix meaning paralysis.
		Build a medical term meaning paralysis of the tongue:
	glossoplegia (glos-<u>o</u>-ple-je-ah)	_____ _____
5-43		Recall that sublingual means under the tongue. Hypoglossal also means under the tongue.
		hypo- is another prefix meaning below or under.
		"gloss/o" is a combining form meaning the tongue.
		-*al* is a suffix meaning pertaining to or a condition of.

BLOCK	DATA AND ANSWERS	DESCRIPTIONS AND QUESTIONS
5-44	hypoglossal (hi´-po-<u>glos</u>-al)	Build another medical word meaning under the tongue: _____ _____
5-45	prefix, below under combining form tongue suffix, pertaining to a condition of	*hypo-* is a _____ meaning _____ or _____. "gloss/o" is a _____ _____ meaning _____. *-al* is a _____ meaning _____ _____ or ___ _____ _____.
5-46	glossosis (glos-<u>o</u>-sis)	*-osis* is another suffix meaning pertaining to or the condition of. "gloss/o" is a combining form meaning tongue. Build a medical term referring to any condition of the tongue: _____ _____
5-47	glossopathy	*-pathy* is a suffix meaning disease. Build a medical term referring to any disease of the tongue: _____
5-48	glossoscope (glos-<u>o</u>-skop)	*-scope* is a suffix meaning an instrument used to examine an object. Build a medical term meaning an instrument for examining the tongue: _____ _____
5-49		"cheil/o" is a combining form meaning lips. *-osis* is a suffix meaning condition. *-pathy* is a suffix meaning disease.

BLOCK	DATA AND ANSWERS	DESCRIPTIONS AND QUESTIONS
5-50		Build medical terms meaning:
	cheilosis (kih-<u>lo</u>-sis)	any condition of the lips: _____ _____
	cheilopathy (kih-<u>lop</u>-ath-e)	any disease of the lips: _____ _____
5-51		"cheil/o" is a combining form meaning lips. *-itis* is a suffix meaning inflammation. *-tomy* is a suffix meaning incision.
5-52		Build medical terms meaning:
	cheilitis (kih-li-<u>ti</u>-tis)	inflammation of the lips: _____ _____
	cheilotomy (kih-<u>lo</u>-to-me)	incision into the lips: _____ _____
5-53		"cheil/o" is a combining form meaning lips. *-plasty* is a suffix meaning plastic repair of. Build a medical term meaning plastic repair of lips:
	cheiloplasty (kih-lo-<u>plas</u>-te)	_____ _____
5-54	cheilostomatoplasty (<u>kih</u>-lo-sto-mat-o-plas-te)	Compound words contain more than one root word, e.g., "cheilostomatoplasty," meaning plastic surgery of the lips and mouth. "cheil/o" is a combining form meaning lips. "stomato" is a root word meaning mouth. "stomat/o" is the combining form. "plasty" is a root word meaning plastic repair or surgery.

BLOCK	DATA AND ANSWERS	DESCRIPTIONS AND QUESTIONS
5-55	Cheilostomatoplasty	_____ is plastic surgery of the lips and mouth.
5-56	buccal (<u>buk</u>-al) bucca (<u>buk</u>-ah)	Buccal means pertaining to the cheek. "bucca" is a word root meaning cheek. -al is a suffix meaning pertaining to or directed toward.
5-57	Buccal -al	_____ means pertaining to the cheek. _____ is a suffix meaning pertaining to.
5-58	pharyngocele (fah-<u>rin</u>-jo-sel)	Pharyngocele is herniation of the throat. Pharynx is the throat. "pharyng/o" is a combining form meaning throat. -cele is a suffix meaning herniation.
5-59	Pharyngocele herniation	_____ is herniation of the throat. -cele is a suffix meaning _____.
5-60		Review: "pharyng/o" is a combining form meaning throat. -algia is a suffix meaning pain. -dynia is a suffix meaning pain. -plegia is a suffix meaning paralysis.
5-61	pharyngalgia (fah-ring-<u>al</u>-je-ah) pharyngodynia (fah-rin-jo-<u>de</u>-ne-ah) pharyngoplegia (fah-rin-jo-<u>ple</u>-je-ah)	Build two medical terms meaning pain in the throat: 1. _____ _____ 2. _____ _____ Build a medical term meaning paralysis of the pharyngeal muscles: _____ _____

BLOCK	DATA AND ANSWERS	DESCRIPTIONS AND QUESTIONS
5-62	*-dynia* *-algia* *-plegia*	_____ is a suffix meaning pain. _____ is another suffix meaning pain. _____ is a suffix meaning paralysis.
5-63		Review: *-itis* is a suffix meaning inflammation. *-ectomy* is a suffix meaning excision. "pharyng/o" is a combining form meaning pharynx.
5-64	pharyngitis (fah'-rin-ji-tis) pharyngectomy (fah'-rin-jek-to-me)	Build medical terms meaning: inflammation of the pharynx: _____ _____ excision of part of the pharynx: _____ _____
5-65	uvula (u-vu-lah)	The pharynx is separated from the mouth by the soft palate, which has a V-shaped extension called a uvula (a word root). "uvul/a" is a combination form meaning uvula. *-itis* is a suffix meaning inflammation. *-ectomy* is a suffix meaning removal or excision.
5-66	uvulitis (u-vu-li-tis) uvulectomy (u'-vu-lek-to-me)	Build medical terms meaning: inflammation of the uvula: _____ _____ excision of the uvula: _____ _____

BLOCK	DATA AND ANSWERS	DESCRIPTIONS AND QUESTIONS
5-67	esophagus (eh-<u>sof</u>-ag-us)	The esophagus is the passage extending from the pharynx (throat) to the stomach. This tube is made up of muscle and membranes (film lining). "esophag/o" is the combining form.
5-68	esophagoscope (eh-<u>sof</u>-ag-o-skop)	A scope is an instrument used for visual examination. It is a word root and can also be a suffix (-*scope*). Build a medical term meaning instrument used for visual examination of the esophagus: _____ _____.
5-69	esophagostenosis (eh-sof-ah-go-<u>sten</u>-o′-sis)	Esophagostenosis is narrowing of the esophagus. "esophag/o" is a combining word meaning esophagus. -*stenosis* is a suffix meaning the condition of narrowing.
5-70	combining form esophagus suffix, the condition of narrowing narrowing of the esophagus	"esophag/o" is a _____ _____ meaning _____. -*stenosis* is a _____ meaning _____ _____ ____ _____. Esophagostenosis is _____ ____ _____ _____.
5-71	-*dynia*, -*algia* -*itis* -*cele*	_____ and _____ are both suffixes meaning pain. _____ is a suffix meaning inflammation. _____ is a suffix meaning herniation.

BLOCK	DATA AND ANSWERS	DESCRIPTIONS AND QUESTIONS
5-72		Build two medical terms meaning pain in the esophagus:
	esophagodynia (eh-sof-ah-go-<u>din</u>-e-ah)	1. _____ _____
	esophagalgia (eh-sof-fah-<u>ga</u>-ge-ah)	2. _____ _____
5-73		Build medical terms meaning:
	esophagitis (eh-sof-ah-<u>ji</u>-tis)	inflammation of the esophagus: _____ _____
	esophagocele (eh-sof-ah-<u>go</u>-sel)	herniation of the esophagus: _____ _____
5-74		"gastr" is a root word meaning stomach. "gastr/o" is the combining form. -*itis* is a suffix meaning inflammation.
5-75		Build a medical term meaning inflammation of the stomach:
	gastritis (gas-<u>tri</u>-tis)	_____ _____
5-76	gastroenteritis (gas'-tro-en-teh-<u>ri</u>-tis)	Gastroenteritis is inflammation of the stomach and small intestines. "enter/o" is a combining form meaning small intestine. "gastr/o" and "enter/o" together create "gastroenter/o," a combining form meaning stomach and intestine. -*itis* is a suffix meaning inflammation.
5-77	"enter/o" "gastr/o" inflammation of the stomach and small intestines	_____ is a combining form meaning small intestine. _____ is a combining form meaning stomach. Gastroenteritis is _____ _____ _____ _____ _____ _____ _____.

BLOCK	DATA AND ANSWERS	DESCRIPTIONS AND QUESTIONS
5-78	gastroenterocolitis (gas'-tro-en-teh-ro-ko-<u>li</u>-tis)	"Gastroenterocolitis" is a compound word meaning inflammation of the stomach, small intestine, and colon (large intestine). The combining forms are gastr/o (stomach), enter/o (small intestine), and col/o (colon or large intestine).
5-79	Gastroenterocolitis	_____ is inflammation of the stomach, small intestine, and colon.
5-80	gastroscope (gas-tro-<u>skop</u>)	A scope is an instrument used for visual examination. It is a word root and can also be a suffix (-*scope*). "gastr/o" is a combining form meaning stomach. Build a medical term meaning instrument used for visual examination of the stomach: _____ _____
5-81	duodenum (doo-o-<u>de</u>-num)	The duodenum is the first segment of the small intestine. "duoden/o" is a combining form meaning duodenum.
5-82		"gastr/o" is a combining form meaning stomach. -*itis* is a suffix meaning inflammation.
5-83	"gastr/o" "duoden/o" -*itis* Gastroduodenitis	_____ is a combining form meaning stomach. _____ is a combining form meaning duodenum. _____ is a suffix meaning inflammation. _____ refers to inflammation of the stomach and duodenum.
5-84	gastrectomy (gas-<u>trek</u>-to-me)	"gastr/o" is a combining form meaning stomach. -*ectomy* is a suffix referring to excision or removal. Build a medical term meaning excision of part or all of the stomach: _____ _____

BLOCK	DATA AND ANSWERS	DESCRIPTIONS AND QUESTIONS
5-85	gastrojejunostomy (gas′-tro-je-ju-<u>nos</u>-to-me)	A gastrojejunostomy is a surgical procedure to make an opening between the stomach and jejunum. The sequence of structures is: stomach, duodenum, and then jejunum. "gastr/o" is a combining form referring to the stomach. "jejun/o" is a combining form meaning jejunum.
5-86		A stoma is a mouth or opening. The plural form is either stomas or stomata. "stomat/o" is the combining form. -*stomy* is a suffix referring to a surgical procedure to make a mouth or opening.
5-87	Gastrojejunostomy	_____ is an operation to make an opening between the stomach and jejunum.
5-88	gastrostomy (gas-<u>tros</u>-to-me)	Gastrostomy is the surgical creation of an opening through the abdominal wall into the stomach. "gastr/o" is a combining form meaning stomach. -*stomy* is a suffix referring to a surgical procedure to make an opening.
5-89	"gastr/o" -*stomy* Gastrostomy	_____ is a combining form referring to the stomach. _____ is a suffix referring to a surgical procedure to make an opening. _____ is the surgical creation of an opening through the abdominal wall into the stomach.

BOX 5.1
Allied Health Professions

Registered Nurses, Licensed Practical Nurses, Licensed Vocational Nurses, and Nursing, Psychiatric, and Home Health Aides

Registered nurses (RNs), regardless of specialty or work setting, treat patients, educate patients and the public about various medical conditions, and provide advice and emotional support to patients' family members. RNs record patients' medical histories and symptoms, help perform diagnostic tests and analyze results, operate medical machinery, administer treatment and medications, and assist with patient follow-up and rehabilitation.

RNs teach patients and their families how to manage their illness or injury, explaining post-treatment home care needs; diet, nutrition, and exercise programs; and self-administration of medication and physical therapy. Some RNs work to promote general health by educating the public about warning signs and symptoms of disease. RNs also might run general health screening or immunization clinics, blood drives, and public seminars on various conditions.

Under the direction of physicians and registered nurses, *licensed practical nurses* (LPNs) or *licensed vocational nurses* (LVNs) care for people who are sick, injured, convalescent, or disabled. The nature of direction and supervision required varies by state and job setting.

LPNs care for patients in many ways. Often, they provide basic bedside care. Many LPNs measure and record patients' vital signs, such as height, weight, temperature, blood pressure, pulse, and respiration. They also prepare and give injections and enemas, monitor catheters, dress wounds, and give alcohol rubs and massages. To help keep patients comfortable, they assist with bathing, dressing, and personal hygiene, turning in bed, standing, and walking. They might also feed patients who need help eating. Experienced LPNs may supervise nursing assistants and aides.

Nursing and psychiatric aides help care for physically or mentally ill, injured, disabled, or infirm individuals in hospitals, nursing care facilities, and mental health settings. *Home health aides* have duties that are similar, but they work in patients' homes or residential care facilities. Nursing aides and home health aides are among the occupations commonly referred to as *direct care workers*, due to their role in working with patients who need long-term care. The specific care they give depends on their specialty.

The following are some resources for further information:

- National League for Nursing, www.nln.org

- American Association of Colleges of Nursing, www.aacn.nche.edu

- American Nurses Association, http://nursingworld.org

- National Association for Practical Nurse Education and Service, www.napnes.org

- National Federation of Licensed Practical Nurses, www.nflpn.org

- National Association for Home Care and Hospice, www.nahc.org

- Visiting Nurse Associations of America, www.vnaa.org

- The Center for the Health Professions, www.futurehealth.ucsf.edu

Source: P.S. Stanfield, N. Cross, Y. H. Hui, eds. *Introduction to the Health Professions*, 5th ed. (Sudbury, MA: Jones & Bartlett, 2009).

BLOCK	DATA AND ANSWERS	DESCRIPTIONS AND QUESTIONS
5-90		Review:
		"gastr/o" is a combining form meaning stomach.
		-dynia is a suffix meaning pain.
		-algia is another suffix meaning pain.
5-91		Build two medical terms meaning pain in the stomach:
	gastrodynia (gas'-tro-<u>de</u>-ne-ah)	1. _____
		_____
	gastralgia (gas-tral-je-ah)	2. _____
		_____
5-92	gastroma (gas-<u>tro</u>-mah)	A gastroma is a tumor of the stomach.
		-oma is a suffix meaning tumor.
	"gastr/o"	_____ is a combining form meaning stomach.
	-oma	_____ is a suffix meaning tumor.
	Gastroma	_____ is a tumor of the stomach.
5-93		The small intestine is divided into three parts: duodenum, jejunum, and ileum. The combining forms are "duoden/o," "jejun/o," and "ile/o," respectively.
	duodenum (doo-o-<u>de</u>-num)	The duodenum is the first segment, and it is joined to the stomach and the second section, the jejunum.
	jejunum (je-<u>ju</u>-num) ileum (<u>il</u>-e-um)	The jejunum in turn is joined to the distal (last) segment of the small intestine, called the ileum, which is connected to the colon (large intestine).
		Thus, anatomically, the sequence is stomach to duodenum to jejunum to ileum to colon.
		"enter" is a word root meaning small intestine.
		"enter/o" is the combining form.

BLOCK	DATA AND ANSWERS	DESCRIPTIONS AND QUESTIONS
5-94		Can you make the combining forms for the medical terms in the preceding block?
	"duoden/o"	_____ refers to the first segment of the small intestine.
	"jejun/o"	_____ refers to the second section of the small intestine.
	"ile/o"	_____ refers to the distal portion of the small intestine, which leads to the large intestine or colon.
	"enter/o"	_____ refers to the small intestine.
5-95		Write the meanings of the following word components:
	small intestine	"enter/o":_____ _____
	duodenum	"duoden/o": _____
	jejunum	"jejun/o":_____
	ileum	"ile/o": _____
	inflammation	-itis: _____
	excision	-ectomy: _____
	incision	-tomy: _____
5-96		Build medical terms meaning:
	duodenitis (doo-o-den-i-tis)	inflammation of the duodenum: _____ _____
	ilectomy (il-e-ek-to-me)	excision of part of the ileum: _____ _____
	jejunotomy (je-ju-not-o-me)	incision into the jejunum: _____ _____
	enteritis (en'-teh-ri-tis)	inflammation of the small intestine: _____ _____

BLOCK	DATA AND ANSWERS	DESCRIPTIONS AND QUESTIONS
5-97	duodenohepatic (doo-o- <u>den</u>-o-hep-ah-tik)	Duodenohepatic is a compound word meaning liver and duodenum or affecting the liver and duodenum. "duoden/o" is a combining form referring to the duodenum. "hepat/o" is a combining form referring to the liver. *-ic* is a suffix meaning pertaining to or affecting.
5-98	"duoden/o" "hepat/o" Duodenohepatic	_____ is a combining form meaning duodenum. _____ is a combining form meaning liver. _____ is pertaining to the duodenum and the liver.
5-99	jejunorrhaphy (je-joo-<u>nor</u>-ah-fe)	"jejun/o" is a combining form referring to the middle section of the small intestine, the jejunum. *-rrhaphy* is a suffix meaning suture. Build a medical term meaning suture of the jejunum: _____ _____
5-100	ileorectal (il'-e-o-<u>rek</u>-tal)	"Ileorectal" means pertaining to the ileum and the rectum. The ileum is the distal (last) segment of the small intestine. The rectum connects the large intestine to the outside. "ile/o" is a combining form meaning ileum. "rect/o" is a combining form meaning rectum. *-al* is a suffix meaning pertaining to.

BLOCK	DATA AND ANSWERS	DESCRIPTIONS AND QUESTIONS
5-101	combining form ileum	"ile/o" is a _____ _____ meaning _____.
	combining form rectum	"rect/o" is a _____ _____ meaning _____.
	suffix, pertaining to	-al is a _____ meaning _____ _____.
	pertaining to the ileum and rectum	Ileorectal means _____ _____ _____ _____ _____ _____.
5-102		Review:
		-stomy is a suffix referring to a surgical procedure to create a mouth or opening.
		Build a medical term meaning creation of an artificial opening (through the abdominal wall) into the ileum:
	ileostomy (il-e-os-to-me)	_____ _____
		(Clinically, this opening is used for the passage of stool. This surgery is performed for ulcerative colitis, Crohn's disease, or cancer of the colon.)
5-103	combining form ileum	"ile/o" is a _____ _____ referring to _____.
	suffix inflammation	-itis is a _____ referring to _____.
	an inflammation of the ileum	Ileitis is _____ _____ _____ _____ _____.
5-104	enterocystocele (en'-teh-ro-sis-to-sel)	Enterocystocele is a hernia of the intestine and bladder.
		"enter/o" is a combining form meaning intestine.
		"cyst/o" is a combining form meaning bladder.
		-cele is a suffix meaning hernia.

BLOCK	DATA AND ANSWERS	DESCRIPTIONS AND QUESTIONS
5-105	combining form small intestine combining form bladder suffix, hernia a hernia of the intestine and bladder	"enter/o" is a _____ _____ meaning _____ _____. "cyst/o" is a _____ _____ meaning _____. -cele is a _____ meaning _____. Enterocystocele is ___ _____ _____ _____ _____ _____ _____.
5-106	enteroptosis (en-teh-rop'-to-sis)	Enteroptosis is a falling, or downward displacement, of intestines. -ptosis is a suffix meaning falling.
5-107	"enter/o" -ptosis Enteroptosis	_____ is a combining form meaning intestine. _____ is a suffix meaning falling. _____ is a falling, or downward displacement, of intestines.
5-108	cecum (se-kum)	The cecum is the first part of the large intestine. "cec" is a root word meaning cecum. "cec/o" is the combining form.
5-109	cecectomy (se-sek-to-me)	-ectomy is a suffix meaning excision or removal. Build a medical term meaning excision of cecum: _____ _____
5-110	ileocecal (il'-e-o-se-kal)	Ileocecal means pertaining to the ileum and cecum. "ile/o" is the combining form of ileum. "cec/o" is the combining form of cecum.
5-111	Ileocecal	_____ is pertaining to the ileum and cecum.

BLOCK	DATA AND ANSWERS	DESCRIPTIONS AND QUESTIONS
5-112	colon (ko̲-lun) rectum (re̲k-tum)	The colon is the part of the large intestine extending from the cecum to the rectum. It is divided as follows: ascending (up), transverse (across), descending (down). The distal (last or farthest) portion of the descending colon forms a curve and becomes the rectum. The curved part of the descending colon is called the sigmoid colon. The appendix is a small structure near the juncture of the ileum and cecum (ileocecal valve).
	anus (a̲-nus)	The anus opens to the outside for evacuation of solid waste.
5-113		The word colon (meaning large intestine) has two different combining forms: "colon/o" and "col/o". Their application depends on the partner or another word component.
5-114		Review the following suffixes: *-itis* means inflammation. *-pathy* means a disease of. *-rrhagia* means hemorrhage.
5-115	colonitis colitis Colonopathy Colonorrhagia	Inflammation of the colon is called _____ or _____. _____ refers to any disease of the colon. _____ is hemorrhage from the colon.

BLOCK	DATA AND ANSWERS	DESCRIPTIONS AND QUESTIONS
5-116	stoma (sto-mah)	Stoma means mouth or opening. (In medicine, it is usually an artificial opening. When created in the large intestine, it is brought to the surface of the abdomen for evacuating the bowels.) -*stomy* is a suffix referring to an operation to create a mouth or opening.
5-117	Colostomy	"col/o" is a combining form referring to the colon. _____ is the creation of an artificial opening in the large intestine.
5-118	cecoileostomy (se-ko-il-e-os-to'-me)	Cecoileostomy is the creation of an opening between the cecum and the ileum. "cec/o" is a combining form meaning cecum. "ile/o" is a combining form meaning ileum. "cecoile/o" is a combining form meaning cecum and ileum. -*stomy* is a suffix meaning an operation to create a mouth or opening.
5-119	cecoileostomy (se-ko-il-e-os-to'-me)	Build a medical term referring to creating an opening between cecum and ileum: _____ _____
5-120	sigmoidectomy (sig'-moy-dek-to-me) sigmoid (sig-moyd)	Sigmoidectomy is surgical excision or removal of the sigmoid colon. Recall that the curved part of the descending colon is called the sigmoid colon. "sigmoid/o" is a combining form. -*ectomy* is surgical excision or removal.
5-121	Sigmoidectomy	_____ is surgical excision or removal of the sigmoid colon.

BLOCK	DATA AND ANSWERS	DESCRIPTIONS AND QUESTIONS
5-122	"ile/o"	_ile/o_ is a combining form meaning ileum.
	"col/o"	_col/o_ is a combining form meaning colon.
	-itis	_itis_ is a suffix meaning inflammation.
	Ileocolitis	_Ileocolitis_ is inflammation of ileum and colon.
5-123	anorectal (a-no-<u>rek</u>-tal)	Anorectal means pertaining to the opening of the rectum.
		"anus" is a word root referring to the opening to the outside from the rectum.
		"an/o" is a combining form meaning anus.
		"rect/o" is a combining form meaning rectum.
		_-al_ is a suffix meaning pertaining to.
5-124	combining form anus, opening	"an/o" is a _combining_ _form_ meaning _anus_ or _opening_.
	combining form rectum	"rect/o" is a _combining_ _form_ meaning _rectum_.
	suffix, pertaining to	_-al_ is a _suffix_ meaning _pertaining to_.
	pertaining to the opening of the rectum or anus	Anorectal means _pertaining to the opening of the rectum or anus_.
5-125	proctology (prok-<u>tol</u>-o-je)	Proctology is a branch of medicine concerned with disorders of the rectum and anus.
		"proct/o" is a combining form referring to disorders of the rectum and anus.
		-logy is a suffix meaning the study of.
	Proctology	_Proctology_ is the branch of medicine concerned with disorders of the rectum and anus.

BLOCK	DATA AND ANSWERS	DESCRIPTIONS AND QUESTIONS
5-126	proctologist (prok-<u>tol</u>-o-jist)	*-logist* is a suffix meaning a specialist engaged in the study of. Build a medical term meaning a physician who specializes in proctology: _____ _____
5-127	colostomy (ko-<u>los</u>-to-me)	"col/o" is a combining word referring to the colon. *-stomy* is a suffix referring to a surgical procedure to make a mouth or opening. A colostomy is the formation of an abdominal anus by bringing a loop of the colon to the surface of the abdomen. Build a medical term meaning to form an abdominal opening to the colon: _____ _____
5-128	sigmoidoscopy (sig-moy-<u>dos</u>-ko-pe) "sigmoid/o" *-scopy* Sigmoidoscopy	Sigmoidoscopy is the viewing of the sigmoid colon with an instrument. *-scopy* is a suffix referring to viewing with an instrument. _____ is a combining form meaning sigmoid colon. _____ is a suffix referring to viewing with an instrument. _____ is the viewing of the sigmoid colon with an instrument.

BLOCK	DATA AND ANSWERS	DESCRIPTIONS AND QUESTIONS
5-129	colectomy (ko-lek-to-me) colostomy (ko-los-to-me)	Recall the suffixes: -ectomy is a suffix meaning excision. -stomy is a suffix referring to a surgical procedure to make an opening. Build a medical term referring to excision of the colon: _____ _____ Build a medical term referring to creating an artificial opening through the abdominal wall into the colon to be used for the passage of stool: _____ _____
5-130	diverticulum (di'-ver-tik-u-lum), diverticula (di-ver-tik-u-lah)	The diverticulum is a pouch in the muscle wall of the colon. Diverticula is the plural form of diverticulum. "diverticul/o" is a combining form meaning diverticulum or diverticula. -ectomy is a suffix meaning excision. -itis is a suffix meaning inflammation.
5-131	diverticulectomy (di'-ver-tik-u-lek-to-me) diverticulitis (di'-ver-tik-u-li-tis)	Build medical terms meaning: excision of the diverticulum: _____ _____ inflammation of the diverticulum: _____ _____
5-132	proctoplasty (prok-to-plas-te)	Proctoplasty is surgical repair of the rectum. "proct/o" is a combining form meaning rectum. -plasty is a suffix meaning surgical repair.

BLOCK	DATA AND ANSWERS	DESCRIPTIONS AND QUESTIONS
5-133		Review:
		-scope is a suffix referring to an instrument for viewing.
		-scopy is a suffix referring to the use of an instrument to view.
		-itis is a suffix meaning inflammation.
5-134	combining form rectum	"proct/o" is a _____ _____ meaning _____.
		Build medical terms meaning:
		instrument used for visual examination of the rectum:
	proctoscope (prok-<u>to</u>-skop)	_____ _____
		visual examination of the rectum with a instrument:
	proctoscopy (prok-<u>tos</u>-ko-pe)	_____ _____
	proctitis (prok-<u>ti</u>-tis)	inflammation of the rectum: _____ _____
5-135	proctocele (prok-<u>to</u>-sel) "proct/o" *-cele* Proctocele	Proctocele is a hernia of the rectum. _____ is a combining form meaning rectum. _____ is a suffix meaning hernia. _____ is a hernia of the rectum.
5-136		*-ptosis* is a suffix meaning prolapse, dropping, or falling.
		"proct/o" is a combining form meaning rectum.
		Build a medical term meaning prolapse of the rectum:
	proctoptosis (prok-top-<u>to</u>-sis)	_____ _____

BLOCK	DATA AND ANSWERS	DESCRIPTIONS AND QUESTIONS
5-137	anal (a̱-nal)	The anus is an opening from the rectum to the outside. "an/o" is the combining form of anus. -al is a suffix meaning pertaining to. Anal means pertaining to the anus. -plasty is a suffix meaning surgical repair of the anus.
5-138	Anal anoplasty (an-o̱-plas-te)	_____ means pertaining to the anus. Build a medical term meaning surgical repair of the anus: _____ _____
5-139	hemorrhoidectomy (hem′-o-roy-de̱k-to-me) hemorrhoid (he̱m-o-royd)	A hemorrhoidectomy is the surgical removal of hemorrhoids. "hemorrhoid" is a word root meaning an enlarged varicose vein in the mucous membrane just outside the rectum. "hemorrhoid/o" is the combining form. -ectomy is a suffix referring to excision or surgical removal.
5-140	hemorrhoid -ectomy Hemorrhoidectomy	A _____ is an enlarged varicose vein outside the rectum. _____ is a suffix meaning removal. _____ is surgical removal of hemorrhoids.
5-141	appendectomy (ap′-pen-de̱k-to-me)	An appendectomy is excision or removal of the appendix. "append" is a root word meaning appendix. "append/o" is the combining form.
5-142	appendectomy	_____ is excision or removal of the appendix.

BLOCK	DATA AND ANSWERS	DESCRIPTIONS AND QUESTIONS
5-143	proctodynia (prok′-to-<u>de</u>-ne-ah)	"proct/o" is a combining form meaning rectum. *-dynia* is a suffix meaning pain. Build a medical term meaning pain in the rectum: _____ _____
5-144	colopexy (ko′-lo-<u>pek</u>-se)	Colopexy is a surgical intervention to correct or "fix" the colon in place. *-pexy* is a suffix meaning fixation.
5-145	"col/o" *-pexy* Colopexy	_____ is a combining form meaning colon. _____ is a suffix meaning fixation. _____ is surgical fixation of the colon.
5-146	pancreas (<u>pan</u>-kre-us), liver (liv-er), gallbladder (<u>gawl</u>-blad-er)	We have reviewed the entire digestive tract from mouth to anus. The next section covers major accessory organs that are vital to the functioning of the GI tract, including the pancreas, the liver, and the gallbladder. Of these three organs, only the gallbladder is expendable. Humans cannot live without a pancreas or a liver.
5-147	pancreatitis (pan′-kre-ah-<u>ti</u>-tis) pancreatectomy (pan′-kre-ah-<u>tek</u>-to-me)	"pancreat/o" is a combining form meaning pancreas. *-itis* is a suffix meaning inflammation. *-ectomy* is a suffix meaning excision or surgical removal. Build medical terms meaning: inflammation of the pancreas: _____ _____ removal of all or part of the pancreas: _____ _____

BLOCK	DATA AND ANSWERS	DESCRIPTIONS AND QUESTIONS
5-148		*-ic* is a suffix meaning pertaining to.
		Build a medical term meaning pertaining to the pancreas:
	pancreatic (pan′-kre-<u>at</u>-ik)	_____ _____
5-149	pancreatopathy (pan′-kre-ah-<u>top</u>-ah-the)	Pancreatopathy is disease of the pancreas.
	combining form	"pancreat/o" is a _____ _____
	pancreas	meaning _____.
	suffix, disease	*-pathy* is a _____ meaning _____.
	disease of the	Pancreatopathy is _____ _____ _____
	pancreas	_____.
5-150		"hepat/o" is a combining form meaning the liver.
		-megaly is a suffix meaning enlarged.
		-malacia is a suffix meaning softening.
		Build medical terms meaning:
	hepatomegaly	enlargement of the liver: _____
	(hep-at′-o-<u>meg</u>-ah-le)	_____
	hepatomalacia	softening of the liver: _____
	(hep-at′-o-mal-<u>a</u>-se-ah)	_____
5-151	combining form	"hepat/o" is a _____ _____ meaning
	liver	_____.
	suffix, softening	*-malacia* is a _____ meaning _____.
	softening of the	Hepatomalacia is _____ _____ _____
	liver	_____.
5-152	"hepat/o"	_____is a combining form meaning liver.
	-megaly	_____ is a suffix meaning enlarged.
	Hepatomegaly	_____ refers to an enlarged liver.

BLOCK	DATA AND ANSWERS	DESCRIPTIONS AND QUESTIONS
5-153	combining form liver	"hepat/o" is a _____ _____ meaning _____.
	suffix, surgical incision	-tomy is a _____ meaning _____ _____.
	a surgical incision of the liver	Hepatotomy is ___ _____ _____ _____ _____ _____.
5-154		-itis is a suffix meaning inflammation.
		Build a medical term meaning inflammation of the liver:
	hepatitis (hep′-ah-<u>ti</u>-tis)	_____ _____
5-155	hepatoma (hep-ah-<u>to</u>-mah)	Hepatoma is tumor of the liver.
	"hepat/o"	_____ is a combining form meaning liver.
	-oma	_____ is a suffix meaning tumor.
5-156	cirrhosis (sih-<u>ro</u>-sis)	Cirrhosis is a group of chronic diseases of the liver. Among other severe manifestations of the disease is jaundice, the yellowing of the skin and membranes. This symptom gives it the name cirrhosis, as explained in the next block.
5-157		"cirrh/o" is a combining form meaning yellow.
		-osis is a suffix meaning abnormal condition.
		Build a medical term meaning abnormal yellow condition:
	cirrhosis (sih-<u>ro</u>-sis)	_____ _____
5-158	hyperbilirubinemia (hi′-per-bil-i-<u>ru</u>-bin-e-me-ah)	Hyperbilirubinemia means excessive bilirubin (a chemical made by the liver) in blood as a result of liver dysfunction or malfunction.
		hyper- is a prefix meaning excessive or over.
		"bilirubin" is a root word meaning bilirubin.
		-emia is a suffix meaning blood.

BLOCK	DATA AND ANSWERS	DESCRIPTIONS AND QUESTIONS
5-159	*hyper-*	_____ is a prefix meaning excessive.
	"bilirubin"	_____ is a root word meaning bilirubin.
	-emia	_____ is a suffix meaning blood.
	hyperbilirubinemia	Excessive bilirubin in blood as a result of liver dysfunction is called _____.
5-160	cholecyst (<u>ko</u>-leh-sist)	Cholecyst means gallbladder.
		"chol/e" is a combining form meaning gall. Note that "e" is the vowel used in the combining form.
		-cyst is a suffix meaning a fluid-filled sac or bladder.
		"cholecyst/o" is a combining form meaning gallbladder.
		Combine these terms with prefixes and suffixes you have learned to build medical terms about the gallbladder.
5-161		"cholecyst/o" is a combining form meaning gallbladder.
		-itis is a suffix meaning inflammation.
		Build a medical term meaning inflammation of the gallbladder:
	cholecystitis (ko'-leh-sis-<u>ti</u>-tis)	_____ _____
5-162	cholelithiasis (ko'-leh-li-<u>thi</u>-ah-sis)	Cholelithiasis is the condition of having gallstones.
		"chol/e" is a combining form meaning bile.
		"lith" is a root word meaning stone. (Under certain circumstances, *-lith* can be a suffix.)
		-iasis is a suffix meaning condition.
5-163	Cholelithiasis	_____ is the condition of having gallstones.

BLOCK	DATA AND ANSWERS	DESCRIPTIONS AND QUESTIONS
5-164	cholecystectomy (ko'-leh-sis-<u>tek</u>-to-me)	"cholecyst/o" is a combining form meaning gallbladder. -*ectomy* is a suffix meaning excision or surgical removal. Build a medical term meaning removal of the gallbladder: _____ _____
5-165	hypercholia (hi'-per-<u>ko</u>-le-ah)	Hypercholia is excessive secretion of bile. Bile is a chemical manufactured by the gallbladder. *hyper-* is a prefix meaning over or increased amount. "cholia" is a word root meaning pertaining to bile. "chol/e" is the combining form. -*ia* is a suffix meaning pertaining to.
5-166	"cholia" -*ia* *hyper-* Hypercholia	_____ is a word root meaning pertaining to the bile. _____ is a suffix meaning pertaining to. _____ is a prefix meaning excessive. _____ is excessive secretion of bile.
5-167	cholesterosis (ko-les'-te-<u>ro</u>-sis)	Cholesterosis is an abnormal deposit of cholesterol in the gallbladder. Cholesterol is a chemical manufactured by the liver. Part of it is metabolized in the gallbladder and found in the bile. "chol/e" is a combining form meaning bile. "sterol" is a word root for a special fat chemical. "cholester/o" is a combining form meaning cholesterol. -*osis* is a suffix meaning abnormal condition, usually excessive.

BLOCK	DATA AND ANSWERS	DESCRIPTIONS AND QUESTIONS
5-168	"chol/e"	_____ is a combining form meaning bile.
	"sterol"	_____ is a word root meaning a special fat chemical.
	"cholester/o"	_____ is a combining form meaning cholesterol.
	-osis	_____ is a suffix meaning abnormal condition, usually excessive.
	Cholesterosis	_____ is an abnormal deposit of cholesterol in the gallbladder.
5-169	cholemia (<u>ko</u>-le-me-ah)	Cholemia is blood in the bile or gall (both substances manufactured by the gallbladder).
		"chol/e" is a combining form meaning bile or gall.
		-emia is a suffix meaning blood.
5-170	combining form bile, gall	"chol/e" is a _____ _____ meaning _____ or _____.
	suffix, blood	*-emia* is a _____ meaning _____.
	blood in the bile or gall	Cholemia is _____ ____ _____ _____ _____ _____.
5-171	biliary (bil-e-<u>ah</u>-re) system	The biliary system is responsible for the metabolism and physiology of bile substances manufactured by the gallbladder.
		Biliary is a medical term meaning pertaining to the biliary system.
		"bil/i" is a combining form meaning biliary system. Note that "i" is the vowel used in the combining form.
		-ary is a suffix meaning pertaining to.

BLOCK	DATA AND ANSWERS	DESCRIPTIONS AND QUESTIONS
5-172	combining form biliary system suffix, pertaining to Biliary	"bil/i" is a _____ _____ meaning _____ _____. -*ary* is a _____ meaning _____ _____. _____ is a medical term meaning pertaining to the biliary system.
5-173	cholangioma (ko-lan-<u>jeo</u>-mah)	A cholangioma is a tumor of the bile vessel. "ang/i" is a combining form meaning vessel. "cholangi/o" is a combining form meaning bile vessel. -*oma* is a suffix meaning tumor.
5-174	combining form bile vessel suffix, tumor tumor of the bile vessel	"cholangi/o" is a _____ _____ meaning _____ _____. -*oma* is a _____ meaning _____. A cholangioma is a _____ _____ _____ _____ _____.
5-175	choledocholithotomy (ko′-led-o-ko-li-<u>thot</u>-o-me)	Choledocholithotomy is incision into the bile duct for removal of gallstones. "choledoch/o" is a combining form meaning bile duct. "lith/o" is a combining form meaning stone. -*tomy* is a suffix meaning incision.
5-176	"choledoch/o" "lith/o" -*tomy* Choledocholithotomy	_____ is a combining form meaning bile duct. _____ is a combining form meaning stone. _____ is a suffix meaning incision. _____ is incision into the bile duct for removal of gallstones.

BLOCK	DATA AND ANSWERS	DESCRIPTIONS AND QUESTIONS
5-177		We have finished the entire digestive system and its associated organs.
		We now proceed to those medical terms frequently encountered when dealing with conditions of the GI tract.
5-178	peritoneum (peh′-rih-<u>to</u>-ne-um)	The peritoneum is the lining of the abdominal cavity.
	peritoneal (per′-rih-<u>to</u>-ne-al)	Peritoneal means pertaining to peritoneum.
		"peritone/o" is a combining form meaning peritoneum.
		-al is a suffix meaning pertaining to.
5-179	"peritone/o"	_____ is a combining form meaning peritoneum.
	-al	_____ is a suffix meaning pertaining to.
	Peritoneal	_____ means pertaining to the peritoneum.
5-180	abdominal (ab-<u>dom</u>-in-al)	Build a medical term meaning pertaining to the abdomen: _____ _____
5-181	abdominocentesis (ab-dom′-in-o-<u>sen</u>-te-sis)	Abdominocentesis is surgical puncture of the abdomen.
		"abdomin/o" is a combining form meaning abdomen.
		-centesis is a suffix meaning puncture.
5-182	"abdomin/o"	_____ is a combining form meaning abdomen.
	-centesis	_____ is a suffix meaning puncture.
	Abdominocentesis	_____ is surgical puncture of the abdomen.

BLOCK	DATA AND ANSWERS	DESCRIPTIONS AND QUESTIONS
5-183	bradypepsia (brah'-de-pep-se-ah)	*brady-* is a prefix meaning slow. *-pepsia* is a suffix meaning digestion. Build a medical term meaning slow digestion: _____ _____
5-184	dyspepsia (dis-pep-se-ah)	*dys-* is a prefix meaning difficult. Build a medical term meaning difficult digestion: _____ _____
5-185	dysphagia (dis-fa-je-ah)	*-phagia* is a suffix meaning swallow. Build a medical term meaning difficulty in swallowing: _____ _____
5-186	apepsia (a-pep-se-ah)	*a-* is a prefix meaning no or none. Build a medical term meaning without digestion: _____ _____
5-187	aphagia (a-fa-je-ah)	*-phagia* is a suffix meaning to swallow or eat. Build a medical term meaning inability to swallow: _____ _____
5-188	postprandial (post-pran-de-al)	Postprandial means after meals. *post-* is a prefix meaning after. *-prandial* is a suffix meaning pertaining to a meal.
5-189	*post-* *-prandial* Postprandial	_____ is a prefix meaning after. _____ is a suffix meaning pertaining to a meal. _____ means after meals.

BLOCK	DATA AND ANSWERS	DESCRIPTIONS AND QUESTIONS
5-190		This chapter reviewed the gastrointestinal system. The next chapter focuses on the respiratory system.

BOX 5.2
Abbreviations

ac	before meals (ante cibum)
Ba	barium
BE	barium enema
bid	twice a day
CT SCAN	computerized tomography (scan)
EGD	esophagogastroduodenoscopy
GI	gastrointestinal
GTT	glucose tolerance test
HAV	hepatitis A virus
IBS	irritable bowel syndrome
IVC	intravenouscholangiography
LES	lower esophageal sphincter
LFT	liver function tests
N&V	nausea and vomiting
NG	nasogastric
NPO (npo)	nothing by mouth
pc	after meals (post cibum)
PPBS	postprandial blood sugar
SBF	small bowel follow-through
S & D	stomach and duodenum
UGI series	upper gastrointestinal series

Progress Check

A. Multiple Choice

1. A suffix meaning excision or surgical removal is:
- **a.** -itis
- **b.** -algia
- **c.** -ectomy
- **d.** -ia

2. A prefix meaning difficult is:
- **a.** dys-
- **b.** inter-
- **c.** hypo-
- **d.** supra-

3. A combining form meaning large intestine is:
- **a.** gloss/o
- **b.** enter/o
- **c.** duod/o
- **d.** col/o

4. A suffix meaning pain is:
- **a.** -dysia
- **b.** -phagia
- **c.** -algia
- **d.** -ic

5. A prefix meaning no or none is:
- **a.** sub-
- **b.** dynia-
- **c.** algia-
- **d.** a-

6. A suffix meaning creating a new opening is:
- **a.** -pathy
- **b.** -stomy
- **c.** -dontia
- **d.** -tomy

7. A word root meaning stomach is:
- **a.** lingu
- **b.** cheilo
- **c.** stoma
- **d.** gastr

B. Building Medical Terms

Use the following word components to build medical terms matching the definitions given on the next page. Some answers may have two words.

-al	esophag	pancreat/o
-algia	esophag/o	-pathy
cheil	esophage	rect
cheil/o	gastr	rect/o
cheilo	gastr/o	-rectal
col	gastric	-rrphagia
colo	gastro	scope
duoden	hepat	-scopy
duoden/o	hepat/o	sigmoid
-dynia	-itis	stoma
dys-	lingu	sub-
enter	-lith	
enter/o	pancreat	

1. instrument for viewing and examining the sigmoid colon

2. bleeding of the small intestine

3. liver inflammation

4. pancreatic stone

5. pertaining to the colon and rectum

6. pertaining to the stomach and esophagus

7. surgical repair of the lips

8. viewing of the esophagus, stomach, and duodenum with an instrument

C. Definitions and Word Components

	TERM	DEFINITION	PREFIX	WORD ROOT	VOWEL	WORD ROOT	VOWEL	SUFFIX
1.	cheilostomatoplasty							
2.	gastrorrhagia							
3.	esophageal							
4.	colopexy							
5.	proctologist							
6.	hepatomegaly							
7.	odontalgia							
8.	oligodontia							

	TERM	DEFINITION	PREFIX	WORD ROOT	VOWEL	WORD ROOT	VOWEL	SUFFIX
9.	gingivectomy							
10.	glossosis							
11.	sialolith							
12.	esophagostenosis							

D. Abbreviations

	ABBREVIATIONS	MEANING
1.	ac	
2.	Ba	
3.	BE	
4.	bid	
5.	CT SCAN	
6.	EGD	
7.	GI	
8.	GTT	

	ABBREVIATIONS	MEANING
9.	HAV	
10.	IBS	
11.	IVC	
12.	LES	
13.	LFT	
14.	N&V	
15.	NG	
16.	NPO (npo)	
17.	pc	
18.	PPBS	
19.	SBF	
20.	S & D	
21.	UGI series	

The Respiratory System

BLOCK	DATA AND ANSWERS	DESCRIPTIONS AND QUESTIONS
6-1	respiration (<u>res</u>-pih-ra′-shun)	Respiration is the exchange of oxygen and carbon dioxide between the atmosphere and the body cells. Lungs are the organs of the body in which the exchange takes place. They are, therefore, called the respiratory organs.
		We will study the medical terminology for the respiratory system by following the body anatomy for the passage of air to the lung, moving from the nose, to the space behind nose and throat, to the voice organ, to the windpipe and its branches, and finally to the sacs or parts of the lung.
		Please refer to **Figures 6.1**, **6.2**, and **6.3** as well as **Table 6.1** (which contains the word roots, combining forms, prefixes, and suffixes relevant to this subject) as we proceed with each block. The figures will facilitate the progress from one block to the next. We will begin with the nose, the major organ where air enters our body.
6-2	nasal cavity (<u>na</u>-zal <u>kav</u>-it-e), nares (<u>nah</u>-rez) septum (<u>sap</u>-tum)	Nasal means nose (nares). Cavity means space. The nasal cavity is the space inside the nose, which is separated by a partition known as a septum.
	the space inside the nose	The nares is _____ _____ _____ _____ _____.
	septum	The partition that divides the nares is known as a _____.

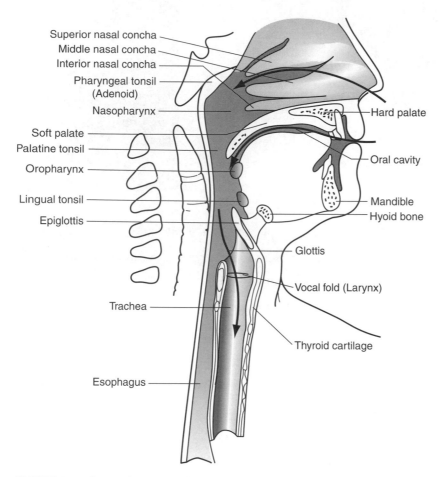

FIGURE 6.1 Sagittal section of the head and neck, showing the respiratory passage down to the bifurcation of the trachea

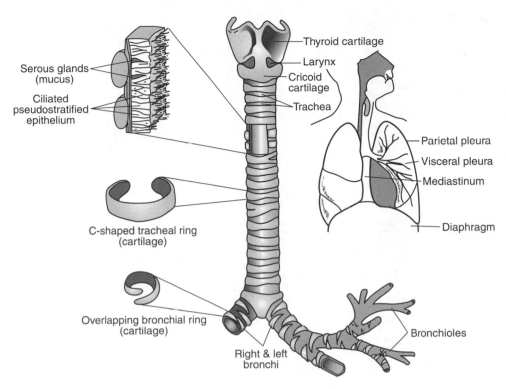

FIGURE 6.2 Human larynx, trachea, and bronchi (anterior aspect)

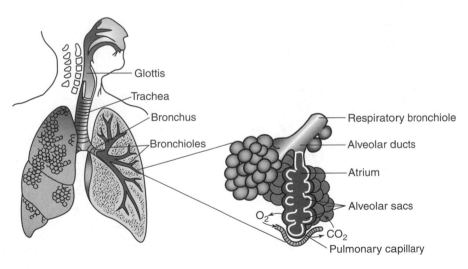

FIGURE 6.3 Internal structure of the lungs

TABLE 6.1 Word Components in this Chapter

WORD ROOTS	COMBINING FORMS	PREFIXES
atel	atel/o	a-
bronchi	bronch/o	an-
centesis	coccidioid/o	brady-
conis	coni/o	dys-
cyan	cyan/o	endo-
ectasis	gastr/o	eu-
gastr	laryn/o	ex-
laryn	laryng/o	hemo-
laryng	lob/o	histo-
lob	myc/o	per-
meter	nas/o	tachy-
myc	orth/o	**SUFFIXES**
mycosis	ox/o	-al
nas	pharyn/o	-centensis
orth	pharyng/o	-ectasis
ox	pleur/o	-ectomy
pharyn	pne/o	-ia
pharyng	pneum/o	-itis
plasma	pneumon/o	-meter
pleura	rhin/o	-osis
pneum	sinus/o	-pathy
pneumon	spir/o	-pnea
pnea	sten/o	-ptysis
ptysis	steth/o	-rrhagia
rhin	thorac/o	-rrhea
sinus	trache/o	-scope
steth	tubercul/o	-spasm
scope		-stomy
spasm		-tomy
spir		
thorax		
tracheal		
tussis		

BLOCK	DATA AND ANSWERS	DESCRIPTIONS AND QUESTIONS
6-3	"nas/o", "rhin/o"	"nas/o" is a combining form meaning nasal cavity. "rhin/o" is another combining form referring to the nasal cavity. Two combining forms relating to the nasal cavity are _nas/o_ and _rhin/o_ .
6-4	nasogastric (na-zo-<u>gas</u>-trik)	"nas/o" is a combining form meaning the nose. "gastric" is a root word meaning stomach. Build a medical word (with pronunciation) meaning related to nose and stomach: _nasogastric_
6-5	nasogastric	In medicine, nasogastric refers to the route from nose to stomach. When a tube is inserted through the nose into the stomach for feeding, it is called a _nasogastric_ tube for feeding.
6-6	rhinorrhagia (<u>ri</u>-no-raj'-e-ah)	-rrhagia is a suffix meaning bursting forth of blood (bleeding or hemorrhaging). "rhin/o" is a combining form meaning nose. Build a term meaning bursting forth of blood from the nose (nose bleed): _rhinorrhagia_
6-7	Rhinorrhea (<u>ri</u>-no-re-ah)	-rrhea means discharge or flow. _Rhinorrhea_ is a medical term meaning discharge from the nose.
6-8	rhinitis (ri-<u>ni</u>-tis)	Rhinitis is inflammation of the nasal membrane. "rhin/o" is a combining form meaning nose. -itis is a suffix meaning inflammation.

BLOCK	DATA AND ANSWERS	DESCRIPTIONS AND QUESTIONS
6-9	an inflammation of the nose membrane combining form nose suffix inflammation	Rhinitis is _____ _____ _____ _____ _____ _____. "rhin/o" is a _____ _____ meaning _____. -*itis* is a _____ meaning _____.
6-10	sinusitis (sĭ′-nu-<u>si</u>-tis)	Sinusitis is sinus inflammation. Sinuses are the hollow spaces within the nasal cavity. "sinus/o" is a combining form referring to the sinus. -*itis* is a suffix meaning inflammation.
6-11	inflammation of the sinus hollow space or cavity of the nose inflammation	Sinusitis is _____ _____ _____ _____. "sinus/o" is a combining form meaning _____ _____ _____ _____ _____ _____ _____. -*itis* is a suffix meaning _____.
6-12	rhinostenosis (<u>ri</u>-no-sten-o′-sis)	Rhinostenosis is the condition of a narrowed nasal passage or cavity. "rhin/o" is a combining form meaning nasal passage or cavity. "sten/o" is a combining form meaning narrowing. -*osis* is a suffix meaning condition. -*stenosis* is a suffix meaning the condition of narrowing.
6-13	Rhinostenosis	_____ is the condition of a narrowed nasal passage.

BLOCK	DATA AND ANSWERS	DESCRIPTIONS AND QUESTIONS
6-14	rhinoplasty (ri-no-plas′-te)	Rhinoplasty is plastic surgery of the nose. "rhin/o" is a combining form meaning the nose. *-plasty* is a suffix meaning surgical repair.
6-15	plastic surgery of the nose nose surgical repair	Rhinoplasty is _____ _____ _____ _____ _____. "rhin/o" is a combining form meaning _____. *-plasty* is a suffix meaning _____ _____.
6-16	pharynx (far-ingks) pharynx	The pharynx refers to the throat and space (cavity) behind the nose cavity, the mouth, and the throat. The combined space behind the nasal cavity, the mouth, and the throat is the _____.
6-17	pharyngitis (far′-in-ji-tis)	Pharyngitis is inflammation of the pharynx. "pharyng/o" is a combining forms meaning pharynx. *-itis* is a suffix meaning inflammation.
6-18	inflammation of the pharynx	Pharyngitis is _____ _____ _____ _____.
6-19	nasopharyngitis (na-zo-far-in-ji-tis)	Review: "nas/o" is a combining form meaning nasal cavity. "pharyng/o" is a combining forms meaning pharynx. Build a medical term meaning inflammation of the nose and pharynx: _____ _____
6-20	Pharyngopathy (far-in-jo-path′-e)	*-pathy* is a suffix meaning disease. _____ _____ is a term referring to any disease of the pharynx.

BLOCK	DATA AND ANSWERS	DESCRIPTIONS AND QUESTIONS
6-21	nasopharyngeal (<u>na</u>-zo-far-in-<u>ji</u>-)	Nasopharyngeal means pertaining to the nose and pharynx. -al is a suffix meaning pertaining to.
6-22	Nasopharyngeal	_Nasopharyngeal_ means pertaining to the nose and pharynx.
6-23	larynx (<u>lar</u>-inks) larynx	Larynx is the organ containing the vocal cords. Vocal cords are housed in a voice organ known as the _larynx_.
6-24	laryngitis (lar'-in-<u>ji</u>-tis)	Laryngitis is inflammation of the larynx. "larynx" is a root word meaning the voice organ or voice box. "laryng/o" is the combining form.
6-25	inflammation of the larynx combining form voice box suffix, inflammation	Laryngitis is _inflammation_ of _the larynx_. "laryng/o" is a _root_ _word_ meaning _voice box_. -itis is a _suffix_ meaning _inflammation_.
6-26	laryngotracheobronchitis (lah-rin'-jo-<u>tra</u>-ke-o-brong-<u>ki</u>-tis)	Laryngotracheobronchitis is a compound word meaning inflammation of the larynx, trachea, and bronchi. This is an unusual medical term in that it is composed of three combining forms and one suffix. Of course, we could also consider this term as made up of one large combining form and one suffix.
6-27	"laryng/o" "trache/o", "bronch/o" -itis Laryngotracheobronchitis	Laryngotracheobronchitis is inflammation of the larynx, trachea, and bronchi. Name the three combining forms: _laryng/o_, _trache/o_, and _bronch/o_. Name the suffix: _itis_ _laryngotracheobronchitis_ is inflammation of the larynx, trachea, and bronchi.

BLOCK	DATA AND ANSWERS	DESCRIPTIONS AND QUESTIONS
6-28	laryngoplasty (<u>lar</u>-in-jo-plas′-te)	Laryngoplasty is surgical repair of a tear in the larynx. "laryng/o" is a combining form meaning the larynx. -*plasty* is a suffix meaning surgical repair.
6-29	Laryngoplasty	_____ is surgical repair of a tear in the larynx.
6-30	trachea (tra-<u>ke</u>-ah) Trachea	The trachea is the tube connecting the throat to the lungs. The trachea is commonly referred to as the windpipe. _____ is the medical term for windpipe. "trache/o" is a combining form meaning trachea. "pharyng/o" is a combining word meaning pharynx. -*tomy* is a suffix meaning incision. -*stomy* is a suffix referring to the making of an opening in a body wall (usually the abdomen) to permit passage through the wall from the inside to the outside.
6-31	tracheotomy (<u>tra</u>-ke-ot-o-me) tracheostomy (<u>tra</u>-ke-os-to-me)	Build medical terms meaning: incision into the trachea: _____ _____ to form a new opening into the trachea: _____ _____
6-32	tracheopharyngotomy (tra′-ke-o-<u>lar</u>-ing-ot-o-me) "trache/o" "pharyng/o" -*tomy*	Tracheopharyngotomy is an incision into the trachea and the larynx. Its three word components are: _____ is a combining form meaning the trachea. _____ is a combining word meaning the pharynx. _____ is a suffix meaning incision.

BLOCK	DATA AND ANSWERS	DESCRIPTIONS AND QUESTIONS
6-33	tracheostomy (<u>tra</u>-ke-os-to-me)	Tracheostomy is a two-stage surgical procedure. First, an incision is made into the trachea through the skin and muscle. Next, the incision is modified to form an opening into the trachea for various purposes (e.g., insertion of a tube to facilitate ventilation). "trache/o" is a combining form meaning the trachea. *-stomy* is a suffix meaning an opening.
6-34	Tracheostomy "trache/o" *-stomy*	_____ is the creation of an opening from outside to the trachea. _____ is a combining form meaning trachea. _____ is a suffix meaning opening.
6-35	endotracheal tube (en'-do-<u>tra</u>-ke-al)	Endotracheal means inside the trachea or windpipe. An endotracheal tube is an airway catheter inserted in the trachea (windpipe) during surgery or used as a temporary airway in emergency situations. *endo-* is a prefix meaning within. "trache/o" is a combining form meaning the trachea. *-al* is a suffix meaning pertaining to. Tracheal means pertaining to the trachea (windpipe).
6-36	in, inside pertaining to the windpipe inside the windpipe	*endo-* is a prefix meaning ____ or _____. Tracheal means _____ ____ _____ _____. Endotracheal means _____ _____ _____.

BLOCK	DATA AND ANSWERS	DESCRIPTIONS AND QUESTIONS
6-37	trachea (tra-ke-ah) bronchi (brong-ki) bronchioles (brong-ki-olz)	Recall the following basic anatomy: The windpipe is connected to the trachea, which is divided into two bronchi, each of which is divided into many bronchioles that are distributed in the lung tissues.
6-38	Bronchitis (brong-ki-tis)	*-itis* is a suffix meaning inflammation. _____ _____ is the condition of inflamed bronchi.
6-39	bronchioles	Each bronchus divides into many bronchioles in the lung, like a big tree branch divides into smaller branches. That is, each branch of an inverted Y enters the lungs and subdivides into many small branches. Each branch of an inverted Y or bronchus is divided into small branches known as _____.
6-40	bronchospasm (brong-ko-spazm)	Bronchospasm is contraction of the muscles of the bronchi of the lung. "bronch/o" is a combining form referring to the bronchus or bronchi (plural for bronchus). "spasm" is a word root meaning muscle contraction. *-spasm* is also a suffix.
6-41	"bronch/o" "spasm" spasm of the muscles of the bronchi	_____ is a combining form referring to the bronchus or bronchii (plural for bronchus). _____ is a word root meaning muscle contraction. Bronchospasm is _____ ___ ___ _____ ___ ___ _____.

BLOCK	DATA AND ANSWERS	DESCRIPTIONS AND QUESTIONS
6-42		The process of breathing air into the lung can be described by one of the following three combining forms:
		"pne/o" means breathing.
		"pneum/o" means air.
		"pneumon/o" means lungs.
	"pne/o," "pneum/o" "pneumon/o"	The three combining forms related to breathing are: _____, _____, and _____.
6-43	pneumoconiosis (nu'-mo-ko-ne-o-sis)	Pneumoconiosis is a generic name for a disease of the lungs caused by breathing dust particles into the lungs. There are many types of dust particles.
		"pneum/o" is a combining form meaning lung.
		"conis" is a word root meaning dust.
		"coni/o" is the combining form.
		-osis is a suffix meaning condition.
6-44	Pneumoconiosis	_____ is a lung disease caused by an excessive inhaling of dust.
	"pneum/o"	_____ is a combining form meaning lung.
	"coni/o"	_____ is a combining form meaning dust.
	-osis	_____ is a suffix meaning condition.
6-45	pneumonectomy (nu'-mo-nek-to-me)	Pneumonectomy means to excise a lung.
	pneumopathy (nu'-mo-path-e)	Pneumopathy is a disease of the lungs.
		-tomy is a suffix meaning to incise (open into).
		-pathy is a suffix meaning disease.

BLOCK	DATA AND ANSWERS	DESCRIPTIONS AND QUESTIONS
6-46	Pneumonectomy Pneumopathy -tomy -pathy	_Pneumonectomy_ means to excise a lung. _Pneumopathy_ is a disease of the lungs. _tomy_ is a suffix meaning to incise (open into). _pathy_ is a suffix meaning disease.
6-47	pneumonia (nu-<u>mo</u>-ne-ah) pneumonitis (nu'-mo-<u>ni</u>-tis) Pneumonia, pneumonitis	Pneumonia is a very serious inflammation of the lungs. Pneumonia may also be called pneumonitis. _Pneumonia_ and _pneumonitis_ both mean lung inflammation. -itis is the most common suffix used to mean inflammation.
6-48	pleurisy (ploo-<u>ris</u>-e) pleuritis (ploo-<u>ri</u>-tis)	Pleurisy and pleuritis are two terms meaning inflammation of the pleura. Both terms have the same combining form but different suffixes. "pleura" is a word root meaning the membrane lining the lungs and related organs. "pleur/o" is the combining form. The two suffixes meaning inflammation are -isy (less common) and -itis (more common).
6-49	"pleur/o" -itis, -isy	_pleur/o_ is the combining form meaning the membrane lining the lungs. _itis_ and _isy_ are two suffixes meaning inflammation.
6-50	inflammation of the pleura inflammation of the pleura	Pleurisy is _inflammation_ _of the pleura_. Pleuritis is _inflammation_ _of the pleura_.

BLOCK	DATA AND ANSWERS	DESCRIPTIONS AND QUESTIONS
6-51	pleura (ploo-<u>rah</u>)	Recall that pleura is the term for a double-folded membrane lining the lungs and the thoracic (chest) cavity.
	visceral (<u>vis</u>-sa-rol)	Visceral pleura is the inner membrane lining the lungs.
	parietal (par-<u>iet</u>-al)	Parietal pleura is the outer membrane lining the walls of the thoracic (chest) cavity. Pleural cavity is the space between the two layers (outer and inner) of the membrane or pleura.
6-52	Pleura	_____ is the term for a double-folded membrane lining the lungs and the thoracic (chest) cavity.
	Visceral pleura	_____ _____ is the inner membrane lining the lungs.
	Parietal pleura	_____ _____ is the outer membrane lining the walls of the thoracic (chest) cavity.
6-53	Pleural cavity	_____ _____ is the space between the two layers (outer and inner) of the membrane or pleura.
	pleuritis	Inflammation of the pleura is _____ or
	pleurisy	_____.
6-54		Next, you will be learning various medical words associated with infection of the lung.
		COPD is the abbreviation for chronic obstructive pulmonary disease. Sometimes the abbreviation is COLD, for chronic obstructive lung disease.
		Two major lung infections are chronic bronchitis and asthma.

BLOCK	DATA AND ANSWERS	DESCRIPTIONS AND QUESTIONS
6-55	COPD	The abbreviation for chronic obstructive pulmonary disease is _____.
	COLD	The abbreviation for chronic obstructive lung disease is _____.
		Name two chronic obstructive pulmonary or lung diseases:
	chronic bronchitis	1. _____ _____
	asthma	2. _____
6-56		"myc/o" is a combining form meaning fungus.
		-*osis* is a suffix meaning condition or disease.
		Build a medical term meaning any condition or disease caused
	mycosis (mi-<u>co</u>-sis)	by a fungus: _____ _____
6-57	coccidioidomycosis (kok′-sid-e-oy-do-mi-<u>ko</u>-sis)	Coccidioidomycosis is a respiratory infection caused by inhalation of *Coccidioides immitis*, a fungus, in the form of a spore, with symptoms varying in severity from those of a common cold to those of influenza; also called valley fever.
6-58		"coccidioid/o" is a combining form referring to the fungus *Coccidioides immitis*.
		"mycosis" is a word root meaning disease caused by a fungus.
6-59	Coccidioidomycosis	_____ is the respiratory infection caused by the inhalation of a fungus spore.
6-60		Recall that "pneumon/o" is a combining form meaning the lungs.
	Pneumonomycosis (nu-mo′-no-mi-<u>ko</u>-sis)	_____ _____ is a respiratory infection of the lungs caused by a fungus.

BLOCK	DATA AND ANSWERS	DESCRIPTIONS AND QUESTIONS
6-61	laryngomycosis (lar'-in-jo-mi-<u>ko</u>-sis) pharyngomycosis (fah'-rin-jo-mi-<u>ko</u>-sis)	Review: "laryng/o" is a combining form meaning larynx (throat). "pharyng/o" is a combining form meaning pharynx. "mycosis" is a word root meaning disease caused by a fungus. Build medical terms meaning: a fungal disease of the larynx: _____ _____ a fungal disease of the pharynx: _____ _____
6-62	diptheria (<u>dip</u>-the-re-ah)	Diptheria is an acute bacterial infection affecting primarily the membranes of the nose, throat, or larynx. The disease is accompanied by fever and pain.
6-63	Diptheria	_____ is the clinical condition of fever, pain, and a specific infection of the nose and throat membrane.
6-64		The next section discusses disorders associated with the respiratory system. The medical terms are not presented in any particular grouping, such as nose or infection, as in earlier sections. Rather, the terms are randomly selected and studied because they represent many potential clinical disorders.
6-65	hemothorax (he'-mo-<u>tho</u>-raks)	Hemothorax is blood in the pleural thoracic cavity. *hemo-* is a prefix meaning blood. "thorax" is a root word referring to the cavity or space inside the rib cage and surrounding area.

BLOCK	DATA AND ANSWERS	DESCRIPTIONS AND QUESTIONS
6-66	blood in the pleural thoracic cavity	Hemothorax is _____ ____ _____ _____ _____ _____.
	prefix, blood	*hemo-* is a _____ meaning _____.
	root word, the cavity or space inside the rib cage and surrounding area	"thorax" is a _____ _____ referring to _____ _____ ____ _____ _____ _____ _____ _____ _____ _____ _____.

BOX 6.1
Allied Health Professions

Respiratory Therapists and Respiratory Therapy Technicians

The term *respiratory therapist* used here includes both respiratory therapists and respiratory therapy technicians. Respiratory care therapists work to evaluate, treat, and care for patients with breathing disorders. They work under the direction of a physician.

Most respiratory therapists work with hospital patients in three distinct phases of care: diagnosis, treatment, and patient management. In the area of diagnosis, therapists test the capacity of the lungs and analyze the oxygen and carbon dioxide concentrations and potential of hydrogen (blood pH), a measure of the acidity or alkalinity level of the blood. To measure *lung capacity*, the therapist has the patient breathe into a tube connected to an instrument that measures the volume and flow of air during inhalation and exhalation. By comparing the reading with the norm for the patient's age, height, weight, and sex, the therapist can determine whether lung deficiencies exist.

To analyze oxygen, carbon dioxide, and pH levels, therapists need an *arterial blood sample*, for which they generally draw arterial blood. This procedure requires greater skill than is the case for routine tests, for which blood is drawn from a vein. Inserting a needle into a patient's artery and drawing blood must be done with great care; any slip can damage the artery and interrupt the flow of oxygen-rich blood to the tissues. Once the sample is drawn, it is placed in a gas analyzer, and the results are relayed to the physician.

The following are some resources for further information:

- American Association for Respiratory Care, www.aarc.org
- National Board for Respiratory Care, www.nbrc.org

Source: P.S. Stanfield, N. Cross, Y.H. Hui, eds. *Introduction to the Health Professions*, 5th ed (Sudbury, MA: Jones & Bartlett, 2009).

BLOCK	DATA AND ANSWERS	DESCRIPTIONS AND QUESTIONS
6-67	thoracotomy (tho'-rah-<u>sot</u>-o-me)	Review: -*tomy* is a suffix meaning to make an opening or incision. "thorac/o" is a combining form meaning chest. An incision in the chest is called a _thoracotomy_ _____.
6-68	histoplasmosis (his-to-plaz-<u>mo</u>-sis)	Histoplasmosis is a fungal infection of the lungs resembling tuberculosis. It may or may not have symptoms.
6-69		*histo-* is a prefix meaning tissue. "plasma" is a word root meaning the liquid part of the blood. "plasm/o" is the combining form. -*osis* is a suffix meaning condition.
6-70	histoplasmosis *histo-* "plasma", "plasm/o" -*osis*	One form of lung infection by a fungus is _histoplasmosis_. _histo_ is a prefix referring to tissue. The word root for the liquid part of the blood is _plasma_. Its combining form is _plasm/o_. A suffix meaning condition is _osis_.
6-71	influenza (in'-floo-en-<u>zah</u>) Influenza	Influenza is an acute viral infection of the respiratory tract, serious for the very young and old. _influenza_ is the clinical condition when the respiratory tract suffers an acute infection from a virus.

BLOCK	DATA AND ANSWERS	DESCRIPTIONS AND QUESTIONS
6-72	pertussis (per-<u>tus</u>-is)	Pertussis is the medical term for whooping cough. It is a respiratory infection caused by the bacteria *Bordetella pertussis*, marked by a peculiar cough ending in a prolonged crowing or whooping respiration. *per-* is a prefix meaning through. "tussis" is a word root meaning cough.
6-73	whooping cough *per-*, through "tussis," cough	The medical term pertussis means _____ _____. Its prefix is _____, meaning _____. The word root is _____, meaning _____.
6-74	tuberculosis (too-ber'-ku-<u>lo</u>-sis)	Tuberculosis (TB) is an infectious disease of the lung, caused by *Mycobacterium tuberculosis* and marked by small swellings (abscesses) in tissues of the lung. "tubercul/o" is a combining form referring to the bacteria *Mycobacterium tuberculosis*. *-osis* is a suffix meaning disease or condition.
6-75	an infectious disease of the lung caused by *Mycobacterium tuberculosis* and marked by small swellings (abscesses) in tissues of the lung	Tuberculosis is _____ _____ _____ _____ _____ _____, _____ ____ _____ _____ _____ _____ _____ _____ _____ _____ ____ _____ _____ _____ _____.
6-76	combining form *Mycobacterium tuberculosis* suffix, disease condition	"tubercul/o" is a _____ _____ referring to the microorganism _____ _____. *-osis* is a _____ meaning _____ or _____.

BLOCK	DATA AND ANSWERS	DESCRIPTIONS AND QUESTIONS
6-77		The next section explores the medical terminology associated with the various clinical disorders of the respiratory system.
6-78	asphyxiation (as-fik-<u>se</u>-a-shun) asphyxiation asphyxiated (as-fik-se-a-ted)	Asphyxiation means suffocation. The medical term for suffocation is _____. We can say a person is suffocated, *or* we can say a person is _____ _____.
6-79	asthma (az-<u>mah</u>) asthma suffocation	Asthma is a condition marked by recurrent attacks of spasm and swelling of airways, with wheezing, usually caused by allergy. A person who is allergic to pollen exhibits many symptoms. One may be gasping for breath characterized by spasms. This clinical condition is known as _____. A person with asthma may experience a feeling of asphyxiation. Another word for asphyxiation is _____.
6-80	atelectasis (at´-eh-<u>lek</u>-ta-sis)	Atelectasis has two meanings: an incomplete expansion of the lungs at birth, or collapse of the adult lung. "atel/o" is a combining form meaning imperfect. -*ectasis* is a suffix meaning expansion.
6-81	atelectasis the collapse of an adult lung	When a child is born with a lung that does not expand properly, the condition is known as _____. The same term applies when _____ _____ _____ _____ _____ _____ occurs.
6-82	"atel/o" -*ectasis*	_____ is a combining form meaning imperfect. _____ is a suffix meaning expansion.

BLOCK	DATA AND ANSWERS	DESCRIPTIONS AND QUESTIONS
6-83	bronchiectasis (<u>brong</u>-ke-ek-ta′-sis)	Bronchiectasis is chronic dilatation (or expansion) of one or more bronchi or a branch of the respiratory tract. "bronch/o" is a combining form meaning bronchi, a branch of the respiratory tract. *-ectasis* is a suffix meaning expansion.
6-84	bronchiectasis "bronch/o" *-ectasis*	When a branch of the respiratory tract is expanded or dilated, the condition is known as _____. The two word components are _____ and _____.
6-85		Many lung diseases are identified by whether the patient is breathing too fast, too slow, or not at all. There are three prefixes that describe these conditions: *tachy-* means fast. *brady-* means slow. *a-* means without or none.
6-86	tachypnea (tak-<u>ip</u>-ne-ah) Bradypnea (bra-<u>dip</u>-ne-ah) apnea (<u>ap</u>-ne-ah)	"pnea" is a word root meaning breathing. *-pnea* also is a suffix. The condition of fast breathing is known as _____ _____. _____ _____ is the term for slow breathing. A person who has temporarily ceased to breathe is said to have _____ _____.

BLOCK	DATA AND ANSWERS	DESCRIPTIONS AND QUESTIONS
6-87	thoracocentesis (tho′-rah-<u>co</u>-sen-te′-sis) spirometer (<u>spi</u>-rom-et-er) laryngoscope (lar-in′-<u>jo</u>-skop)	Thoracocentesis is surgical puncture of the chest for removal of fluid. A spirometer is an instrument used to measure volume of air. A laryngoscope is an instrument used to examine the larynx.
6-88		"centesis" is a root word meaning surgical puncture. -centesis also is a suffix. "meter" is a root word meaning an instrument used to measure. -meter also is a suffix. "scope" is a root word meaning an instrument used to examine. -scope also is a suffix.
6-89		Note the following three combining forms: "thorac/o" means chest cavity. "spir/o" means to breathe. "laryn/o" means the larynx.
6-90	"centesis" "meter" "scope"	_____ is a word root meaning surgical puncture. _____ is a word root referring to an instrument used to measure. _____ is a word root referring to an instrument used to examine.
6-91	"thorac/o" "spir/o" "laryn/o"	_____ is a combining form meaning the chest cavity. _____ is a combining form meaning to breathe. _____ is a combining form meaning the larynx.

BLOCK	DATA AND ANSWERS	DESCRIPTIONS AND QUESTIONS
6-92	Thoracocentesis	_____ is surgical puncture of the chest for removal of fluid.
	spirometer	A _____ is an instrument used to measure volume of air.
	laryngoscope	A _____ is an instrument used to examine the larynx.
6-93	cyanosis (si′-ah-<u>no</u>-sis)	Cyanosis is a bluish discoloration of skin and mucous membranes caused by insufficient oxygen in the blood. "cyan/o" is a combining form meaning blue. -osis is a suffix meaning condition.
6-94	Cyanosis	_____ is bluish skin due to a lack of oxygen.
	"cyan/o"	_____ is a combining form meaning blue.
	-osis	_____ is a suffix meaning condition.
6-95	expectoration (ek-spek-to′-<u>ra</u>-shun)	Expectoration is the expulsion of mucus or phlegm from the throat or lungs.
	expectorant (ek-spek-<u>to</u>-rant)	An expectorant is an agent that promotes expectoration.
	expectoration	The expulsion of phlegm from the throat or lungs is _____.
	expectorant	The substance that can facilitate the expulsion of mucus from the throat or lungs _____.
6-96	hemoptysis (he-mop-<u>tih</u>-sis)	Hemoptysis is the spitting of blood or of blood-stained sputum (from the lungs). "hem/o" is a combining form meaning blood. It also can be a prefix (hemo-). -ptysis is a suffix meaning spitting.

BLOCK	DATA AND ANSWERS	DESCRIPTIONS AND QUESTIONS
6-97	Hemoptysis	_____ is the spitting of blood.
	"hem/o"	_____ is a combining form meaning blood.
	-ptysis	_____ is a suffix meaning spitting.
6-98	exhalation (ex-hel'-a-shum)	Exhalation is the process of breathing out.
	dyspnea (disp-ne-ah)	Dyspnea is labored or difficult breathing.
		dys- is a prefix meaning bad or difficult.
		-pnea is a suffix meaning breathing.
6-99	Dyspnea	_____ is breathing difficulty.
	dys-	_____ is a prefix meaning bad or difficult.
	breathing	*-pnea* is a suffix meaning _____.
6-100	eupnea (up-ne-a)	Eupnea refers to normal breathing.
		eu- is a prefix meaning good or normal.
		-pnea is a suffix meaning breathing.
6-101	*Eu-*	_____ is a prefix meaning good or normal.
	Eupnea	_____ is normal breathing.
6-102	Dyspnea	_____ is labored or difficult breathing.
	Eupnea	_____ is normal breathing.
	Hemoptysis	_____ is spitting up blood.
	Exhalation	_____ is the process of breathing out.

BLOCK	DATA AND ANSWERS	DESCRIPTIONS AND QUESTIONS
6-103		Review:
	eu-	_____ is a prefix meaning good or normal.
	dys-	_____ is a prefix meaning bad.
	brady-	_____ is a prefix meaning slow.
	-ptysis	_____ is a suffix meaning spitting.
	-osis	_____ is a suffix meaning condition.
	-ectasis	_____ is a suffix meaning expansion.
	"pneum/o"	_____ is a combining form meaning air.
	"thorac/o"	_____ is a combining form meaning chest.
	"sten/o"	_____ is a combining form meaning narrowing.
6-104	lobectomy (lo-<u>bek</u>-to-me)	Lobectomy is the removal of part of the lung (a lobe), usually because it has a cancerous tumor in it.
		"lob/o" is a combining form referring to a lobe or a defined part of an organ, such as a lung in this case.
		-ectomy is a suffix meaning excision (removal).
6-105	a lobe or a defined part of an organ	"lob/o" is a combining form meaning ___ _____ _____ __ _____ _____ _____ _____ _____.
	excision	*-ectomy* is a suffix meaning _____ or
	removal	_____
6-106	lobectomy	A _____ is the excision of a lobe (or part) of the lung.
6-107	orthopnea (or-<u>thop</u>-ne-ah)	Orthopnea is the condition of difficult breathing except in the upright, normal, or straight position.
		"orth/o" is a combining form meaning upright, normal, or straight.
		-pnea is a suffix meaning breath or respiration.

BLOCK	DATA AND ANSWERS	DESCRIPTIONS AND QUESTIONS
6-108	difficulty in breathing except in the upright position upright normal, straight respiration breath	Orthopnea is the condition of _____ ___ _____ _____ ___ _____ _____ _____. "orth/o" is a combining form meaning _____, _____, or _____. -*pnea* is a suffix meaning _____ or _____.
6-109	orthopnea "orth/o"	A person who must sit in an upright position in order to breathe has a condition known as _____. The combining form meaning upright or straight is _____.
6-110	percussion (per-<u>kush</u>-un) auscultation (<u>aw</u>-skul-ta′-shun)	Percussion (P) means striking. Ausculation (A) means listening for sounds. P & A refers to striking the body (e.g., chest) with short, sharp blows of the fingers and listening for the sounds produced through a stethoscope.
6-111		The word stethoscope has two parts: "steth/o" is a combining form meaning chest. "scope" is a root word meaning an instrument used to examine. -*scope* also is a suffix. A stethoscope is an instrument used by doctors to listen to sounds in the body.

BLOCK	DATA AND ANSWERS	DESCRIPTIONS AND QUESTIONS
6-112	striking listening to the sounds of the body striking body with fingers and listening to the sounds of the body with a stethoscope	Percussion is _____. Ausculation is _____ ____ _____ _____ ____ _____ _____. P & A is _____ _____ _____ _____ _____ _____ ____ _____ _____ ____ _____ _____ __ _____.
6-113	an instrument used by doctors to listen to sounds of the body chest an instrument used to examine	A stethoscope is _____ _____ _____ ____ _____ ____ _____ ____ _____ ____ _____ _____. "steth/o" is a combining form meaning _____. "scope" is a root word meaning _____ _____ _____ ____ _____.
6-114	perfusion (per-fu-zhun)	Perfusion is the passage of a fluid through the blood vessels of a specific organ to supply nutrients and oxygen.
6-115	the passage of a fluid through the blood vessels of a specific organ to supply nutrients and oxygen	Perfusion is _____ _____ _____ __ _____ _____ _____ _____ _____ ____ __ _____ _____ ____ _____ _____ _____ _____.
6-116	rales (rahlz), rhonchi (rong-ki) rales rhonchi	Rales and rhonchi refer to abnormal respiratory sounds heard on auscultation (via a stethoscope), indicating some pathologic condition. Name two medical terms for the abnormal respiratory sound heard by a doctor during the chest examination: 1. _____ 2. _____

BLOCK	DATA AND ANSWERS	DESCRIPTIONS AND QUESTIONS
6-117	respirator (res-pi-<u>ra</u>-tor), ventilator (ven-ti-<u>la</u>-tor)	A respirator or ventilator is a device used to give artificial respiration or to improve breathing.
6-118	a device used to give oxygen or to improve breathing respirator, ventilator	A ventilator or respirator is ___ _____ _____ _____ _____ _____ ____ ____ _____ _____. A person who has difficulty breathing may need medical assistance. The machine used to improve breathing is a _____ or _____.
6-119	sputum (<u>spu</u>-tum)	Sputum is matter expelled from the lungs through the respiratory tract (e.g., bronchioles, bronchi, trachea) to the mouth.
6-120	matter expelled from the lungs through the respiratory tract (e.g., bronchioles, bronchi, trachea) to the mouth	Sputum is _matter_ _expelled_ _from_ _the_ _lungs_ _through_ _the_ _respiratory_ _tract_ _(e.g.,)_ _bronchioles_ _____ _____ _to_ _the_ _mouth_.
6-121	 respiratory	You have now completed study of the body parts and structures that make possible the exchange of oxygen and carbon dioxide in the lungs, and some of the conditions that can affect breathing. Collectively, these body parts and structures make up the _respiratory_ system.

BOX 6.2	
Abbreviations	
ABG(s)	arterial blood gas(es)
ARF	acute respiratory failure
CXR	chest x-ray
LLL	left lobe of the lung
Pao$_2$	partial pressure of oxygen dissolved in the blood
PFT(s)	pulmonary function test(s)
R	respiration
RDS	respiratory distress signal
RUL	right upper lobe of the lung
TB	tuberculosis
TPR	temperature, pulse, and respiration

Progress Check

A. Multiple Choice

1. A word root meaning a fungal disease is:
   a. spir
   b. myc
   c. mast
   d. tracheal

2. A word root meaning chest is:
   a. steth
   b. ox
   c. pharyn
   d. his

3. A word root meaning expansion is:
   a. nas
   b. gastr
   c. ectasis
   d. lob

4. A word root meaning incomplete or imperfect is:
   a. meter
   b. cyan
   c. atel
   d. bronchi

5. A combining form meaning straight is:
   a. pneum/o
   b. tubercul/o
   c. orch/o
   d. orth/o

6. A combining form meaning membrane lining the lung is:
   a. pneumon/o
   b. pleur/o
   c. mes/o
   d. sinus

7. A combining form meaning chest is:
   a. meningi/o
   b. thorac/o
   c. cyan/o
   d. pathy/o

8. A combining form meaning dust is:
   a. oste/o
   b. coni/o
   c. dist/o
   d. ox/o

9. A prefix meaning slow is:
   a. brady-
   b. primi-
   c. quad-
   d. histo-

10. A prefix meaning rapid is:
    a. retro-
    b. tans-
    c. tachy-
    d. ultra-

11. A suffix meaning to create a mouth or opening is:
    a. -pathy
    b. -stomy
    c. -pnea
    d. -osis

12. A suffix meaning condition or process is:

    a. -ia

    b. -ical

    c. -gen

    d. -al

13. A suffix meaning spitting is:

    a. -itis

    b. -ptysis

    c. -rrhagia

    d. -spasm

14. A suffix meaning excision or removal is:

    a. -rrhea

    b. -globin

    c. -emia

    d. -ectomy

B. Building Medical Terms

Use the following word components to build medical terms matching the definitions given.

-al	myc	rhin
bronch	myc/o	rhin/o
bronch/o	nas	spasm
-centesis	nas/o	-spasm
coccidioid	orth	sten
coccidioid/o	orth/o	sten/o
end/o	-osis	thorac
endo-	pharyng	thorac/o
gastr	pharyng/o	-tomy
gastr/o	pleur	trache
-ic	pleur/o	trache/o
-itis	-pnea	

1. condition of the narrowed nasal passage or cavity

2. inflammation of the nose and pharynx

3. inflammation of the membrane lining the lung and related organs

4. surgical puncture of the chest for removal of fluid

5. incision into the trachea and the larynx

6. respiratory infection caused by inhalation of a fungus spore

7. condition of difficult breathing except in the upright position

8. pertaining to the nose and stomach, usually referring to the passage from nose to stomach

9. pertaining to the inside of the windpipe

10. contraction of the muscles of the bronchi of the lung

C.   Definitions and Word Components

	TERM	DEFINITION	PREFIX	WORD ROOT	VOWEL	WORD ROOT	VOWEL	SUFFIX
1.	tracheopharyngotomy							
2.	pneumoconiosis							
3.	histoplasmosis							
4.	nasopharyngeal							
5.	hemoptysis							
6.	atelectasis							
7.	sinusitis							
8.	pertussis							
9.	tuberculosis							
10.	bronchiectasis							

D. Abbreviations

	ABBREVIATION	MEANING
1.	ABG(s)	
2.	ARF	
3.	CXR	
4.	LLL	
5.	Pao_2	
6.	PFT(s)	
7.	R	
8.	RDS	
9.	RUL	
10.	TB	
11.	TPR	

The Cardiovascular System

BLOCK	DATA AND ANSWERS	DESCRIPTIONS AND QUESTIONS
7-1		The cardiovascular system includes the heart and blood vessels, which are the arteries, veins, and capillaries. The function of the heart is to pump blood. This action maintains the circulation of oxygen and all other nutrients to every body cell, via the blood vessels, and returns carbon dioxide and wastes from the cells. Thus, the four parts of the cardiovascular system are: heart, arteries, veins, and capillaries.
		The heart has four chambers. The two collecting chambers are the right and left atria. The two pumping chambers are the right and left ventricles (some times called "little belly"). The apex is the pointed end (bottom) of the heart. The heart has a system of valves that keep the blood from flowing back.
		Table 7.1 lists the medical word components covered in this chapter.
		See **Figures 7.1 through 7.5**. Refer to these figures frequently as you progress with each block.

TABLE 7.1   Word Components in this Chapter

WORD ROOTS	COMBINING FORMS	PREFIXES
adeno	aden/o	a-
agranul	agranul/o	bi-
ang	angi/o	endo-
angi	arter/o	hyper-
aort	arteriol/o	hypo-
apex	ather/o	inter-
arter	bas/o	intra-
arteriol	blast/o	mano-
ather	card/o	mono-
atri	cardi/o	peri-
capill	embol/o	poly-
card	eosin/o	supra-
cardi	erythr/o	tri-
cuspid	erythrocyt/o	SUFFIXES
cyte	fibrin/o	-cytes
edema	granul/o	-ectomy
erythrocyte	gem/o	-edema
embol	hemat/o	-gen
eosin	leuk/o	-genic
gem	lymph/o	-graph
genesis	lymphaden/o	-graphy
globin	lymphoid/o	-iasis
granu	man/o	-ic
lith	my/o	-itis
manometer	neutr/o	-lysis
meter	phleb/o	-megaly
mono	sider/o	-meter
phil	sphygm/o	-oid
phleb	thromb/o	-oma
saphenous	thrombocyt/o	-osis
scler	ven/o	-tomy
sepsis	ventricul/o	-pathy
tension		-penia
thrombocyt		-poiesis
valves		-rrhaphy
varix		-sepsis
ventricul		-stasis
ven		-stenosis

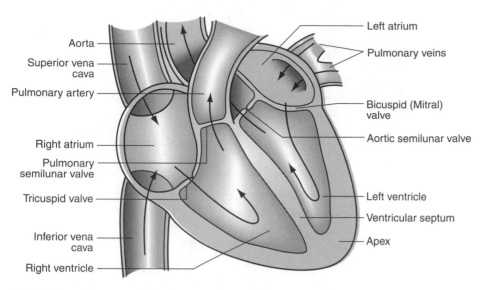

FIGURE 7.1 Diagram of the heart (arrows indicate the direction of blood flow)

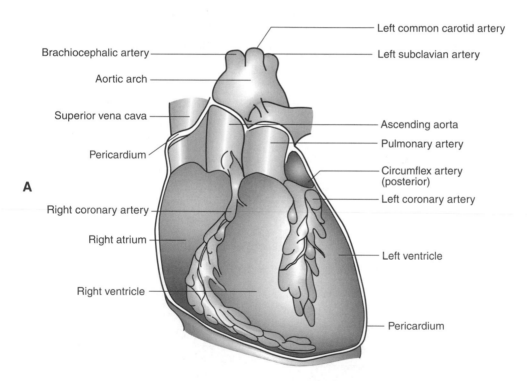

FIGURE 7.2 Anterior (A) and posterior (B) structures of the heart

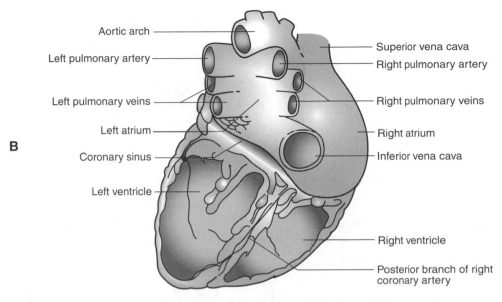

B

Aortic arch

Left pulmonary artery

Left pulmonary veins

Left atrium

Coronary sinus

Left ventricle

Superior vena cava

Right pulmonary artery

Right pulmonary veins

Right atrium

Inferior vena cava

Right ventricle

Posterior branch of right coronary artery

FIGURE 7.2 Anterior (A) and posterior (B) structures of the heart (continued)

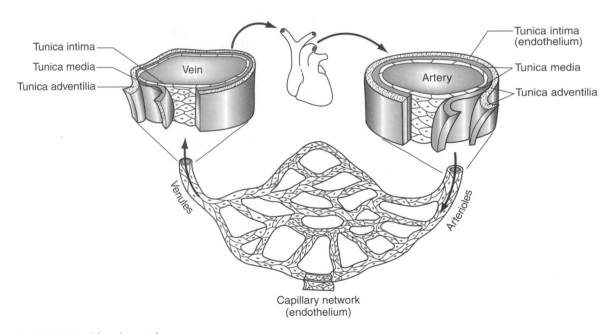

Tunica intima

Tunica media

Tunica adventilia

Vein

Artery

Tunica intima (endothelium)

Tunica media

Tunica adventilia

Venules

Arterioles

Capillary network (endothelium)

FIGURE 7.3 Blood vessels

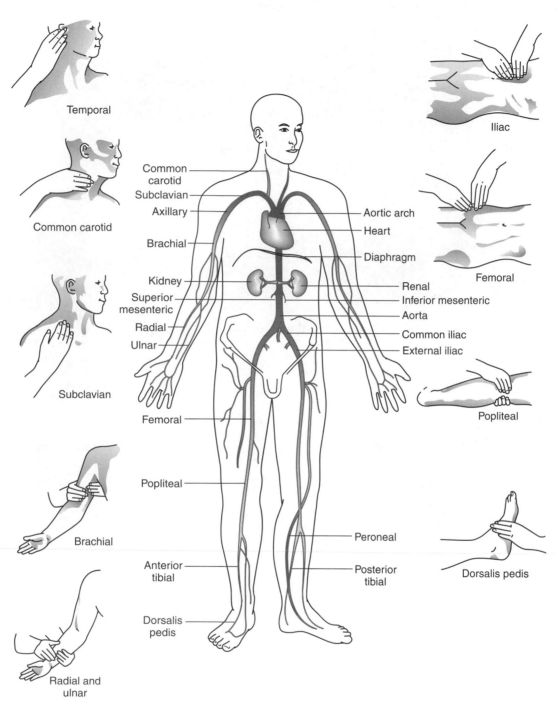

FIGURE 7.4 Major arteries of the body

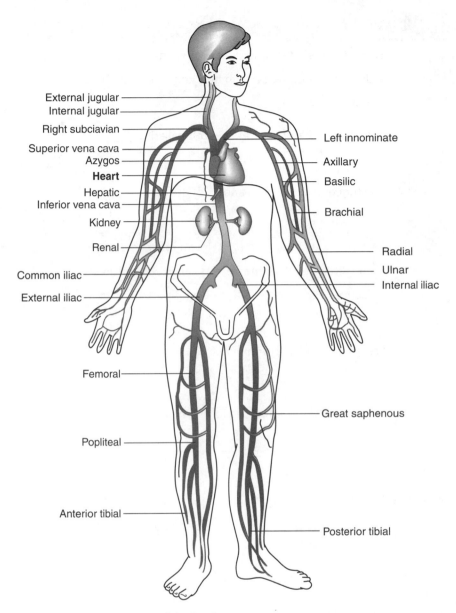

External jugular
Internal jugular
Right subciavian
Superior vena cava
Azygos
Heart
Hepatic
Inferior vena cava
Kidney
Renal
Common iliac
External iliac
Femoral
Popliteal
Anterior tibial

Left innominate
Axillary
Basilic
Brachial
Radial
Ulnar
Internal iliac
Great saphenous
Posterior tibial

FIGURE 7.5 Major veins of the body

BLOCK	DATA AND ANSWERS	DESCRIPTIONS AND QUESTIONS
7-2	atrium (a̲-tre-um) atria (a̲-tre-ah) an atrium collect blood	Each of the two (left and right) upper chambers of the heart is called an atrium. These chambers collect blood. The plural of atrium is atria. Each upper chamber of the heart is called _____ _____. The function of these chambers of the heart is to _____ _____.
7-3	ventricle (ven̲-trih-kul)	Each of the two (left and right) lower chambers (sometimes called "little belly") of the heart is called a ventricle. The adjective form is ventricular, meaning pertaining to the ventricle. "ventricul/o" is the combining form. -ar means pertaining to.
7-4	apex (a-pe̲ks) the pointed end (of the heart)	The apex is the pointed end (of the heart). The apex is _____ _____ _____ _____ _____ _____.
7-5	heart, arteries, veins capillaries pump blood collect blood	The four parts of the cardiovascular system are the _____, _____, _____, and _____. The function of the heart is to _____ _____. The function of the chambers of the heart is to _____ _____. The circulation of blood through the vessels carries oxygen and other nutrients to the cells and receives carbon dioxide and wastes from the cells.

BLOCK	DATA AND ANSWERS	DESCRIPTIONS AND QUESTIONS
7-6	the apex	The pointed end of the heart is called _____ _____.
	arteries, veins capillaries	The blood vessels are called _____, _____, and _____.
	valves	The _____ prevent backflow of blood in each heart chamber.
7-7	oxygen, other nutrients carbon dioxide wastes	The circulation of blood through the vessels carries _____ and _____ _____ to the cells and receives _____ _____ and _____ from the cells.
7-8	periatrial (peh-re-a-tre-al)	Periatrial means around the atria. *peri-* is a prefix meaning around. "atrial" is a word root meaning the upper chambers of the heart.
7-9	Periatrial	*peri-* is a prefix meaning around. _____ means around the atria.
7-10	interatrial (in-ter-a-tre-al)	Interatrial means between the atria. *inter-* is a prefix meaning between. "atrial" is the plural word root for the two chambers of the heart (atrium, singular). (Some consider the word a medical adjective, and some consider it a suffix. Both terms can be used to describe the two atria.)
7-11	between the atria prefix, between word root, adjective suffix, two chambers of the heart	Interatrial means _____ _____ _____. *inter-* is a _____ meaning _____. "atrial" is a _____ _____, an _____, or a _____ meaning _____ _____ _____ _____ _____.

BLOCK	DATA AND ANSWERS	DESCRIPTIONS AND QUESTIONS
7-12	valve (valv)	Another term associated with the heart is valve.
		A valve is a membrane in a passage that prevents backflow.
		The heart has many such valves.
	a membrane in a passage to prevent backflow	A valve is ___ _____ ____ __ _____ ____ _____ _____.
7-13	supravalvular (soo'-prah-val-<u>vu</u>-lar)	Supravalvular means above a valve.
		Intervalvular means between the valves.
	intervalvular (in'-ter-val-<u>vu</u>-lar)	The adjective form of valve is valvular.
		supra- is a prefix meaning above.
		inter- is a prefix meaning between.
7-14	*inter-*	_____ is a prefix meaning between.
	supra-	_____ is a prefix meaning above.
	Supravalvular	_____ means above a valve.
	Intervalvular	_____ means between valves.
7-15	tricuspid (tri-<u>kus</u>-pid)	A tricuspid valve is situated between the right atrium and the right ventricle of the heart.
		tri- is a prefix meaning three.
		"cuspid" is a root word meaning having points or cusps.
7-16	tricuspid	A _____ valve is located between the right atrium and the right ventricle of the heart.
7-17	bicuspid (bi-<u>kus</u>-pid)	A bicuspid valve is situated between the left atrium and the left ventricle of the heart.
		bi- is a prefix meaning two.
		"cuspid" is a root word meaning having points or cusps.

BLOCK	DATA AND ANSWERS	DESCRIPTIONS AND QUESTIONS
7-18	mitral (mi-<u>tral</u>)	A bicuspid valve is sometimes called a mitral valve because it is shaped like a miter.
		"mitral" is a word root referring to an object shaped like a miter.
7-19	Bicuspid	_____ means having two points or cusps.
	the valve situated between the left atrium and the left ventricle of the heart	A bicuspid valve is _____ _____ _____ _____ _____ _____ _____ _____ _____ _____ _____ ____ _____ _____.
	mitral	A bicuspid valve is sometimes called a _____ valve
	miter	because it is shaped like a _____.
7-20		Now that we have studied some medical terms related to the parts of the heart, we will concentrate on some terms associated with diseases of the heart.
		"cardi" is a word root meaning heart.
		"cardi/o" is the combining form.
		"card/i" is another combining form for heart, though its usage is less common.
		peri- is a prefix meaning around.
		-tomy is a suffix meaning incision.
		-ectomy is a suffix meaning excision.

BOX 7.1
Allied Health Professions

Cardiovascular Technologists and Technicians, Nuclear Medicine Technologists, Surgical Technologists, Emergency Medical Technicians, and Paramedics

Cardiovascular technologists and technicians assist physicians in diagnosing and treating cardiac (heart) and peripheral vascular (blood vessel) ailments. They schedule appointments, perform ultrasound or cardiovascular procedures, review doctors' interpretations and patient files, and monitor patients' heart rates. They also operate and maintain testing equipment, explain test procedures, and compare test results to a standard to identify problems. Other day-to-day activities vary significantly between specialties.

Surgical technologists, also called scrubs and surgical or operating room technicians, assist in surgical operations under the supervision of surgeons, registered nurses, or other surgical personnel. Surgical technologists are members of operating room teams, which most commonly include surgeons, anesthesiologists, and circulating nurses.

Before an operation, *surgical technologists* help prepare the operating room by setting up surgical instruments and equipment, sterile drapes, and sterile solutions. They assemble both sterile and nonsterile equipment, as well as check and adjust it to ensure it is working properly. Technologists also get patients ready for surgery by washing, shaving, and disinfecting incision sites. They transport patients to the operating room, help position them on the operating table, and cover them with sterile surgical drapes. Technologists also observe patients' vital signs, check charts, and help the surgical team put on sterile gowns and gloves.

Nuclear medicine technologists operate cameras that detect and map the radioactive drug in a patient's body to create diagnostic images. After explaining test procedures to patients, technologists prepare a dosage of the radiopharmaceutical and administer it by mouth, injection, inhalation, or other means. They position patients and start a gamma scintillation camera, or "scanner," which creates images of the distribution of a radiopharmaceutical as it localizes in, and emits signals from, the patient's body. The images are produced on a computer screen or on film for a physician to interpret.

Paramedics, or *emergency medical technicians (EMTs)*, have a career that is often very dramatic, calling for immediate, calm application of the EMT's skills amid sometimes dangerous conditions. The September 11, 2001, attack on the World Trade Center was the most dramatic and deadly situation that paramedics, along with teams of firefighters and police, have ever faced, and they lived up to their potential and training with great heroism. If you watched the terrible events unfolding at that scene, you saw many of them in action as their ambulances drove through dangerous smoke, fire, and rubble to help rescue and transport the critically injured to hospitals. Their bravery in the face of peril speaks well of the crucial role played by paramedics in times of crisis as well as in everyday life.

The following are some resources for further information:

- Alliance of Cardiovascular Professionals, www.acp-online.org

- American Society of Radiologic Technologists, www.asrt.org

- Society of Nuclear Medicine Technologists, www.snm.org

For a list of accredited programs in nuclear medicine technology, contact:

- Joint Review Committee on Educational Programs in Nuclear Medicine Technology, www.jrcnmt.org

- National Association of Emergency Medical Technicians, www.naemt.org

Source: P.S. Stanfield, N. Cross, Y.H. Hui, eds. *Introduction to the Health Professions*, 5th ed (Sudbury, MA: Jones & Bartlett, 2009).

BLOCK	DATA AND ANSWERS	DESCRIPTIONS AND QUESTIONS
7-21	"cardi," root word	_____ is a _____ _____ meaning heart.
	peri-, prefix	_____ is a _____ meaning around.
	-tomy, suffix	_____ is a _____ meaning incision.
	-ectomy, suffix	_____ is a _____ meaning excision.
7-22	membranes (mem-branz)	The layers of soft tissue that line an organ are called membranes.
		peri- is a prefix meaning around.
		endo- is a prefix meaning within.
		"cardium" is a root word meaning the heart.
7-23	pericardium (per´-ih-kar-de-um)	Build medical terms (with pronunciations) meaning:
		the membrane that lines the outside of the heart:
		_____
		_____
	endocardium (en´-do-kar-de-um)	the membrane that lines the inside of the heart:
		_____
		_____
7-24	myocardium (mi´-o-kar-de-um)	Myocardium is the middle, thickest layer of muscle of the heart wall.
		"my/o" is a combining form meaning muscle.
		"cardium" is a word root meaning heart.
		"cardi" also is a word root meaning heart.
7-25	myocardium	Heart muscle is called _____.
	"my/o"	_____ is a combining form meaning muscle.
	"cardium"	The two word roots for heart are _____ and
	"cardi"	_____.

BLOCK	DATA AND ANSWERS	DESCRIPTIONS AND QUESTIONS
7-26	cardiogenic (kar'-de-o-<u>jen</u>-ik)	Cardiogenic means originating in or from the heart. "cardi/o" is a combining form meaning heart. Genesis is a medical word meaning beginning, origin, or produce. "gen" is the word root. "gen/o" is the combining form. -*ic* is a suffix meaning pertaining to.
7-27	"cardi/o," combining form "gen/o," combining form -*ic*, suffix Cardiogenic	_____ is a _____ _____ meaning heart. _____ is a _____ _____ meaning beginning, origin, or produce. _____ is a _____ meaning pertaining to. _____ means originating in or from the heart.
7-28	pericarditis (per'-ih-<u>kar</u>-di-tis)	The pericardium is a fibrous sac enclosing the heart and the great vessel. *peri-* is a prefix meaning around or about. -*itis* is a suffix meaning inflammation. Build a medical term meaning the inflammation of the fibrous sac around the heart: _____ _____
7-29	pericardectomy (per-i-kar-<u>dek</u>-to-me)	A pericardectomy is removal of the membrane around the heart. The pericardium is the membrane around the heart. *peri-* is a prefix meaning around. -*ectomy* is a suffix meaning to remove (excise).

BLOCK	DATA AND ANSWERS	DESCRIPTIONS AND QUESTIONS
7-30	*peri-*, prefix	_____ is a _____ meaning around.
	pericardium	The _____ is the membrane around the heart.
	to remove (excise)	*-ectomy* is a suffix meaning _____ _____ _____.
	Pericardectomy	_____ is removal of the membrane around the heart.
7-31		"cardi/o" is a combining form meaning heart.
		-megaly is a suffix meaning enlarged.
		Build a medical term meaning enlarged heart:
	cardiomegaly (kar′-de-o-<u>meg</u>-ah-le)	_____
7-32	cardiolysis (car-de-oh-<u>lih</u>-sis)	Cardiolysis is the freeing of pericardial adhesions.
		"cardi/o" is a combining form meaning heart.
		-lysis is a suffix meaning to separate.
7-33	Cardiolysis	_____ is freeing the pericardium from adhesions.
7-34	cardiomyopathy (car′-di-o-mi-<u>op</u>-path-e)	Cardiomyopathy refers to any disease of the heart muscle.
		"cardi/o" is a combining form meaning the heart
		"my/o" is a combining form meaning muscle.
		-pathy is a suffix meaning disease.
7-35	*-pathy*, suffix	_____ is a _____ meaning disease.
	"my/o," combining form	_____ is a _____ _____ meaning muscle.
	Cardiomyopathy	_____ is any disease of the heart muscle.

BLOCK	DATA AND ANSWERS	DESCRIPTIONS AND QUESTIONS
7-36	intracardiac (in-trah-kar-de-ak)	Intracardiac means within or inside the heart. Cardiac is an adjective meaning pertaining to the heart. *intra-* is a prefix meaning within or inside.
7-37	within or inside the heart	Intracardiac is _____ _____ _____ _____ _____.
7-38	endocarditis (en'-do-kar-di-tis)	Endocarditis is inflammation of the lining of the heart. *endo-* is a prefix meaning within. "cardi/o" is another combining form for heart. *-itis* is a suffix meaning inflammation.
7-39	prefix, within combining form heart *-itis*, suffix Endocarditis	*endo-* is a _____ meaning _____. "card/o" is a _____ _____ meaning _____. _____ is a _____ meaning inflammation. _____ is an inflammation of the lining of the heart.
7-40	myocarditis (mi'-o-kar-di-tis)	Myocarditis is inflammation of the heart muscle. "my/o" is a combining form meaning muscles. "cardi/o" is another combining form meaning the heart. *-itis* is a suffix meaning inflammation.
7-41	inflammation of the heart muscle	Myocarditis is _____ _____ _____ _____ _____.
7-42	cardiotomy (kar-de-ot-o-me)	Recall that the combining form for heart is "cardi/o." *-tomy* is a suffix meaning to open into (incise). Build a medical term meaning incision of the heart: _____ _____

BLOCK	DATA AND ANSWERS	DESCRIPTIONS AND QUESTIONS
7-43		*-rrhaphy* is a suffix meaning to suture.
	suture of the heart	Cardiorrhaphy is _____ _____ _____ _____.
7-44	combining form heart	"cardi/o" is a _____ _____ meaning _____.
	suffix, suture	*-rrhaphy* is a _____ meaning _____.
7-45	pericardectomy (per-i-kar-<u>dek</u>-to-me)	Pericardectomy is the removal of the membrane around the heart.
		peri- is a prefix meaning around.
		The pericardium is the membrane around the heart.
		-ectomy is a suffix meaning excision or removal.
		-tomy is a suffix meaning incision or cut into.
7-46	Pericardectomy	_____ is the removal of the membrane around the heart.
	Pericardium	_____ is the membrane around the heart.
	-ectomy	_____ is a suffix meaning excision.
	-tomy	_____ is a suffix meaning incision or cut into.
7-47	thrombectomy (throm-<u>bek</u>-to-me)	Thrombectomy is removal (excision) of a blood clot.
		"thromb/o" is a combining form meaning blood clot.
		-ectomy is a suffix meaning removal (excision).
7-48	Thrombectomy	_____ is removal (excision) of a blood clot.
	"thromb/o"	_____ is a combining form meaning blood clot.
	-ectomy	_____ is a suffix for removal (excision).

BLOCK	DATA AND ANSWERS	DESCRIPTIONS AND QUESTIONS
7-49		The next section covers the medical terms for arteries and associated diseases.
7-50	artery (<u>ar</u>-ter-e) a vessel through which oxygenated blood flows away from the heart	An artery is a vessel through which oxygenated blood flows away from the heart. It has two combining forms: "arter/o" and "arteri/o." Both are used in some medical terminology books. Some use only one of the two. This book uses both. An artery is ___ _____ _____ _____ _____ _____ _____ _____ _____ _____ _____.
7-51	aorta (a-<u>or</u>-tah) the largest artery in the body, the left ventricle of the heart	The aorta is the largest artery in the body. It originates from the left ventricle of the heart. The aorta is _____ _____ _____ ____ _____ _____. It originates from _____ _____ _____ _____ _____ _____.
7-52	arteriole (<u>ar</u>-te-re-ol) arteriole	An arteriole is a small artery. In the body an artery leads into an arteriole. The combining form is "arteriol/o." An _____ is a small artery.
7-53	endarteritis (end'-ar-ter-i-tis)	Endarteritis is inflammation of the inner lining of a(n) artery. "end/o" is a combining form meaning within. "arter/o" is a combining form meaning artery. -itis is a suffix meaning inflammation.
7-54	inflammation of the inner lining of an artery	Endarteritis is _____ _____ _____ _____ _____ _____ _____ _____.

BLOCK	DATA AND ANSWERS	DESCRIPTIONS AND QUESTIONS
7-55	arteriosclerosis (ar-te′-re-o-skleh-ro-sis)	Arteriosclerosis is hardening of an artery. "arteri/o" is a combining form meaning artery. "scler" is a root word meaning hardening. -osis is a suffix meaning condition.
7-56	Arteriosclerosis "arteri/o" "scler" -osis	_____ is hardening of an artery. _____ is a combining form meaning artery. _____ is a root word meaning hardening. _____ is a suffix meaning condition.
7-57	aortostenosis (a-or′-to-steh-no-sis)	Aortostenosis is narrowing of the aorta. The aorta is the largest artery in the body. "aort/o" is the combining form. -stenosis is a suffix meaning narrowing.
7-58	narrowing of the aorta combining form aorta suffix, narrowing	Aortostenosis is _____ _____ _____ _____. "aort/o" is a _____ _____ meaning _____. -stenosis is a _____ meaning _____.
7-59	arteriolitis (ar-ter′-i-o-li-tis)	"arteriol/o" is a combining form meaning little artery (arteriole). -itis is a suffix meaning inflammation. Build a medical term meaning inflammation of an arteriole: _____ _____

BLOCK	DATA AND ANSWERS	DESCRIPTIONS AND QUESTIONS
7-60	atherosclerosis (ath-er-o-skleh-<u>ro</u>-sis)	Atherosclerosis is a condition of the arteries characterized by the buildup of fatty substances on the lumen of a vessel, causing it to become hardened. "ather/o" is a combining form meaning fatty deposit (fatty degeneration). "scler" is a root word meaning hardening. -osis is a suffix meaning condition of. Lumen is the channel or cavity inside a vessel.
7-61	combining form fatty deposit (fatty degeneration) root word hardening suffix, condition of the channel or cavity inside a vessel Atherosclerosis	"ather/o" is a _____ _____ meaning _____ _____ _____ _____. "scler" is a _____ _____ meaning _____. -osis is a _____ meaning _____ _____. Lumen is _____ _____ _____ _____ _____ __ _____. _____ is a condition of the arteries characterized by the buildup of fatty substances on the lumen of a vessel, causing it to become hardened.
7-62	endarterectomy (en-dar'-te-<u>rek</u>-to-me)	Endarterectomy is the removal of the lining of an artery. "end/o" is a combining form meaning within. "arter/o" is a combining form meaning artery. -ectomy is a suffix meaning excision.

BLOCK	DATA AND ANSWERS	DESCRIPTIONS AND QUESTIONS
7-63	removal of the lining of an artery	Endarterectomy is _____ _____ _____ _____ _____ _____ _____.
	combining form within	"end/o" is a _____ _____ meaning _____.
	combining form artery	"arter/o" is a _____ _____ meaning _____.
	suffix, excision	-*ectomy* is a _____ meaning _____.
7-64	polyarteritis (pol-e-<u>ar</u>-ter-i'-tis)	Polyarteritis is a disease involving inflammation of many arteries.
		poly- is a prefix meaning many.
		"arter/o" is a combining form meaning artery.
		-*itis* is a suffix meaning inflammation.
7-65	prefix, many	*poly-* is a _____ meaning _____.
	combining form artery	"arter/o" is a _____ _____ meaning _____.
	suffix inflammation	-*itis* is a _____ meaning _____.
7-66	coronary (<u>kor</u>-o-ner'-e)	Coronary arteries originate at the base of the aorta and supply the heart muscle with blood.
	coronary	The arteries that stem from the base of the aorta and supply blood to the heart muscle are called _____ arteries.
7-67	occlusion (<u>o</u>-kloo-zhun)	Occlusion refers to an obstruction or a closing off—e.g., occlusion of coronary arteries. This can cause heart attack.
	occluded	If the arteries that supply oxygen to the heart muscles are blocked or _____, the person can have a heart attack.

BLOCK	DATA AND ANSWERS	DESCRIPTIONS AND QUESTIONS
7-68	veins (vanz)	The next section covers medical terms pertaining to the veins. Veins are blood vessels through which blood flows toward the heart, carrying little oxygen.
7-69	blood vessels through which blood flows toward the heart carrying little oxygen	Veins are _____ _____ _____ _____ _____ _____ _____ _____ _____, _____ _____ _____
7-70	venule (ven-ul) venule	A venule is a small vein. In the body a venule leads into a vein. The name for a small vein is _____.
7-71	vena cava (ve-na ka-vah)	The vena cava is the largest vein in the body. The superior vena cava drains blood from the head, neck, upper limbs, and thorax. The inferior vena cava drains blood from the lower limbs, pelvic, and abdominal area. Superior indicates a position above (the heart). Inferior indicates a position below (the heart).
7-72	the vena cava inferior vena cava to drain blood from the neck upper limbs, and thorax	The largest vein in the body is called _____ _____ _____. When blood is drained from regions below the heart, the vein is called _____ _____ _____. The function of the superior vena cava is _____ _____ _____ _____ _____ _____, _____ _____, _____ _____.

BLOCK	DATA AND ANSWERS	DESCRIPTIONS AND QUESTIONS
7-73	common carotid (<u>kah</u>-rot-id)	The common carotid is the large artery that supplies blood to the head.
	jugular (<u>jug</u>-u-lar)	The jugular is the large vein that drains blood from the head.
	to drain blood from the head	The function of the jugular vein is _____ _____ _____ _____ _____ _____.
	to supply blood to the head	The function of the common carotid is _____ _____ _____ _____ _____ _____.
7-74	saphenous (sah-<u>fe</u>-nus)	The saphenous is the longest vein in the body, which runs the length of the leg.
	the longest vein in the body, which runs the length of the leg	Define saphenous: _____ _____ _____ ____ _____ _____, _____ _____ _____ _____ _____ _____ _____
7-75		"phleb/o" and "ven/o" are both combining forms meaning vein.
		-rrhaphy is a suffix meaning suture.
		Build two medical terms meaning suturing of a vein:
	phleborrhaphy (fle-<u>bor</u>-ah-fe)	1. _____ _____
	venorrhaphy (ve-nor-rah-fe)	2. _____ _____
7-76	phlebotomy (fle-<u>bot</u>-o-me)	Phlebotomy means opening of a vein.
		"phleb/o" is the combining form.
		-tomy is a suffix meaning opening (incision).

BLOCK	DATA AND ANSWERS	DESCRIPTIONS AND QUESTIONS
7-77	opening of a vein combining form vein suffix, opening (incision)	Phlebotomy is _____ _____ __ _____. "phleb/o" is a _____ _____ meaning _____. -*tomy* is a _____ meaning _____ _____.
7-78	venotomy (ve-<u>not</u>-om-e)	Recall that "ven/o" is another combining form meaning vein. Use this word part to build a medical word meaning opening of a vein: _____ _____
7-79	combining form vein suffix, opening (incision)	"phleb/o" (ven/o) is a _____ _____ meaning _____. -*tomy* is a _____ meaning _____ _____.
7-80	phlebotomist (fleh-<u>bot</u>-o-mist) a person who drains blood from a vein	A phlebotomist is a person who drains blood from a vein. A phlebotomist is ___ _____ _____ _____ _____ _____ __ _____.
7-81	phlebolithiasis (fleh-bo-li-thia-sis')	Phlebolithiasis is the development of calculi (stones) in a vein. "phleb/o" is a combining form meaning vein. "lith" is a word root meaning stone (calculi). -*iasis* is a suffix meaning condition.
7-82	Phlebolithiasis "phleb/o" lith -*iasis*	_____ is the development of calculi (stones) in a vein. _____ is a combining form meaning vein. _____ is a word root meaning stone. _____ is a suffix meaning condition.

BLOCK	DATA AND ANSWERS	DESCRIPTIONS AND QUESTIONS
7-83	venograph (ve-<u>no</u>-graf)	Recall that "ven/o" is a combining form meaning vein. *-graph* is a suffix meaning record. A medical term meaning to make a record (e.g., x-ray) for a vein is _____ _____.
7-84		"thrombus" is a root word meaning blood clot. "vein" is a root word meaning vein. "ven/o" and "phleb/o" are both combining forms meaning vein. *-rrhaphy* is a suffix meaning suture. *-graph* is a suffix meaning record.
7-85	root word "phleb/o" "ven/o" "thrombus" *-rrhaphy* *-graph*	"vein" is a _____ _____. Two combining forms meaning vein are _____ and _____. _____ is a root word meaning blood clot. _____ is a suffix meaning suture. _____ is a suffix meaning record.
7-86	phlebolysis (fle-bok-<u>li</u>-sis)	Phlebolysis is washing or irrigation of a vein by injecting fluid. "phleb/o" is a combining form meaning vein. *-lysis* is a suffix meaning washing or irrigation.
7-87	washing or irrigation of the vein by injecting fluid combining form vein suffix, washing irrigation	Phlebolysis is _____ _____ _____ ____ _____ _____ ____ _____ _____. "phleb/o" is a _____ _____ meaning _____. *-lysis* is a _____ meaning _____ or _____.

BLOCK	DATA AND ANSWERS	DESCRIPTIONS AND QUESTIONS
7-88	varicose (var-ih-kus) vein, varix (var-ics)	A varicose vein is called a varix.
	a varicose vein	A varix is ___ _____ _____.
7-89		-oid is a suffix meaning resembling.
	varicoid (var-ih-koyd)	Varicoid means resembling a varix (varicose vein).
	resembling a varix	Varicoid means _____ __ _____.
7-90	capillary (kap-il-ler-e)	You have studied the heart, arteries, and veins. The next structure is the capillary. A capillary is a minute, hairlike blood vessel. It forms the meeting ground between arterioles and venules. It permits arteries to meet with veins to complete the flow of blood in the body.
	a minute, hairlike vessel connecting arterioles and venules	A capillary is ___ _____, _____ _____ _____ _____ _____ _____.
7-91		Materials are exchanged between the blood and the tissues through microscopic vessels called capillaries.
	capillaries (kap-il-ler-ez)	Vessels that make the exchange are called _____ _____.
7-92	circulation (ser-ku-la-shun)	Blood circulation is made possible by a combined effort of the heart, the arteries, the veins, the capillaries, and other structures within the body.
		Circulation refers to the circuitous movement of blood, forming a complete circle of heart, blood vessels, and heart.
	systemic (sis-tem-ik)	Systemic means pertaining to a system. A systemic circulation pertains to movement of blood through the body as a whole.

BLOCK	DATA AND ANSWERS	DESCRIPTIONS AND QUESTIONS
7-93	the circuitous movement of blood forming a complete circle of heart, blood vessels and heart	Circulation is _____ _____ _____ ____ _____, _____ __ _____ _____ ____ _____, _____ _____, _____ _____.
7-94	systemic	The circulation of blood through the entire body is called _____ circulation.
7-95	pulmonary (<u>pul</u>-mo-ner'-e)	Pulmonary is a medical term referring to the lungs. Pulmonary circulation refers to the movement of blood through the lungs and the arteries of the lungs.
	portal (<u>por</u>-tal)	Portal refers to an entrance to an organ. Portal circulation is the entry of blood from the digestive tract through the portal vein to the liver.
7-96	the movement of blood through the lungs and the arteries of the lungs	Pulmonary circulation is _____ _____ ____ _____ _____ _____ _____ _____ _____ _____ _____ _____ _____.
	portal	The circulation of blood from the digestive tract to the liver is known as _____ circulation.
7-97		The next few blocks are devoted to medical terms associated with blood components and blood pressure.
7-98	plasma (plas-<u>mah</u>)	Plasma is the amber-colored fluid portion of the blood or lymph without the blood cells. (When whole blood is undisturbed in a tube, clotting cells settle in the bottom with the plasma is on top.)
	serum (<u>se</u>-rum)	Serum is the clear portion of the blood separated from solid elements.

BLOCK	DATA AND ANSWERS	DESCRIPTIONS AND QUESTIONS
7-99	the amber-colored fluid portion of the blood or lymph, without the blood cells	Plasma is _____ _____ _____ _____ _____ _____ _____ _____ _____, _____ _____ _____ _____.
	the clear portion of the blood separated from solid elements	Serum is _____ _____ _____ _____ _____ _____ _____ _____ _____ _____.
7-100	hemoglobin (he-mo-<u>glo</u>-bin)	Hemoglobin is blood protein. It is the iron-containing pigment of erythrocytes. Erythrocytes are red blood cells (RBCs). "hem/o" is a combining form meaning blood. "globin" is a root word meaning protein.
7-101	a blood protein containing iron	Hemoglobin is ___ _____ _____ _____ _____.
	combining form blood	"hem/o" is a _____ _____ meaning _____.
	word root protein	"globin" is a _____ _____ meaning _____.
	Erythrocytes	_____ are red blood cells (RBCs).
7-102		"hem/o" is a combining form meaning blood. -*poiesis* is a suffix meaning making (producing). Build a medical term meaning making (producing) blood:
	hemopoiesis (he'-mo-<u>poy</u>-e-sis)	_____ _____

BLOCK	DATA AND ANSWERS	DESCRIPTIONS AND QUESTIONS
7-103	sphygmomanometer (sfig'-<u>mo</u>-mah-nom'-eh-ter)	A sphygmomanometer is an instrument used to measure blood pressure. "sphygm/o" is a combining form meaning pulse. "manometer" is a word root meaning measuring instrument. "man/o" is a combining form meaning pressure. *mano-* also is a prefix. "meter" is a word root meaning measure. *-meter* also is a suffix.
7-104	*mano-* *-meter*	_____ is a prefix meaning pressure. _____ is a suffix meaning measure.
7-105	"man/o" "meter" word root measuring instrument	_____ is a combining form meaning pressure. _____ is a word root meaning measure. "manometer" is a _____ _____ meaning _____ _____.
7-106	sphygmomanometer	A _____ is an instrument that measures blood pressure.
7-107	hypertension (hi'-per-<u>ten</u>-shun) hypotension (hi'-po-<u>ten</u>-shun)	Hypertension is persistently high blood pressure. Its causes may or may not be identifiable. Hypotension is persistently low blood pressure. Its causes may or may not be identifiable. *hyper-* is a prefix meaning high. *hypo-* is a prefix meaning low. "tension" is a word root meaning pressure.
7-108	Hypertension *hyper-* "tension"	_____ is high blood pressure. _____ is a prefix meaning high. _____ is a word root meaning pressure.

BLOCK	DATA AND ANSWERS	DESCRIPTIONS AND QUESTIONS
7-109	hypotension	A person with blood pressure lower than normal has _____.
	hypo-	_____ is a prefix meaning decreased or below normal.
7-110	systole (<u>sis</u>-to-le)	The contraction phase of the heart cycle is called systole. It is the top number of a blood pressure reading.
	diastole (di-<u>as</u>-to-le)	The relaxation phase of the heart cycle is called diastole. It is the bottom number of a blood pressure reading.
7-111	Systole	_____ is the heart's contraction phase.
	Diastole	_____ is the heart's relaxation phase.
7-112		The next section covers medical terms associated with diseases of the blood.
	hemangioma (he-man-<u>je</u>-<u>o</u>-mah)	A hemangioma is a tumor of the blood vessels.
	hemostasis (he'-mo-<u>sta</u>-sis)	Hemostasis is the arrest (stopping) of bleeding by vasoconstriction or by surgical means.
		"hem/o" is a combining form meaning blood.
		"angi/o" is a combining form meaning vessel.
		-oma is a suffix meaning tumor.
		-stasis is a suffix meaning stopping (not moving).
7-113	"hem/o"	_____ is a combining form meaning blood.
	"angi/o"	_____ is a combining form meaning vessel.
	-oma	_____ is a suffix meaning tumor.
	-stasis	_____ is a suffix meaning stopping (not moving).

BLOCK	DATA AND ANSWERS	DESCRIPTIONS AND QUESTIONS
7-114	hemangioma Hemostasis	A _____ is a tumor of the blood vessels. _____ is the arrest (stopping) of bleeding by vasoconstriction or by surgical means.
7-115	stopping blood by vasoconstriction or by surgical means combining form blood suffix, stopping (not moving)	Hemostasis is _____ _____. ____ _____ ____ ____ _____ _____. "hem/o" is a _____ _____ meaning _____. -stasis is a _____ meaning _____ _____ _____.
7-116	ischemia (is-<u>ke</u>-me-ah)	Ischemia is the condition of a temporary loss of blood to organs.
7-117	Ischemia	_____ is a temporary lack of blood supply.
7-118	hemosiderosis (he-mo-sid-<u>er</u>-<u>o</u>-sis)	Hemosiderosis is a condition in which there is an increased concentration of iron stored in tissues. "hem/o" is a combining form meaning blood vessels. "sider/o" is a combining form meaning iron. -osis is a suffix meaning condition.
7-119	increased iron concentration combining form blood combining form iron suffix, condition	Hemosiderosis is a condition of _____ _____ _____. "hem/o" is a _____ _____ meaning _____. "sider/o" is a _____ _____ meaning _____. -osis is a _____ meaning _____.

BLOCK	DATA AND ANSWERS	DESCRIPTIONS AND QUESTIONS
7-120	hematosepsis (he-mat-o-<u>sep</u>-sis)	Hematosepsis is the presence of pathogenic microorganisms or their toxins in the blood. "hemat/o" is a combining form meaning blood. "sepsis" is a root word meaning toxic or pathogenic (disease-producing). -*sepsis* is a suffix meaning toxic or pathogenic (disease-producing).
7-121	Hematosepsis "hemat/o," "hem/o" "sepsis"	_____ is the presence of toxins or pathogens in the blood. _____ and _____ are both combining forms meaning blood. _____ is a root word meaning toxic or pathogenic.
7-122	fibrinogen (fi-brin-o-jen)	Fibrinogen is a component (protein) in the blood that can promote blood clotting (coagulation). "fibrin/o" is a combining form meaning a small fiber. -*gen* is a suffix meaning genus, which means beginning or producing.
7-123	Fibrinogen "fibrin/o" -*gen*	_____ is a substance in the blood that facilitates blood clotting. _____ is a combining form meaning fibrin. _____ is a suffix meaning beginning or producing.

BLOCK	DATA AND ANSWERS	DESCRIPTIONS AND QUESTIONS
7-124	thrombectomy (throm-<u>bek</u>-to-me) Thrombectomy "thromb/o" *-ectomy*	Thrombectomy is removal (excision) of a blood clot. _____ is removal (excision) of a blood clot. _____ is a combining form meaning blood clot. _____ is a suffix meaning removal (excision).
7-125	embolectomy (em-bo-<u>lek</u>-to-me)	Embolectomy is the removal of a clot or plug in a vessel. "embol/o" is a combining form meaning embolus, which is a clot or plug in a vessel. *-ectomy* is a suffix meaning excision or removal.
7-126	Embolectomy "embol/o" *-ectomy*	_____ is the removal of a clot or plug in a vessel. _____ is a combining form for embolus, which is a clot or plug in a vessel. _____ is a suffix meaning excision or removal.
7-127		There are several types of cells in the blood: e.g., red blood cells (RBCs), white blood cells (WBCs), and platelets.
7-128	erythrocytes (e-<u>rith</u>-ro-sits)	Erythrocytes are mature red blood cells (RBCs).
7-129		"erythr/o" is a combining form meaning red. "cyte" is a word root meaning cell. It is also a suffix, *-cyte*.
7-130	erythrocytolysis (er-rith'-ro-si-<u>toh</u>-lih-sis)	Erythrocytolysis is the destruction of red blood cells.

BLOCK	DATA AND ANSWERS	DESCRIPTIONS AND QUESTIONS
7-131		"erythr/o" is a combining form meaning red.
		"cyte" is a word root meaning cell.
		"erythrocyt/o" is the combining form for red cells.
		-lysis is a suffix meaning destruction.
7-132	Erythrocytolysis	_____ refers to red cell destruction.
	"erythr/o"	_____ is a combining form meaning red.
	"erythrocyt/o"	_____ is a combining form meaning red cells.
	-lysis	_____ is a suffix meaning destruction.
7-133	Erythrocytes	_____ are mature red blood cells.
	the destruction of red cells	Erythrocytolysis is _____ _____ _____ _____ _____.
7-134	erythroblastosis (eh-rith-ro-<u>blas</u>-to'-sis)	Erythroblastosis means immature or primitive red blood cell.
		"blast/o" is a combining form meaning primitive or immature cell.
		"erythr/o" is a combining form meaning red (cell).
		-osis is a suffix meaning condition.
	Erythroblastosis	_____ means immature or primitive red blood cell.
7-135	leucocytes (loo-<u>ko</u>-sits)	A leukocyte is a white blood cell or a colorless blood cell that protects the body against harmful microorganisms. There are five types of white blood cells (WBCs).
		"leuk/o" is a combining form meaning white.
		"cyte" is a word root meaning cell.

BLOCK	DATA AND ANSWERS	DESCRIPTIONS AND QUESTIONS
7-136	Leukocytes	_____ are white blood cells.
	five	There are _____ types of white blood cells.
	WBC	The acronym for a leukocyte is _____.
7-137	granulocytes (gran-u-lo-sitz)	Granulocytes are any cells containing granules, especially granular leukocytes, which are formed in the bone marrow. Granulocytes form one group of white blood cells. There are three types of granulocytes.
		"granul/o" is a combining form meaning granules, small grainlike substances.
		"cytes" is a word root meaning cells.
7-138	any white blood cells containing granules	Granulocytes are _____ _____ _____ _____ _____ _____.
	three	There are _____ types of granulocytes.
	combining form	"granul/o" is a _____ _____ meaning
	granules	_____.
	word root, cells	"cytes" is a _____ _____ meaning _____.
7-139	neutrophils (nu-tro-filz)	Neutrophils are the first type of granulocytes. They stain easily with neutral (not acidic and not alkaline) dyes.
		"neutr/o" is a combining form meaning neutral.
		"phil" is a word root meaning to love (i.e., granulocytes love being neutral).

BLOCK	DATA AND ANSWERS	DESCRIPTIONS AND QUESTIONS
7-140	white blood cells (with granules) that stain easily with neutral dyes	Neutrophils are _____ _____ _____ _____ _____ _____ _____ _____ _____ _____ _____.
	combining form neutral	"neutr/o" is a _____ _____ meaning _____.
	word root, to love	"phil" is a _____ _____ meaning _____ _____.
7-141	eosinophils (ē-o-sin-o'-filz)	Eosinophils are the second type of granulocyte. They stain easily with acidic dyes and increase in allergic conditions.
		"eosin/o" is a combining form meaning acidic.
7-142	white blood cells (with granules) that stain easily with acidic dyes	Eosinophils are _____ _____ _____ _____ _____ _____ _____ _____ _____ _____.
	combining form acidic	"eosin/o" is a _____ _____ meaning _____.
	word root, to love	"phil" is a _____ _____ meaning _____ _____.
7-143		An alkaline substance is called a base (adjective = basic).
	basophils (bā-so-filz)	Basophils are the third type of granulocytes.
		They stain easily with basic dyes. Their function is unclear.
		"bas/o" is a combining form meaning alkaline or basic.
7-144	white blood cells (with granules) that stain easily with basic/alkaline dyes	Basophils are _____ _____ _____ _____ _____ _____ _____ _____ _____ _____ _____.
	combining form basic	"bas/o" is a _____ _____ meaning _____.
	word root, to love	"phil" is a _____ _____ meaning _____ _____.

BLOCK	DATA AND ANSWERS	DESCRIPTIONS AND QUESTIONS
7-145	agranulocytes (ah-gran-u-lo-sitz')	Agranulocytes are cells that contain no granules. They form another group of white blood cells. There are two types of agranulocytes. They are produced by the spleen and lymph nodes. "granule" is a word root meaning a small grainlike substance. "agranul/o" is a combining form meaning no granules. *a-* is a prefix meaning none. "cytes" is a word root meaning cells. *-cytes* also is a suffix.
7-146	white blood cells containing no granules two	Agranulocytes are _____ _____ _____ _____ _____ _____. There are _____ types of agranulocytes.
7-147	combining form no granules word root, cells *-cytes*	"agranul/o" is a _____ _____ meaning _____ _____. "cytes" is a _____ _____ meaning _____. _____ is a suffix meaning cells.
7-148	lymphocytes (lĭm-fo-sitz)	Lymphocytes are the first type of agranulocytes. They participate in immunity-producing antibodies to destroy foreign materials. "lymph/o" is a combining form meaning lymph cells.
7-149	agranulocytes that participate in immunity-producing antibodies to destroy foreign materials combining form lymph cells	Lymphocytes are _____ _____ _____ ___ _____ _____ _____ _____ _____ _____. "lymph/o" is a _____ _____ meaning _____ _____.

BLOCK	DATA AND ANSWERS	DESCRIPTIONS AND QUESTIONS
7-150	monocytes (<u>mon</u>-o-sitz) agranulocytes that destroy foreign invaders in the body	The second type of agranulocytes are the monocytes. They destroy foreign invaders in the body. "mono" is a word root meaning one. *mono-* also is a prefix. "cytes" is a word root meaning cells. *-cytes* also is also a suffix. Monocytes are _____ _____ _____ _____ _____ ___ _____ _____.
7-151	thrombocyte (throm-<u>bo</u>-sit) platelet (plate-<u>let</u>)	A thrombocyte is a disk-shaped structure in the blood that facilitates blood coagulation. Thrombocytes may be called blood platelets. "thromb/o" is a combining form meaning a clot. "cytes" is a word root meaning cells. "Platelet" is a medical word meaning flat and small.
7-152	thrombocyte platelet "thromb/o"	A component in the blood that can facilitate the clotting of blood is called a _____ or a blood _____. _____ is a combining form meaning clot.
7-153	thrombocytolysis (throm′-bo-si-<u>tol</u>-lih-sis)	Thrombocytolysis is the destruction of blood platelets. *-lysis* is a suffix meaning destruction.
7-154	the destruction of blood platelets combining form clot suffix, destruction "cytes"	Thrombocytolysis is _____ _____ _____ _____ _____. "thromb/o" is a _____ _____ meaning _____. *-lysis* is a _____ meaning _____. _____ is a word root meaning cells.

BLOCK	DATA AND ANSWERS	DESCRIPTIONS AND QUESTIONS
7-155	thrombocytopenia (throm'-bo-si-to-<u>pe</u>-ne-ah)	Thrombocytopenia is a decrease in the number of platelets in blood circulation. A thrombocyte is a blood platelet. "thrombocyt/o" is a combining form meaning blood platelet. *-penia* is a suffix meaning decreased or below normal.
7-156	Thrombocytopenia "thrombocyt/o" *-penia*	_____ is a platelet (thrombocyte) decrease in blood. _____ is a combining form meaning platelet. _____ is a suffix meaning decrease.
7-157	thrombophlebitis (throm'-bo-fleh-<u>bi</u>-tis)	Thrombophlebitis is inflammation of a vein caused by the formation of a thrombus (blood clot) in the blood. "thromb/o" is a combining form meaning blood clot. "phleb" is a word root meaning vein. "phleb/o" is the combining form. *-itis* is a suffix meaning inflammation.
7-158	"thromb/o" "phleb" *-itis* inflammation of a vein from the formation of a thrombus (blood clot)	_____ is a combining form meaning blood clot. _____ is a word root meaning vein. _____ is a suffix meaning inflammation. Thrombophlebitis is _____ ____ __ _____ _____ _____ _____ _____ __ _____ _____ _____.

BLOCK	DATA AND ANSWERS	DESCRIPTIONS AND QUESTIONS
7-159		Another important component of the blood is its fluid.
	lymph (limf) lymphatic vessels (lim-<u>fat</u>-ik <u>ves</u>-selz)	Lymph fluid comes from the blood. It filters into the spaces between the cells and returns to the blood via lymphatic vessels. The spleen is the largest lymphatic organ of the body. The lymph is sometimes known as lymph fluid. Lymph is a clear, transparent fluid formed in tissue spaces all over the body and transported through a system of vessels called lymphatic vessels.
		The next several blocks pertain to the lymphatic system.
7-160		The fluid formed in tissue spaces is called
	lymph, lymph fluid	_____ or _____ _____.
		The fluid is transported throughout the body by a network
	lymphatic vessels	called _____ _____.
7-161	lymph nodes (limf nodz)	Lymph nodes are small organs along the course of the lymphatic vessels that serve to filter or remove foreign or noxious agents (e.g., bacteria) from the lymph fluid.
	Lymph nodes	_____ _____ are the small organs that filter the lymph.
7-162	lymphopathy (lim-<u>fop</u>-ah-the)	Lymphopathy is a medical term meaning disease of the lymphatic system.
		"lymph/o" is a combining form meaning the lymphatic system.
		-pathy is a suffix meaning disease.
7-163	combining form the lymphatic system	"lymph/o" is a _____ _____ meaning _____ _____ _____.
	-pathy	_____ is a suffix meaning disease.
	Lymphopathy	_____ is disease of the lymphatic system.

BLOCK	DATA AND ANSWERS	DESCRIPTIONS AND QUESTIONS
7-164	lymphoidectomy (lim´-foy-<u>dek</u>-o-me)	Lymphoidectomy is excision of lymphoid tissue. "lymph/o" is a combining form meaning lymphatic tissue. -oid is a suffix meaning resembling. "lymphoid/o" is a combining form meaning lymphoid tissue. -ectomy is a suffix meaning excision.
7-165	Lymphoidectomy suffix "lymphoid/o" -ectomy	_____ is excision of lymphoid tissue. -oid is a _____ meaning resembling. _____ is a combining form meaning lymphoid tissue. _____ is a suffix meaning excision.
7-166	lymphadenotomy (lim-fah-<u>den</u>-ot-o-me)	Lymphadenotomy is incision of a lymph node. "lymph/o" is a combining form meaning lymphatic tissue. "aden/o" is a combining form meaning gland (node). -tomy is a suffix meaning incision.
7-167	"aden/o," combining form "lymphoid/o" -tomy incision of a lymph node	_____ is a _____ _____ meaning gland. _____ is a combining form meaning lymphoid tissue. _____ is a suffix meaning incision. Lymphadenotomy is _____ ____ __ _____ _____.

BLOCK	DATA AND ANSWERS	DESCRIPTIONS AND QUESTIONS
7-168	lymphedema (limf-eh-de-mah)	Lymphedema is swelling due to obstruction of the flow of lymph. "lymph/o" is a combining form meaning lymph tissues. "edema" is a word root meaning abnormal accumulation of fluid in intercellular body spaces. -edema also can be a suffix.
7-169	Lymphedema	_____ is swelling due to obstruction of the flow of lymph.
7-170	lymphangioma (lim-fan-je-o-mah)	Lymphangioma is a tumor composed of lymphatic vessels. "lymph/o" is a combining form meaning lymphatic tissues. "ang" or "angi" is a word root meaning vessel or channel. -oma is a suffix meaning tumor.
7-171	a tumor composed of lymphatic vessels "ang," "angi" combining form lymphatic tissues -oma	Lymphangioma is ___ _____ _____ _____ _____ _____. _____ or _____ is a word root meaning vessel or channel. "lymph/o" is a _____ _____ meaning _____ _____. _____ is a suffix meaning tumor.
7-172	lymphangitis (lim-fan-ji-tis)	Lymphangitis is inflammation of a lymphatic vessel. "lymph/o" is a combining form meaning lymphatic tissues. "ang" is a root word meaning vessels or channels. -itis is a suffix meaning inflammation.

BLOCK	DATA AND ANSWERS	DESCRIPTIONS AND QUESTIONS
7-173	inflammation of a lymphatic vessel "lymph/o" root word *-itis*	Lymphangitis is _____ ____ __ _____ _____. _____ is a combining form meaning lymphatic tissues. "ang" is a _____ _____ meaning vessels or channels. _____ is a suffix meaning inflammation.
7-174	lymphadenectomy (lim′-fah-den-<u>ek</u>-to-me)	Lymphadenectomy is excision of a lymph node. "adeno" is a word root meaning gland. "aden/o" is the combining form. "lymphaden/o" is a combining form meaning lymph node. *-ectomy* is a suffix meaning excision.
7-175	"lymphaden/o" *-ectomy* "adeno" Lymphadenectomy	_____ is a combining form meaning lymph node. _____ is a suffix for excision. _____ is a word root meaning gland. _____ is excision of a lymph node.
7-176	lymphadenography (lim′-fad-eh-<u>nog</u>-rah-fe)	Lymphadenography is an x-ray record (study) of the lymph nodes. "lymph/o" is a combining form meaning lymphatic tissues. "aden/o" is a combining form meaning gland (node). *-graphy* is a suffix meaning a record of an image (formed by x-ray).

BLOCK	DATA AND ANSWERS	DESCRIPTIONS AND QUESTIONS
7-177	Lymphadenography *-graphy*	_____ is an x-ray study of the lymph nodes. _____ is a suffix meaning to record an image.
7-178	spleen (splen)	The spleen is a glandular organ in the upper-left part of the abdominal cavity. One of its many functions is the production of lymphocytes and plasma cells.
7-179	spleen	The _____ is a gland-like organ that produces lymphocytes and plasma cells.
7-180	splenomegaly (sple-no- <u>meg</u>-ah-le)	Splenomegaly is enlargement of the spleen. "splen/o" is a combining form meaning spleen. *-megaly* is a suffix meaning enlarged.
7-181	Splenomegaly "splen/o" *-megaly*	_____ is enlargement of the spleen. _____ is a combining form meaning spleen. _____ is a suffix meaning enlarged.
7-182	splenoid (sple-<u>noyd</u>)	"Splenoid" means resembling the spleen. "splen/o" is a combining form meaning spleen. *-oid* is a suffix meaning resembling.
7-183	Splenoid	_____ means resembling the spleen.
7-184	splenitis (sple-<u>ni</u>-tis)	Splenitis is inflammation of the spleen. *-itis* is a suffix meaning inflammation.
7-185	Splenitis	_____ is inflammation of the spleen.
7-186		This chapter reviewed the cardiovascular system. The next chapter focuses on the nervous system.

BOX 7.2
Abbreviations

AMI	acute myocardial infarction
BP	blood pressure
CCU	coronary care unit
CHD	coronary heart disease
CHF	congestive heart failure
CAT (scan)	computed axial tomography (scan)
DVT	deep vein thrombosis
ECG	electrocardiogram
HDL	high-density lipoprotein
LDL	low-density lipoprotein
MI	myocardial infarction
PDA	patent ductus arteriosus

Progress Check

A. Multiple Choice

1. A word root meaning vessel is:
   a. vagin
   b. angi
   c. adeno
   d. capill

2. A word root meaning red cell is:
   a. globin
   b. scler
   c. cutane
   d. erythrocyt

3. A word root meaning varicose vein is:
   a. varix
   b. cyan
   c. vulv
   d. proct

4. A word root meaning plug is:
   a. cardi
   b. rach
   c. embol
   d. pod

5. A combining form meaning small artery is:
   a. arter/o
   b. arteriol/o
   c. my/o
   d. thromb/o

6. A combining form meaning vein is:
   a. phleb/o
   b. neutr/o

c. gangli/o
d. humer/o

7. A combining form meaning a pulse is:
   a. man/o
   b. lymphoid/o
   c. leuk/o
   d. sphygm/o

8. A combining form meaning iron is:
   a. sider/o
   b. ir/o
   c. sinistr
   d. presby/o

9. A prefix meaning pressure is:
   a. mano-
   b. ambi-
   c. primi-
   d. ultra-

10. A prefix meaning above is:
    a. hyper-
    b. peri-
    c. supra-
    d. extra-

11. A suffix meaning condition is:
    a. -ia
    b. -iasis
    c. -ic
    d. -ule

12. A suffix meaning large is:
    a. -lysis

   b. -meter

   c. -oid

   d. -megaly

13. A suffix meaning decreased or below normal is:

   a. -stasis

   b. -penia

   c. -itis

   d. -oma

14. A suffix meaning formation or production is:

   a. -poiesis

   b. -cytes

   c. -stenosis

   d. -tic

B.   Building Medical Terms

Use the following word components to build medical terms matching the definitions given.

a-	hem	-penia
agranul	hem/o	peri-
blast	hemo-	phleb
blast/o	-iasis	phleb/o
cardi	lith	sider
cardi/o	lith/o	sider/o
cyt	man	sphygm
cyt/o	man/o	sphygm/o
-cytes	-meter	thromb
-ectomy	my	thromb/o
erythr	my/o	varic
erythr/o	-oid	varic/o
-genic	-osis	
granul/o	-pathy	

1. development of calculi (stones) in a vein

2. resembling a varix (varicose vein)

3. instrument used to measure blood pressure

4. removal of the membrane around the heart

5. any disease of the heart muscle

6. immature or primitive red blood cell

7. cells that contain no granules

8. decrease in the number of platelets in blood circulation

9. condition in which there is an increased concentration of iron storage in tissues

10. originating in or from the heart

C. Definitions and Word Components

	TERM	DEFINITION	PREFIX	WORD ROOT	VOWEL	WORD ROOT	VOWEL	SUFFIX
1.	aortostenosis							
2.	lymphadenotomy							
3.	pericardectomy							
4.	arteriosclerosis							
5.	intracardiac							
6.	supravalvular							
7.	thrombocytolysis							
8.	endocarditis							
9.	venorrhaphy							
10.	hemangioma							

D.   Abbreviations

	ABBREVIATION	MEANING
1.	AMI	
2.	BP	
3.	CCU	
4.	CHD	
5.	CHF	
6.	CAT (scan)	
7.	DVT	
8.	ECG	
9.	HDL	
10.	LDL	
11.	MI	
12.	PDA	

The Nervous System

BLOCK	DATA AND ANSWERS	DESCRIPTIONS AND QUESTIONS
8-1		The nervous system has two divisions: the central nervous system (CNS), which includes the brain and spinal cord, and the peripheral nervous system (PNS), which contains 12 pairs of cranial nerves and 31 pairs of spinal nerves.
	cranial (<u>kra</u>-ne-al)	
	neurons (<u>new</u>-rons)	Neurons are the structural and functional units of the nervous system. These specialized cells conduct impulses that allow the body to interact with both internal and external stimuli. There is an interconnecting neuron (interneuron) system that carries messages between the CNS and PNS.
	cerebrospinal (<u>ser</u>-e-bral-spine'-no)	Cerebrospinal fluid circulates continuously around the brain and spinal cord, which is enclosed by the bones of the skull and spinal column.
		See **Figure 8.1** and **Figure 8.2**.
		In this chapter, we will study selected medical terms related to the brain, spinal cord, nerve cells, and the senses.
8-2		Let us begin with the brain.
	cerebrum (<u>cer</u>-eh-bru'-m)	Cerebrum is the largest and upper most part of the brain.
	cerebellum (cer'-eh-<u>bel</u>-lum)	Cerebellum is the part of the brain located in the back.

BLOCK	DATA AND ANSWERS	DESCRIPTIONS AND QUESTIONS
8-3	craniocerebral (<u>kra</u>-ne-o-ser′-e-bral)	Craniocerebral means pertaining to the cranium and cerebrum.
		"cranium" or "crani" is a word root meaning skull bones.
		"crani/o" is the combining form.
		"cerebr" is a word root meaning cerebrum.
		"cerebr/o" is the combining form.
		-al is a suffix meaning pertaining to.

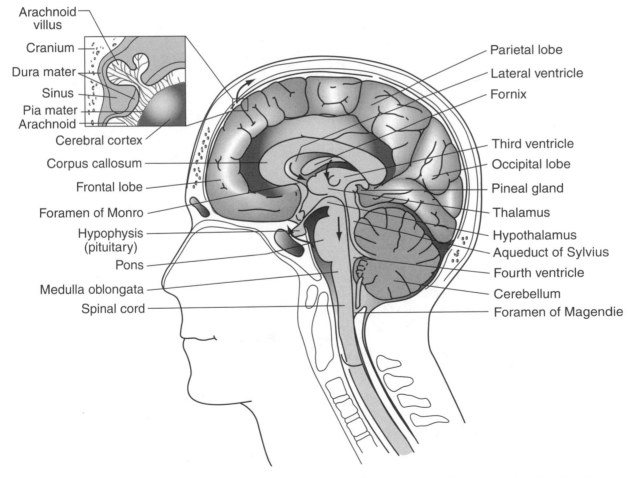

FIGURE 8.1 Midsagittal section of the human brain, showing the circulation of cerebrospinal fluid in the brain and spinal cord

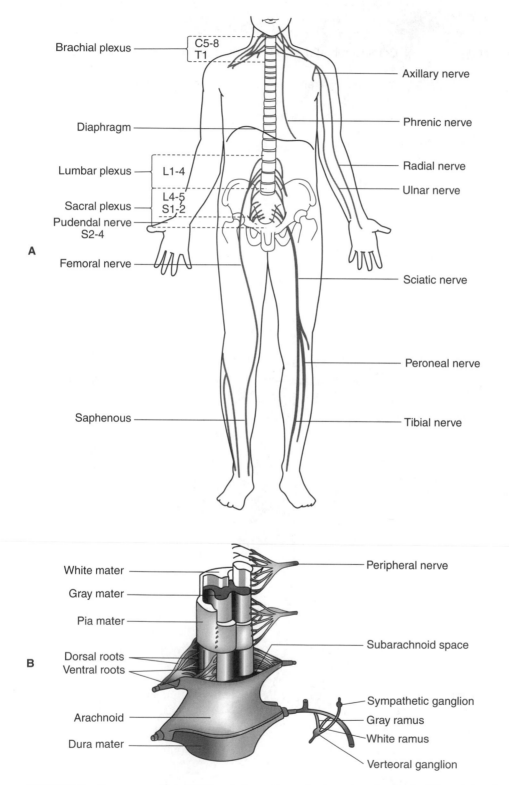

FIGURE 8.2 Sensory and motor tracts from the spinal cord to the brain (A) and the three meningeal layers in association with the sympathetic trunk of the spinal cord (B)

BLOCK	DATA AND ANSWERS	DESCRIPTIONS AND QUESTIONS
8-4	combining form cranium	"crani/o" is a _____ _____ meaning _____.
	combining form cerebrum	"cerebr/o" is a _____ _____ meaning _____.
	suffix, pertaining to	-al is a _____ meaning _____ _____.
	pertaining to the cranium and cerebrum	Craniocerebral means _____ ____ _____ _____ _____ _____.
8-5	lobectomy (lo′-bek-to-me)	Lobectomy is excision of a lobe (of the brain). "lobe" is a word root meaning sides or parts (may refer to any organ with lobes). "lob/o" is the combining form. -ectomy is a suffix meaning removal or excision.
	Lobectomy	_____ is excision of a lobe of the brain.
8-6	meningitis (men′-in-ji-tis)	Meningitis is inflammation of the membrane covering the brain. "meninges" or "mening" is a word root meaning membrane. "mening/o" is the combining form. -itis is a suffix meaning inflammation.
8-7	"meninges," "mening"	_____ or _____ is a word root meaning membrane.
	-itis	_____ is a suffix meaning inflammation.
	Meningitis	_____ is inflammation of the meninges.

BLOCK	DATA AND ANSWERS	DESCRIPTIONS AND QUESTIONS
8-8		The cerebellum is part of the brain, as indicated earlier.
		"cerebell" is a word root meaning the cerebellum.
		"cerebell/o" is the combining form.
		Build a medical term (including pronunciation) meaning
	cerebellitis (cer'-eh-bel-i-tis)	inflammation of cerebellum: _____ _____
8-9	cephalocele (sef'-ah-lo-sel)	Cephalocele is herniation of a part of the cranial contents (i.e., the brain).
		"cephal" is a word root meaning brain.
		"cephal/o" is a combining form meaning brain.
		-cele is a suffix meaning hernia.
	Cephalocele	_____ is herniation of a part of the brain.
8-10	meningocephalocele (men-in'-jo-sef-ah-lo-sel)	Meningocephalocele is herniation of the meninges and brain substance (through a defect of the skull).
		"mening/o" is a combining form meaning membrane (surrounding the brain).
		"cephal/o" is a combining form meaning brain.
		-cele is a suffix meaning herniation.
8-11	herniation of the meninges and brain substance (through a defect of the skull)	Meningocephalocele is _____ _____ _____ _____ _____ _____ _____ _____ ___ _____ ____ _____ _____.

BLOCK	DATA AND ANSWERS	DESCRIPTIONS AND QUESTIONS
8-12	"mening/o" brain -cele	_____ is a combining form meaning the membrane (surrounding the brain). cephal/o is a combining form meaning _____. _____ is a suffix meaning herniation.
8-13	encephalitis (en-sef´-ah- <u>li</u>-tis)	Encephalitis is inflammation of the brain. "encephal" is a word root meaning brain. "encephal/o" is a combining form meaning brain. -itis is a suffix meaning inflammation.
8-14	Encephalitis combining form brain -itis	_____ is inflammation of the brain. "encephal/o" is a _____ _____ meaning _____. _____ is a suffix meaning inflammation.
8-15	cephalalgia (sef´-<u>al</u>-je-ah)	Cephalalgia is pain in the brain or the head (headache). "cephal/o" is a combining form meaning brain or head. -algia is a suffix meaning pain.
8-16	combining form brain or head suffix, pain pain in the brain or the head (headache)	"cephal/o" is a _____ _____ meaning _____ ____ _____. -algia is a _____ meaning _____. Cephalalgia is _____ ___ _____ _____ _____ _____ _____ _____.

BLOCK	DATA AND ANSWERS	DESCRIPTIONS AND QUESTIONS
8-17	meningioma (men-in-je'-o-mah)	Meningioma is a tumor of the meninges. "meninges" is a root word meaning membrane (surrounding the brain). "mening/o" and "meningi/o" are both combining forms of meninges. -*oma* is a suffix meaning tumor.
	a tumor of the meninges	Meningioma is ___ _____ _____ _____ _____.
8-18	"mening/o" "meningi/o"	"meninges" has two combining forms: _____ and _____.
	suffix, tumor	-*oma* is a _____ meaning _____.
8-19	encephalomalacia (en-sef'-al-o-mah-la'-se-ah)	Encephalomalacia is softening of the brain. "encephal/o" is a combining form meaning brain. -*malacia* is a suffix meaning softening.
8-20	"encephal/o"	_____ is a combining form meaning brain.
	-*malacia*	_____ is a suffix meaning softening.
	Encephalomalacia	_____ is softening of the brain.
8-21	encephalosclerosis (en-sef'-ah-lo'-skleh-ro-sis)	Encephalosclerosis is hardening of the brain.
	anencephalia (an'-en-sef'-ah-le-ah)	Anencephalia is a birth defect in which a person has no cerebral hemispheres or cranial vault.

BLOCK	DATA AND ANSWERS	DESCRIPTIONS AND QUESTIONS
8-22		"encephal" is a root word meaning brain.
		"encephal/o" is the combining form.
		"sclerosis" is a word root meaning hardening.
		-sclerosis also is a suffix.
		an- is a prefix meaning no or none.
		-ia is a suffix meaning condition. The condition can be normal or abnormal.
8-23	Encephalosclerosis	_____ is hardening of the brain.
8-24	the absence of cerebral hemispheres and cranial vault	Anencephalia is _____ _____ _____ _____ _____ _____ _____ _____ .
8-25	*an-* "encephal" suffix, condition.	_____ is a prefix meaning no. _____ is a root word meaning brain. *-ia* is a _____ meaning _____.
8-26		The next section describes the medical terms associated with the brain and its nerves.
	hydrencephalo-meningocele (<u>hi</u>-dren′-cef-al-o′-men-in-jo-sel)	Hydrencephalomeningocele is herniation of brain substance and meninges caused by a defect, with accumulation of cerebrospinal fluid in the sac along with brain substance.
		"hydr" is a word root meaning water.
		"hydr/o" is the combining form.
		hydro- also can be a prefix.
		"encephal/o" is a combining form meaning brain.
		Meninges refers to a membrane (covering the brain).
		"mening/o" is the combining form.
		-cele is a suffix meaning hernia.

BLOCK	DATA AND ANSWERS	DESCRIPTIONS AND QUESTIONS
8-27	hydrencephalo- meningocele	_____ _____ is herniation of brain substance and meninges through a defect, with accumulation of cerebrospinal fluid in the sac along with brain substance.
8-28	"hydr" "hydr/o" brain "mening/o" hernia	_____ is a word root meaning water. _____ is a combining form meaning water. "encephal/o" is a combining form meaning _____. _____ is a combining form referring to a membrane (covering the brain). -cele is a suffix meaning _____.
8-29	polioencephalomeningo- myelitis (po-le-o-en-sef'- al-o-men-in'-jo-mi'-<u>el</u>-i- tis)	Polioencephalomeningomyelitis is inflammation of the gray matter of the brain, the membrane, and the spinal cord. "polio" or "poli" is a word root meaning gray. "poli/o" is the combining form. "encephal/o" is a combining form meaning brain. "mening/o" is a combining form meaning membrane. "myel" is a word root for spinal cord. "myel/o" is a combining form meaning spinal cord. -itis is a suffix meaning inflammation.
8-30	Polioencephalo- meningomyelitis	_____ _____ is inflammation of the gray matter of the brain, spinal cord, and meninges.

BLOCK	DATA AND ANSWERS	DESCRIPTIONS AND QUESTIONS
8-31	gray	"polio" is a word root meaning _____.
	"encephal/o"	_____ is a combining form meaning brain.
	membrane	"mening/o" is a combining form meaning _____.
	"myel/o"	_____ is a combining form meaning spinal cord.
	inflammation	*-itis* is a suffix meaning _____.
8-32	electroencephalogram (el'-ek-<u>tro</u>-en-sef-al-o'-gram)	An electroencephalogram is a record (graphic chart) of the electrical impulses of the brain.
		"electric," "electri," and "electr" are word roots for electricity or electrical impulses.
		"electr/o" is the combining form.
		"encephal/o" is a combining form meaning brain.
		-gram is a suffix meaning record (i.e., graphic chart).
8-33	"electr/o"	_____ is a combining form meaning electrical.
	"encephal/o"	_____ is a combining form meaning brain.
	-gram	_____ is a suffix meaning record (graphic chart).
8-34	electroencephalogram	An _____ is a record (graphic chart) of the electrical impulses of the brain.
	electroencephalograph (el'-ek-<u>tro</u>-en-sef'-al-o-graf)	Some medical books use electroencephalograph instead of electroencephalogram. Both have the same clinical meaning (i.e., a diagram or graphic record of the electrical impulses of the brain).

BLOCK	DATA AND ANSWERS	DESCRIPTIONS AND QUESTIONS
8-35	electroencephalography (el′-ek-<u>tro</u>-en-sef′-al-og-raf-e)	Electroencephalography is a medical term meaning the process of recording a graph of the electrical impulses of the brain. "electric" or "electri" is a word root for electricity or electrical impulses. "electr/o" is the combining form. "encephal/o" is a combining form meaning brain. *-graphy* is a suffix meaning the process of recording (a graph)
8-36	combining form electricity or electrical impulses combining form brain suffix, the process of recording a graphic chart	"electr/o" is a _____ _____ meaning _____ ____ _____ _____. "encephal/o" is a _____ _____ meaning _____. *-graphy* is a _____ meaning _____ _____ ____ _____ __ _____ _____.
8-37	electroencephalography	Build a medical term meaning the process of recording a graph of the electrical impulses of the brain: _____.
8-38	pneumoencephalogram (nu′-mo-en′-<u>sef</u>-al-o-gram) pneumoencephalogram	A pneumoencephalogram is a record (X-ray film) of the brain made by using air as the contrast medium. "pneum" is a word root meaning air. "pneum/o" is a combining form meaning air. "encephal/o" is a combining form meaning brain. *-gram* is a suffix meaning record (X-ray film). A _____ is an X-ray film of the brain using air as the contrast medium.

BLOCK	DATA AND ANSWERS	DESCRIPTIONS AND QUESTIONS
8-39	echoencephalography (ek-o-en-sef'-ah-log-rah-fe)	Echoencephalography is the process of recording brain structures by using sound (waves). "echo" is a word root for sound. "ech/o" is a combining form meaning sound. *echo-* also can be prefix. "encephal/o" is a combining form meaning brain. *-graphy* is a suffix meaning the process of recording (sound waves).
8-40	echoencephalography "ech/o" "encephal/o" *-graphy*	_____ is the process of recording brain structures by use of sound (waves). _____ is a combining form meaning sound. _____ is a combining form meaning brain. _____ is a suffix meaning the process of recording (sound waves).
8-41	ventriculogram (ven-trik-u-lo'-gram)	A ventriculogram is an X-ray film of the cerebral ventricles. The brain has compartments or segments called cerebral ventricles. "ventricle" is a word root. "ventricul/o" is a combining form meaning cerebral ventricles. *-gram* is a suffix meaning a record (here, X-ray film).
8-42	ventriculogram	A _____ is an X-ray film of the cerebral ventricles.

BLOCK	DATA AND ANSWERS	DESCRIPTIONS AND QUESTIONS
8-43	myelalgia (<u>mi</u>-e-la-je-ah)	We will now proceed to medical terms related to the spinal cord. Myelalgia is pain in the spinal cord. "myel/o" is a combining form meaning spinal cord (nerve cells). -*algia* is a suffix meaning pain.
8-44	Myelalgia "myel/o," combining form -*algia*	_____ is pain in the spinal cord. _____ is a _____ _____ meaning spinal cord. _____ is a suffix meaning pain.
8-45	rachiomyelitis (<u>rak</u>-e-o'-mye-<u>li</u>-tis)	Rachiomyelitis is inflammation of the spinal canal and cord. "rachi" is a word root for spinal canal. "rachi/o" is a combining form meaning spinal canal. "myel/o" is a combining form meaning spinal cord. -*itis* is a suffix meaning inflammation.
8-46	inflammation of the spinal canal and cord "rachi/o," combining form combining form spinal cord suffix, inflammation	Rachiomyelitis is _____ _____ _____ _____ _____ _____ _____. _____ is a _____ _____ meaning spinal canal. "myel/o" is a _____ _____ meaning _____ _____. -*itis* is a _____ meaning _____.

BLOCK	DATA AND ANSWERS	DESCRIPTIONS AND QUESTIONS
8-47	rachicentesis (rak′-ih-<u>sen</u>-te-sis)	Rachicentesis is surgical puncture of the spinal canal. "rachi/o" is a combining form meaning spinal canal. "centesis" is a root word meaning surgical puncture. -centesis also is also a suffix.
8-48	combining form spinal canal suffix, puncture surgical puncture of the spinal canal	"rachi/o" is a _____ _____ meaning _____ _____. -centesis is a _____ meaning _____. Rachicentesis is _____ _____ _____ _____ _____ _____.
8-49	myelomeningocele (mi′-el-o-men′-in-<u>jo</u>-sel)	Myelomeningocele is herniation of the spinal cord and its membranes caused by a defect in the vertebral column. "myel/o" is a combining form meaning spinal cord. "mening/o" is a combining form meaning membranes. -cele is a suffix meaning herniation.
8-50	Myelomeningocele combining form spinal cord "mening/o" suffix, herniation	_____ is the herniation of the spinal cord and its meninges caused by a defect in the vertebral column. "myel/o" is a _____ _____ meaning _____ _____. _____ is a combining form meaning membranes. -cele is a _____ meaning _____.
8-51	hydromyelocele (hi′-dro-<u>mi</u>-elo-sel)	Hydromyelocele is water in a herniation (a sac) of the spinal cord. "hydr/o" is a combining form meaning water. hydro- also can be a prefix.

BLOCK	DATA AND ANSWERS	DESCRIPTIONS AND QUESTIONS
8-52	water in a herniation (a sac) of the spinal cord "myel/o," combining form water -*cele*, suffix	Hydromyelocele is _____ ____ __ _____ ____ _____ ____ _____ _____ _____. _____ is a _____ _____ meaning spinal cord. "hydr/o" is a combining form meaning _____. _____ is a _____ meaning herniation.
8-53	myeloschisis (<u>mi</u>-el-o-skih-sis)	Myeloschisis is a split or cleft in the spinal cord. "myel/o" is a combining form meaning spinal cord. -*schisis* is a suffix meaning split or cleft.
8-54	-*schisis*, suffix a split or cleft in the spinal cord	_____ is a _____ meaning split or cleft. Myeloschisis is ___ _____ _____ _____ ___ _____ _____ _____.
8-55	poliomyelitis (<u>po</u>-le-o-mi'-el-i-tis)	Poliomyelitis is inflammation of the gray matter or cells of the spinal cord. It results from a viral disease causing inflammation of the nerve cells (gray matter) of the spinal cord. "polio" or "poli" is a word root meaning gray (matter or cells). "poli/o" is the combining form. "myel/o" is a combining form referring to the spinal cord or bone marrow (gray cells). -*itis* is a suffix meaning inflammation.

BLOCK	DATA AND ANSWERS	DESCRIPTIONS AND QUESTIONS
8-56	inflammation of the gray matter or cells of the spinal cord, which results from a viral disease causing inflammation of the nerve cells (gray matter) of the spinal cord	Poliomyelitis is _____ _____ _____ _____ _____ _____ _____ _____ _____ _____ _____ _____ _____ _____ ____ _____ _____ _____ _____ ____ _____ _____ _____ _____ _____ _____ _____ _____ _____.
8-57	"poli/o" spinal cord (gray cells) suffix, inflammation	_____ is a combining form meaning gray (matter or cells). "myel/o" is a combining form referring to the _____ _____ _____ _____. -itis is a _____ meaning _____.
8-58	laminectomy (lam-i-<u>nek</u>-to-me)	Laminectomy is excision of the posterior arch of a vertebra. "lamina" or "lamin" is a word root meaning one of the bony arches of the vertebrae. "lamin/o" is the combining form. -ectomy is a suffix meaning removal or excision.
8-59	one of the bony arches of the vertebrae suffix, excision excision of the posterior arch of a vertebra	"lamin/o" is a combining form meaning _____ _____ _____ _____ _____ _____ _____ _____. -ectomy is a _____ meaning _____. Laminectomy is _____ _____ _____ _____ _____ ____ __ _____.

BLOCK	DATA AND ANSWERS	DESCRIPTIONS AND QUESTIONS
8-60	meningocele (<u>men</u>-in-jo'-sel)	A meningocele is a hernia (protrusion) through the membrane of the nervous system due to a birth defect in the skull or spinal column. "mening/o" is a combining form meaning the meninges or membrane around the nerve cells. -*cele* is a suffix meaning hernia or protrusion.
8-61	a hernia (protrusion) through the membrane of the nervous system due to a birth defect in the skull or spinal column	A meningocele is ___ _____ _____ _____ _____ _____ ____ ____ ___ _____ _____ _____ ____ ___ _____ _____ ___ _____ _____ _____ _____ _____ .
8-62	meningomyelocele (<u>men</u>-in-jo-mi'-el-o'-sel)	Meningomyelocele is protrusion of the meninges and spinal cord through a defect in the vertebrae. "mening/o" is a combining form referring to the meninges or membrane around the nerve cells. "myel/o" is a combining form meaning spinal cord. -*cele* is a suffix meaning hernia or protrusion.
8-63	the _____ meninges or membrane around the nerve cells combining form spinal cord suffix, hernia protrusion	mening/o is a combining form referring to _____ _____ ____ _____ _____ _____ _____ _____ . "myel/o" is a _____ _____ meaning _____ _____ . -*cele* is a _____ meaning _____ or _____ .
8-64	Meningomyelocele	_____ is protrusion of the meninges and spinal cord through a defect in the vertebrae.

BLOCK	DATA AND ANSWERS	DESCRIPTIONS AND QUESTIONS
8-65	myelomalacia (mi′-el-o-mah-la′-se-ah)	Myelomalacia is a softening of the spinal cord. "myel/o" is a combining form meaning spinal cord. *-malacia* is a suffix meaning softening.
8-66	Myelomalacia *-malacia* combining form spinal cord	_____ is a softening of the spinal cord. _____ is a suffix meaning softening. "myel/o" is a _____ _____ meaning _____ _____.
8-67	myelogram (mi-el-o-gram)	A myelogram is a record (X-ray film) of the spinal cord. *-gram* is a suffix meaning record (here, X-ray film).
8-68	myelogram suffix, record (X-ray film) spinal cord	A _____ is a record (X-ray film) of the spinal cord. *-gram* is a _____ meaning _____ _____ _____. "myel/o" is a combining form meaning _____ _____.
8-69	neuroma (nu-ro-mah′) neurectomy (nu′-rek-to-me)	The next few blocks cover medical terms related to nerve cells in general. A neuroma is a tumor of the nerve cells. Neurectomy is excision of a nerve. "neur" is a word root for nerve. "neur/o" is a combining form meaning nerves. *-oma* is a suffix meaning tumor. *-ectomy* is a suffix meaning removal or excision.

BLOCK	DATA AND ANSWERS	DESCRIPTIONS AND QUESTIONS
8-70	"neur/o"	_____ is a combining form meaning nerves.
	-oma	_____ is a suffix meaning tumor.
	-ectomy	_____ is a suffix meaning removal or excision.
	neuroma	A _____ is a tumor of the nerve cells.
	Neurectomy	_____ is excision of a nerve.
8-71		-plasty is a suffix meaning plastic repair.
		Build a medical term meaning plastic repair of a nerve:
	neuroplasty	_____
	(nu'-ro-plas-te)	_____
8-72		-rrhaphy is a suffix meaning suture.
		Build a medical term meaning suture of a nerve:
	neurorrhaphy	_____
	(nu'-ro-raf'-e)	_____
8-73	neurotripsy (nu'-ro-trip-se)	Neurotripsy is surgical crushing of a nerve.
		-tripsy is a suffix meaning crushing (surgical).
8-74	"neur/o"	_____ is a combining form meaning nerve.
	-tripsy	_____ is a suffix meaning crushing.
	-plasty	_____ is a suffix meaning plastic repair.
	-rrhaphy	_____ is a suffix meaning suture.
8-75	neurasthenia (nu-ras-the'-ne-ah)	Neurasthenia is exhaustion (without strength) of the nerves.
		-asthenia is a suffix meaning exhaustion.

BLOCK	DATA AND ANSWERS	DESCRIPTIONS AND QUESTIONS
8-76	combining form nerve suffix exhaustion (without strength) exhaustion (without strength) of the nerves	"neur/o" is a _____ _____ meaning _____. -*asthenia* is a _____ meaning _____ _____ _____. Neurasthenia is _____ _____ _____ ___ _____ _____.
8-77		All of our senses (thinking, sight, touch, smell, taste, feeling, and others) are at least partially controlled by our nervous system (brain, spinal cords, and nerve cells). There are hundreds of medical terms associated with the nervous system and our senses. The next few blocks present some of these medical terms related to our brain, our mind, and our senses.
8-78	psychopathy (<u>si</u>-kop-ah'-the)	Psychopathy is disease of the mind. "psych" is a word root meaning mind. "psych/o" is a combining form meaning mind. -*pathy* is a suffix meaning disease.
8-79	Psychopathy "psych/o" -*pathy*	_____ is disease of the mind. _____ is a combining form meaning mind. _____ is a suffix meaning disease.

BOX 8.1
Allied Health Professions

Physical Therapists, Physical Therapist Assistants, and Aides

Physical therapists provide services that help restore function, improve mobility, relieve pain, and prevent or limit permanent physical disabilities. They restore, maintain, and promote overall fitness and health. Their patients include accident victims and individuals with disabling conditions such as lower-back pain, arthritis, heart disease, fractures, head injuries, and cerebral palsy.

Therapists examine patients' medical histories and then test and measure the patients' strength, range of motion, balance and coordination, posture, muscle performance, respiration, and motor function. Next, physical therapists develop plans describing a treatment strategy and its anticipated outcome.

Physical therapist assistants and aides help physical therapists to provide treatment that improves patient mobility, relieves pain, and prevents or lessens physical disabilities of patients. A physical therapist might ask an assistant to help patients exercise or learn to use crutches, for example, or ask an aide to gather and prepare therapy equipment. Patients include accident victims and individuals with disabling conditions such as lower-back pain, arthritis, heart disease, fractures, head injuries, and cerebral palsy.

Physical therapist assistants perform a variety of tasks. Under the direction and supervision of physical therapists, they provide part of a patient's treatment. This might involve exercises, massages, electrical stimulation, paraffin baths, hot and cold packs, traction, and ultrasound. Physical therapist assistants record the patient's responses to treatment and report the outcome of each treatment to the physical therapist.

Physical therapist aides help make therapy sessions productive under the direct supervision of a physical therapist or physical therapist assistant. They usually are responsible for keeping the treatment area clean and organized and for preparing for each patient's therapy. When patients need assistance moving to or from a treatment area, aides push them in a wheelchair or provide them with a shoulder to lean on. Physical therapist aides are not licensed and do not perform the clinical tasks of a physical therapist assistant in states where licensure is required.

The duties of aides include some clerical tasks, such as ordering depleted supplies, answering the phone, and filling out insurance forms and other paperwork. The extent to which an aide or an assistant performs clerical tasks depends on the size and location of the facility.

A great resource is the American Physical Therapy Association at www.apta.org.

Source: P. S. Stanfield, N. Cross, Y. H. Hui, eds. *Introduction to the Health Professions,* 5th ed. (Sudbury, MA: Jones & Bartlett, 2009).

BLOCK	DATA AND ANSWERS	DESCRIPTIONS AND QUESTIONS
8-80	psychology (si-kol-o-je)	Psychology is the study of the mind (mental processes and behavior).
	psychologist (si-kol-o-jist)	A psychologist is a specialist who studies the mind (mental processes and behavior).
		"psych/o" is a combining form meaning mind.
		-logy is a suffix meaning study of.
		-logist is a suffix meaning a person or specialist.
8-81	psychologist	A _____ is a specialist engaged in the study of the mind.
	Psychology	_____ is the study of the mind (mental processes and behavior).
	"psych/o"	_____ is a combining form meaning mind.
	suffix, study of	*-logy* is a _____ meaning _____ _____.
	-logist	_____ is a suffix meaning a person or specialist.
8-82	psychosis (si-ko-sis)	Psychosis is a disorder of the mind, or psychiatric disorder.
		-osis is a suffix meaning condition. The condition can be normal or abnormal.
8-83	combining form mind	"psych/o" is a _____ _____ meaning _____.
	suffix, condition	*-osis* is a _____ meaning _____.
	a disorder of the mind, or psychiatric disorder	Psychosis is ___ _____ _____ _____ _____, _____ _____ _____.

BLOCK	DATA AND ANSWERS	DESCRIPTIONS AND QUESTIONS
8-84	psychiatry (si-ki-ah-tre)	*-iatry* is a suffix meaning healing or treatment. Build a medical term meaning the branch of medicine that deals with the treatment of mental disorders: _____ _____
8-85	psychosomatic (si-ko-so-mat′-ik) "psych/o" "somat/o" *-ic* Psychosomatic	Psychosomatic means pertaining to the body and mind. "psych/o" is a combining form meaning mind. "somat/o" is a combining form meaning body. *-ic* is a suffix meaning pertaining to. _____ is a combining form meaning mind. _____ is a combining form meaning body. _____ is a suffix meaning pertaining to. _____ is pertaining to the body and mind.
8-86	psychogenic (si-ko-jen′-ik)	Psychogenic means originating within the mind. *-genic* is a suffix meaning originating within.
8-87	combining form mind suffix, originating within originating within the mind	"psych/o" is a _____ _____ meaning _____. *-genic* is a _____ meaning _____ _____. Psychogenic is _____ _____ _____ _____.
8-88	psychotherapy (si-ko-ther′-ah-pe)	"therapy" is a root word meaning treatment. *-therapy* is a suffix meaning treatment. Build a medical term meaning treatment of mental disease: _____ _____

BLOCK	DATA AND ANSWERS	DESCRIPTIONS AND QUESTIONS
8-89	phrenic (<u>fren</u>-ik)	Phrenic means pertaining to the mind.
		"phren" is a word root meaning the mind.
		"phren/o" is a combining form meaning mind.
		-*ic* is a suffix meaning pertaining to.
8-90	"phren/o"	_____ is a combining form meaning mind.
	-*ic*	_____ is a suffix meaning pertaining to.
	Phrenic	_____ is pertaining to the mind.
8-91		"phren/o" is a combining form meaning mind.
		-*pathy* is a suffix meaning disease.
		Build a medical term meaning mental disease:
	phrenopathy	_____
	(fren'-<u>op</u>-ah-the)	_____
8-92	amentia (ah'-<u>men</u>-te-ah)	Amentia is mental deficiency.
		a- is a prefix meaning without or lack of.
		"ment" is a root word meaning the mind.
		"ment/o" is a combining form meaning the mind.
		-*ia* is a suffix meaning pertaining to.
8-93	*a*-	___ is a prefix meaning without or lack of.
	"ment/o"	_____ is a combining form meaning the mind.
	-*ia*	_____ is a suffix meaning pertaining to.
	Amentia	_____ is mental deficiency.

BLOCK	DATA AND ANSWERS	DESCRIPTIONS AND QUESTIONS
8-94	bradyphrenia	*brady-* is a prefix meaning slow. "phrenia" is a root word meaning mind. *-phrenia* also is a suffix. A person whose thinking processes are very slow would have a condition known as _____.
8-95	oligophrenia (ol'-ig-o-fren-e-ah) combining form little, scanty, defective suffix, mind	Oligophrenia is little (defective) mental development. "olig/o" is a combining form meaning little, scanty, or defective. *oligo-* also is a prefix. *-phrenia* is a suffix meaning the mind. "olig/o" is a _____ _____ meaning _____, _____, or _____. *-phrenia* is a _____ meaning _____.
8-96	defective mental development	Oligophrenia is _____ _____ _____.
8-97	egomania (e-'go-ma-ne-ah)	"ego" is a word root meaning self-interest, self-importance, and so on. "eg/o" is a combining form meaning self-interest. *ego-* also is a prefix. *-mania* is a suffix meaning excited state or obsession. Build a medical term meaning obsessed (abnormal) self-interest: _____ _____

BLOCK	DATA AND ANSWERS	DESCRIPTIONS AND QUESTIONS
8-98	dipsomania (dip'-so-<u>ma</u>-ne-ah)	"dips/o" is a combining form meaning thirst. -*mania* is a suffix meaning excited state or obsession. Build a medical term meaning obsessed (uncontrollable) thirst: _____ _____
8-99	megalomania (meg'-ah-lo-<u>ma</u>-ne-ah)	"megal" is a word root meaning large. "megal/o" is a combining form meaning large. -*mania* is a suffix meaning excited state or obsession. Build a medical term meaning delusions of grandeur or obsession with one's own importance: _____ _____
8-100	schizophrenia (skit'-so-<u>fren</u>-e-ah)	Schizophrenia is a major psychosis or mental disorder, characterized by abnormalities in the perception or expression of reality. "schiz" is a word root meaning split. "schiz/o" is a combining form meaning split. -*phrenia* is a suffix meaning mind.
8-101	combining form split -*phrenia*, suffix	"schiz/o" is a _____ _____ meaning _____. _____ is a _____ meaning the mind.
8-102	a major psychosis or mental disorder characterized by abnormalities in the perception or expression of reality	Schizophrenia is ___ _____ _____ _____ _____ _____, _____ _____ _____ _____ _____ _____ _____ _____ _____ _____.

BLOCK	DATA AND ANSWERS	DESCRIPTIONS AND QUESTIONS
8-103	hyperkinesis (hi'-per-<u>kin</u>-e-sis)	Hyperkinesis is excessive movement. *hyper-* is a prefix meaning excessive. *-kinesis* is a suffix meaning movement.
8-104	*hyper-* *-kinesis* Hyperkinesis	_____ is a prefix meaning excessive. _____ is a suffix meaning movement. _____ is excessive movement.
8-105	photophobia (fo'-to-<u>fo</u>-be-ah)	Photophobia is abnormal sensitivity to light. "phot/o" is a combining form meaning light. *photo-* also is a prefix. *-phobia* is a suffix meaning persistent, irrational fear.
8-106	"phot/o" *-phobia*	_____ is a combining form meaning light. _____ is a suffix meaning persistent, irrational fear.
8-107	Photophobia	_____ is abnormal sensitivity to light.
8-108	narcolepsy (nar-<u>ko</u>-lep'-se)	"narc/o" is a combining form meaning sleep. *-lepsy* is a suffix meaning seizure. Build a medical term meaning seized by sudden episodes of sleep: _____ _____
8-109	echolalia	ech/o is a combining form meaning sounds or repetitive sounds. *-lalia* is a suffix meaning talk. Build a medical term meaning repetition of talk (words): _____

BLOCK	DATA AND ANSWERS	DESCRIPTIONS AND QUESTIONS
8-110	dysphasia (dis′-fa̲-se-ah)	*dys-* is a prefix meaning difficulty. *-phasia* is a suffix meaning speech. Build a medical term meaning difficulty in speech: _____ _____
8-111	prefix, difficulty suffix, speech	*dys-* is a _____ meaning _____. *-phasia* is a _____ meaning _____.
8-112	aphasia (ah′-fa̲-se-ah)	Aphasia is loss or impairment of the ability to speak. *a-* is a prefix meaning none or lack of. *-phasia* is a suffix meaning speech.
8-113	*a*, prefix *-phasia*, suffix	___ is a _____ meaning none or lack of. _____ is a _____ meaning speech.
8-114	loss or impairment of the ability to speak	Aphasia is _____ _____ _____ _____ _____ _____ _____ _____.
8-115	anesthesia (an′-es-the̲-se-ah)	Anesthesia means a lack of feeling or sensation. *an-* is a prefix meaning without. "esthes" is a word root for sensation. "esthes/o" is a combining form meaning sensation. *-ia* is a suffix meaning condition. *-esthesia* also can be used as a suffix.
8-116	*an-*, prefix "esthes/o," combining form *-ia*, suffix	_____ is a _____ meaning without. _____ is a _____ _____ meaning sensation. _____ is a _____ meaning condition.
8-117	a lack of feeling or sensation	Anesthesia is ___ _____ _____ _____ _____ _____.

BLOCK	DATA AND ANSWERS	DESCRIPTIONS AND QUESTIONS
8-118	hyperesthesia (hi'-per-es-the-se-ah)	Hyperesthesia is excessive sensitivity.
8-119	hyper- "esthes/o" -ia	_____ is a prefix meaning higher or excessive. _____ is a combining form meaning sensation. _____ is a suffix meaning condition.
8-120	excessive sensitivity	Hyperesthesia is _____ _____.
8-121		**Table 8.1** summarizes the word components you have learned in this chapter about the nervous system. The next chapter focuses on the genitourinary system.

TABLE 8.1   Word Components in this Chapter

WORD ROOTS	COMBINING FORMS	PREFIXES
centesis	cephal/o	a-
cephal	cerebell/o	an-
cerebell	cerebr/o	brady-
cerebr	crani/o	dys-
crani	dips/o	echo-
cranium	ech/o	ego-
dip	eg/o	hydro-
ech	electr/o	hyper-
ego	encephal/o	oligo-
electr	esthes/o	photo-
encephal	hydr/o	SUFFIXES
esthes	lamin/o	-al
hydr	lob/o	-algia
lamin	megal/o	-asthenia
lamina	mening/o	-cele
lob	meningi/o	-centesis
lobe	ment/o	-ectomy
megal	myel/o	-esthesia
mening	narc/o	-genic

TABLE 8.1   Word Components in this Chapter (continued)

WORD ROOTS	COMBINING FORMS	SUFFIXES
meningi	neur/o	-gram
ment	olig/o	-graph
myel	phot/o	-graphy
neur	phren/o	-ia
olig	pneum/o	-iatry
photo	poli/o	-ic
phrenia	psych/o	-itis
poli	rachi/o	-kinesis
polio	schiz/o	-lalia
psych	scler/o	-lepsy
rachi	somat/o	-logist
schiz	vascul/o	-logy
scler	ventricul/o	-malacia
somat		-mania
vascul		-oma
ventricul		-osis
		-pathy
		-phasia
		-phobia
		-phrenia
		-plasty
		-rrhaphy
		-schisis
		-sclerosis
		-tripsy
		-therapy

BOX 8.2
Abbreviations

ANS	autonomic nervous system
CNS	central nervous system
CT	computerized tomography
EEG	electroencephalogram
ICP	intracranial pressure
MRI	magnetic resonance imaging
MS	multiple sclerosis
PNS	peripheral nervous system
REM	rapid eye movement
RT	reading test
SNS	somatic nervous system
TIA	transient ischemic attack

Progress Check

A. Multiple Choice

1. A word root meaning sensation is:
   a. meninges
   b. esthesia
   c. epiglott
   d. mast

2. A word root meaning lower back part of the brain is:
   a. cephal
   b. lobe
   c. dent
   d. cerebell

3. A word root meaning the mind is:
   a. ment
   b. meta
   c. melan
   d. medi

4. A word root meaning hardening is:
   a. lumb
   b. cycl
   c. scler
   d. blephar

5. A combining form meaning skull is:
   a. fibul/o
   b. odont/o
   c. crani/o
   d. cry/o

6. A combining form meaning the posterior arch of a vertebra is:
   a. lamin/o
   b. leiomy/o
   c. kerat/o
   d. ichthy/o

7. A combining form meaning the brain covering is:
   a. sarc/o
   b. xanth/o
   c. steth/o
   d. mening/o

8. A prefix meaning slow is:
   a. diplo-
   b. brady-
   c. dacry-
   d. sym-

9. A prefix meaning sound is:
   a. echo-
   b. ambi-
   c. ecto-
   d. medi-

10. A suffix meaning speech is:
    a. -rrhexia
    b. -ptosis
    c. -plasia
    d. -phasia

11. A suffix meaning seizure is:
    a. -y
    b. -lepsy
    c. -tocia
    d. -spasm

12. A suffix meaning splitting is:
    a. -blast
    b. -ar
    c. -schisis
    d. -stasis

13. A suffix meaning exhaustion (without strength) is:
    a. -asthenia
    b. -taxia
    c. -arche
    d. -crine

B. Building Medical Terms

Use the following word components to build medical terms matching the definitions given.

an-	esthes	mening/o
cele	esthes/o	myel/o
-cele	-gram	myel
cephal	hydro	narc
cephal/o	-ia	narc/o
dips/o	-lepsy	-phasia
dys-	-malacia	-schisis
encephal	-mania	ventricul
encephal/o	mening	ventricul/o

1. difficulty in speech

2. herniation of the meninges and brain substance

3. softening of the brain

4. birth defect in an infant with no cerebral hemispheres and cranial vault

5. water in a herniation (a sac) of the spinal cord

6. X-ray film of the cerebral ventricles

7. obsessed with thirst

8. lack of feeling or sensation

9. cleft in the spinal cord

10. condition seized by sudden episodes of sleep

C. Definitions and Word Components

	TERM	DEFINITION	PREFIX	WORD ROOT	VOWEL	WORD ROOT	VOWEL	SUFFIX
1.	encephalo-sclerosis							
2.	cephalalgia							
3.	electro-encephalogram							
4.	rachiomyelitis							
5.	oligophrenia							
6.	myelo-meningocele							
7.	hyperesthesia							
8.	schizophrenia							
9.	poliomyelitis							
10.	psychosomatic							

D. Abbreviations

	ABBREVIATION	MEANING
1.	ANS	
2.	CNS	
3.	CT	
4.	EEG	
5.	ICP	
6.	MRI	
7.	MS	
8.	PNS	
9.	REM	
10.	RT	
11.	SNS	
12.	TIA	

The Genitourinary System

BLOCK	DATA AND ANSWERS	DESCRIPTIONS AND QUESTIONS
9-1		This chapter is divided into two segments. The first segment studies the urinary system. The second segment studies the male and female genital systems. See **Figure 9.1** and **Figure 9.2**.
	urinary (u-<u>rih</u>-nah′-re) renal (<u>ren</u>-al), pelvis (<u>pal</u>-viss), ureters (u′-<u>re</u>-tars), urethra (u′-<u>re</u>-thrah), nephron (<u>ne</u>-fron)	The urinary system consists of two kidneys, the renal pelvis, two ureters, one bladder, and one urethra, in that order. Within the kidney, the nephron is the structural and functional unit. The upper part of the ureters is an expanded area known as the renal pelvis, leading from the kidney into the ureters. Check the figures for exact locations and supporting structures.
9-2		"ren" and "nephr" are both root words meaning kidney.
		"ren/o" and "nephr/o" are the combining forms.
		"pelvis" is a root word meaning pelvis.
		"pyel/o" is a combining form meaning renal pelvis.
9-3	"ren/o," "nephr/o"	_____ and _____ are both combining forms meaning kidney.
	"pyel/o"	_____ is a combining form meaning renal pelvis.
9-4	urinary (u-<u>rih</u>-nah′-re)	Urinary means pertaining to urine.
		"ur/o" and "urin/o" are combining forms meaning urine.
		-ary is a suffix meaning pertaining to.

BLOCK	DATA AND ANSWERS	DESCRIPTIONS AND QUESTIONS
9-5	"ur/o," "urin/o"	_____ and _____ are combining forms meaning urine.
	-*ary*, suffix	_____ is a _____ meaning pertaining to.
	Urinary	_____ means pertaining to urine.
9-6		The urinary tract forms urine from waste in the blood and eliminates it from the body.
	urology (u'-<u>rol</u>-o-je)	Urology is the branch of medicine related to the male and female urinary tract and male genital system.
		-*logy* is a suffix meaning the study of.

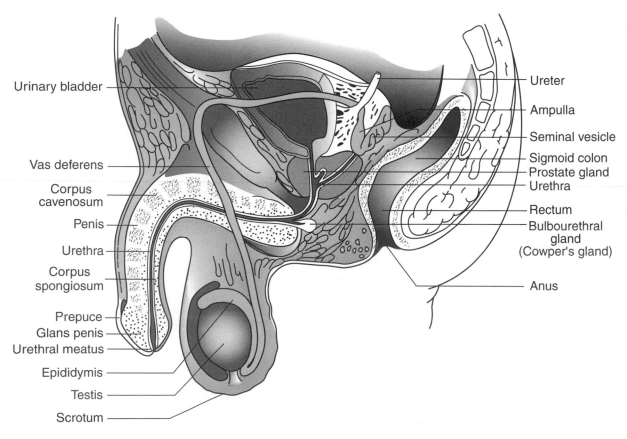

FIGURE 9.1   The male genitourinary system

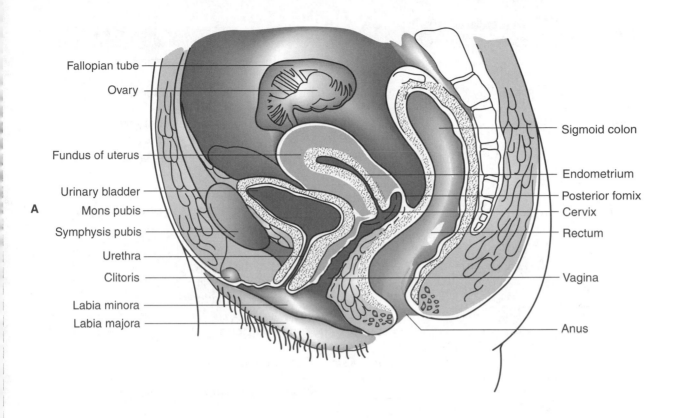

A

Fallopian tube
Ovary
Fundus of uterus
Urinary bladder
Mons pubis
Symphysis pubis
Urethra
Clitoris
Labia minora
Labia majora

Sigmoid colon
Endometrium
Posterior fomix
Cervix
Rectum
Vagina
Anus

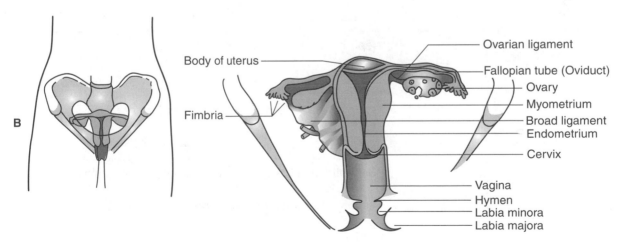

B

Body of uterus
Fimbria

Ovarian ligament
Fallopian tube (Oviduct)
Ovary
Myometrium
Broad ligament
Endometrium
Cervix
Vagina
Hymen
Labia minora
Labia majora

FIGURE 9.2   The female genitourinary system

BLOCK	DATA AND ANSWERS	DESCRIPTIONS AND QUESTIONS
9-7		*-logist* is a suffix meaning a person who specializes.
	urologist (u'-<u>rol</u>-o-jist)	A urologist is a physician specializing in urology.
9-8	Urology	_____ is the study of the urinary tract.
		A person who specializes in the study of the urinary tract is a
	urologist	_____.
9-9		Our first group of medical terms relates to physiology and disorders of the kidney.
	nephroma (ne-<u>fro</u>-mah')	A nephroma is a tumor of the kidney.
		"nephr" is a word root meaning kidney.
		"nephr/o" is the combining form.
		-oma is a suffix meaning tumor.
9-10	"nephr"	_____ is a word root meaning kidney.
	"nephr/o"	_____ is the combining form.
	-oma	_____ is a suffix meaning tumor.
	nephroma	A _____ is a tumor of the kidney.
9-11	nephritis (ne-<u>fri</u>-tis')	Nephritis is inflammation of the kidney.
	"nephr/o"	_____ is a combining form meaning kidney.
	-itis	_____ is a suffix meaning inflammation.
	Nephritis	_____ is inflammation of the kidney.
9-12	nephrolithiasis (nef'-ro-<u>lith</u>-i-ah-sis)	Nephrolithiasis is a condition of stone(s) in the kidney.
		"nephr/o" is a combining form meaning kidney.
		"lith" is a root word meaning stone.
		"lith/o" is the combining form.
		-iasis is a suffix meaning condition. The condition can be normal or abnormal.

BLOCK	DATA AND ANSWERS	DESCRIPTIONS AND QUESTIONS
9-13	combining form kidney	"nephr/o" is a _____ _____ meaning _____.
	combining form stone	"lith/o" is a _____ _____ meaning _____.
	suffix, condition	-iasis is a _____ meaning _____.
	condition of stone(s) in the kidney	Nephrolithiasis is a _____ _____ _____ ___ _____ _____.
9-14		"lith/o" is a combining form meaning stone.
		-tripsy is a suffix meaning surgical crushing.
		Build a medical term (with pronunciation) meaning surgical
	lithotripsy (lith-o-<u>trip</u>-se)	crushing of a stone: _____ _____
9-15	hydronephrosis (hi'-dro- <u>nef</u>-ro-sis)	Hydronephrosis is distention of part of the kidney. (The kidney is distended because of the buildup of urine due to a blockage in the normal disposal route.)
		hydro- is a prefix meaning water (here referring to urine).
		"nephr/o" is a combining form meaning kidney.
		-osis is a suffix meaning condition. The condition can be normal or abnormal.
9-16	hydro-	_____ is a prefix meaning water (urine).
	kidney	"nephr/o" is a combining form meaning _____.
	-osis	_____ is a suffix meaning condition.
	Hydronephrosis	_____ is distention of the kidney.
9-17		-trophy is a suffix meaning development.
		hyper- is a prefix meaning over or excessive.

BLOCK	DATA AND ANSWERS	DESCRIPTIONS AND QUESTIONS
9-18	*hyper-*	_____ is a prefix meaning over or excessive.
	"nephr/o"	_____ is a combining form meaning kidney.
	-trophy	_____ is a suffix meaning development.
		Build a medical term meaning overdevelopment of the kidney:
	nephrohypertrophy (nef-ro-<u>hi</u>-per′-tro-fe)	_____ _____
9-19	nephromegaly (nef′-ro-<u>meg</u>-ah-le)	Nephromegaly is enlargement of a kidney. *-megaly* is a suffix meaning enlargement.
9-20	"nephr/o"	_____ is a combining form meaning kidney.
	-megaly	_____ is a suffix meaning enlargement.
	Nephromegaly	_____ is enlargement of a kidney.
9-21	nephrolysis (nef′-ro-<u>li</u>-sis)	Nephrolysis is the separating (breaking up) of the kidney (from other body structures). *-lysis* is a suffix meaning separation (breaking up) of.
9-22	"nephr/o"	_____ is a combining form meaning kidney.
	-lysis	_____ is a suffix meaning separation.
	Nephrolysis	_____ is the separation or breaking up of the kidney.
9-23	nephrostomy (nef-<u>ros</u>-to′-me)	Nephrostomy is the creation of an artificial opening into the kidney. "nephr/o" is a combining form meaning the kidney. *-stomy* is a suffix meaning creating an (artificial) opening.
	"nephr/o"	_____ is a combining form meaning kidney.
	-stomy	_____ is a suffix meaning opening.
	Nephrostomy	_____ is the creation of an artificial opening into the kidney.

BLOCK	DATA AND ANSWERS	DESCRIPTIONS AND QUESTIONS
9-24	nephropexy (nef-ro-<u>peks</u>-e)	Nephropexy is (surgical) fixation of the kidney. *-pexy* is a suffix meaning fixation.
9-25	combining form kidney suffix, fixation surgical fixation of the kidney	"nephr/o" is a _____ _____ meaning _____. *-pexy* is a _____ meaning _____. Nephropexy is _____ _____ _____ _____ _____.
9-26	nephrectomy (nef-<u>rek</u>-to'-me) suffix, excision excision of a kidney	Nephrectomy is the excision of a kidney. *-ectomy* is a _____ meaning _____. Nephrectomy is _____ _____ __ _____.
9-27	pyelonephritis (pi'-el-o-nef-<u>ri</u>-tis)	We have finished with the kidney, which passes the waste fluid into the ureters (which lead to the bladder). Between the kidney and the ureter is an expanded part of the ureter known as the renal pelvis. Pyelonephritis is inflammation of the renal pelvis and the kidney. The term contains two root words and combining forms, so it is a compound word. "pyel/o" is a combining form meaning renal pelvis. "nephr/o" is a combining form meaning kidney. *-itis* is a suffix meaning inflammation.

BLOCK	DATA AND ANSWERS	DESCRIPTIONS AND QUESTIONS
9-28	"pyel/o" "nephr/o" -*itis* Pyelonephritis	_____ is a combining form meaning renal pelvis. _____ is a combining form meaning kidney. _____ is a suffix meaning inflammation. _____ is inflammation of the renal pelvis and the kidney.
9-29	pyelitis (pi′-el-i-tis)	Pyelitis is inflammation of the renal pelvis. "pyel/o" is a combining form referring to the renal pelvis. -*itis* is a suffix meaning inflammation.
9-30	Pyelitis combining form renal pelvis suffix inflammation	_____ is inflammation of the renal pelvis. "pyel/o" is a _____ _____ meaning _____ _____. -*itis* is a _____ meaning _____.
9-31	pyelolithotomy (pi-el-o-litho-to′-me)	A pyelolithotomy is an incision to remove a stone from the renal pelvis. "pyel/o" is a combining form referring to the renal pelvis. "lith" is a root word meaning stone. "lith/o" is a combining form meaning stone. -*tomy* is a suffix meaning incision.
9-32	"pyel/o" "lith/o" -*tomy* Pyelolithotomy	_____ is a combining form meaning renal pelvis. _____ is a combining form meaning stone. _____ is a suffix meaning incision. _____ is an incision to remove a stone from the renal pelvis.

BLOCK	DATA AND ANSWERS	DESCRIPTIONS AND QUESTIONS
9-33	pyelostomy (pi̲-el-os′-to-me) "pyel/o" -stomy	Pyelostomy is creation of an artificial opening in the renal pelvis. -stomy is a suffix meaning creating an (artificial) opening. _____ is a combining form meaning renal pelvis. _____ is a suffix meaning artificial opening.
9-34	Pyelostomy	_____ is creation of an artificial opening in the renal pelvis.
9-35	pyeloplasty (pi′-el-o-plas̲-te) Pyeloplasty -plasty	Pyeloplasty is plastic repair of the renal pelvis. -plasty is a suffix meaning plastic repair. _____ is plastic repair of the renal pelvis. _____ is a suffix meaning plastic repair.
9-36		The renal pelvis leads into the ureters, which are the tubes leading from the renal pelvis to the bladder.
9-37	ureteritis (u′-re-te-ri̲-tis) Ureteritis	Ureteritis is inflammation of the ureter(s). "ureter" is a root word meaning ureter. -itis is a suffix meaning inflammation. _____ is inflammation of the ureter.
9-38	ureterostenosis (u′-re-ter-o-sten̲-o-sis)	Ureterostenosis is narrowing of the ureter(s). "ureter/o" is a combining form meaning ureter. "sten/o" is a combining form meaning narrowing. -osis is a suffix meaning condition.
9-39	"ureter/o" narrowing -osis Ureterostenosis	_____ is a combining form meaning ureter. "sten/o" is a combining form meaning _____. _____ is a suffix meaning condition. _____ is narrowing of the ureter.

BLOCK	DATA AND ANSWERS	DESCRIPTIONS AND QUESTIONS
9-40	ureterotomy (u'-re-ter-<u>ot</u>-to-me)	Ureterotomy is incision of a ureter.
		"ureter/o" is a combining form meaning ureter.
		-*tomy* is a suffix meaning incision.
	Ureterotomy	_____ is incision of a ureter.
9-41	"ureter/o"	_____ is a combining form meaning ureter.
	incision	-*tomy* is a suffix meaning _____.
9-42	ureterectomy (u'-re-te-<u>rek</u>-to-me)	Ureterectomy is excision of a ureter.
		-*ectomy* is a suffix meaning excision.
	excision of the ureter	Ureterectomy is _____ _____ _____ _____.
	-*ectomy*, suffix	_____ is a _____ meaning excision.
9-43		The ureters lead into the bladder. We will now concentrate on the medical terms for the bladder.
9-44		"cyst" is a root word meaning bladder (urinary). It means a fluid-filled sac.
		"cyst/o" is the combining form.
		"vesic" is another root word for bladder.
		"vesic/o" is the combining form.
	"cyst"	_____ is a root word meaning a fluid-filled sac (bladder).
	"cyst/o," "vesic/o"	_____ and _____ are two combining forms meaning bladder.

BLOCK	DATA AND ANSWERS	DESCRIPTIONS AND QUESTIONS
9-45	cystoplasty (sis'-to-<u>plas</u>-te)	Cystoplasty is plastic repair of the bladder.
		"cyst/o" is a combining form meaning urinary bladder.
		-*plasty* is a suffix meaning plastic repair.
	Cystoplasty	_____ is plastic repair of the bladder.
	"cyst/o," combining form	_____ is a _____ _____ meaning urinary bladder.
	suffix, plastic repair	-*plasty* is a _____ meaning _____ _____.
9-46		"cyst/o" is a combining form meaning urinary bladder.
		-*lith* is a suffix meaning stone.
		Build a medical term meaning stone in the urinary bladder:
	cystolith (<u>sis</u>-to-lith)	_____ _____
9-47	cystocele (<u>sis</u>-to'-sel)	Cystocele is an abnormal condition in which the urinary bladder herniates into the vagina.
		-*cele* is a suffix meaning herniation.
9-48	combining form bladder	"cyst/o" is a _____ _____ meaning _____.
	suffix, herniation	-*cele* is a _____ meaning _____.
	a herniation of the bladder into the vagina	Cystocele is ___ _____ ____ ____ _____ ____ ____ _____.

BLOCK	DATA AND ANSWERS	DESCRIPTIONS AND QUESTIONS
9-49	trachelocystitis (tra'-kel-o-sis-<u>ti</u>-tis)	Trachelocystitis is inflammation of the neck of the urinary bladder. "trachel/o" is a combining form meaning neck. "cyst/o" is a combining form meaning urinary bladder. *-itis* is a suffix meaning inflammation.
	Trachelocystitis	_____ is inflammation of the neck of the bladder.
9-50	"trachel/o," combining form	_____ is a _____ _____ meaning neck.
	combining form	"cyst/o" is a _____ _____ meaning urinary bladder.
	-itis, suffix	_____ is a _____ meaning inflammation.
9-51	vesicotomy (ves'-ih-<u>kot</u>-o-me)	Vesicotomy is incision of the bladder. "vesic/o" is a combining form meaning urinary bladder. *-tomy* is a suffix meaning incision.
9-52	combining form bladder	"vesic/o" is a _____ _____ meaning _____.
	suffix, incision	*-tomy* is a _____ meaning _____.
	incision of the bladder	Vesicotomy is _____ _____ _____ _____.
9-53		"cyst/o" is a combining form meaning urinary bladder. *-tomy* is a suffix meaning incision.
	Cystotomy	_____ is incision of the bladder.
9-54		*-ectomy* is a suffix meaning excision.
	Cystectomy	_____ is excision of the bladder.

BLOCK	DATA AND ANSWERS	DESCRIPTIONS AND QUESTIONS
9-55	cystotrachelotomy (sis'-to-tra-<u>ke</u>-lot-o-me)	Cystotrachelotomy is incision of the neck of the urinary bladder. "cyst/o" is a combining form meaning urinary bladder. "trachel" is a root word meaning neck. "trachel/o" is the combining form. -*tomy* is a suffix meaning incision.
	Cystotrachelotomy	_____ is incision of the neck of the urinary bladder.
9-56	"trachel"	_____ is a root word meaning neck.
	incision	-*tomy* is a suffix meaning _____.
9-57	cystostomy (sis'-<u>tos</u>-to-me)	Cystostomy is the creation of an artificial opening into the bladder.
	"cyst/o"	_____ is a combining form meaning urinary bladder.
	-*stomy*	_____ is a suffix meaning artificial opening.
	Cystostomy	_____ is creation of an artificial opening into the bladder.
9-58	cystorrhaphy (sis'-to-<u>rah</u>-fe)	Cystorrhaphy is suturing or repairing of the bladder.
	combining form bladder	"cyst/o" is a _____ _____ meaning _____.
	suffix, suturing repairing	-*rrhaphy* is a _____ meaning _____ or _____.
	repairing of the bladder	Cystorrhaphy is _____ ____ _____ _____.

BLOCK	DATA AND ANSWERS	DESCRIPTIONS AND QUESTIONS
9-59	urethra (u'-<u>re</u>-thrah)	The urethra carries urine from the ureter to the outside of the human body. "urethr/o" is a combining form meaning urethra.
9-60	urethropexy (u'-re-thro-<u>pek</u>-se) Urethropexy	Urethropexy is surgical fixation of the urethra. -*pexy* is a suffix meaning surgical fixation. _____ is surgical fixation of the urethra.
9-61	urethrostomy (u'-re-thros-<u>to</u>-<u>me</u>) Urethrostomy	Urethrostomy is creation of an artificial opening into the urethra. -*stomy* is a suffix meaning creation of an opening. _____ is creation of an artificial opening into the urethra.
9-62	urethroplasty (u'-re-thro-<u>plas</u>-te)	-*plasty* is a suffix meaning plastic repair. Build a medical term meaning plastic repair of the urethra: _____ _____
9-63	urethrocystitis (u'-re-thro-sis-<u>ti</u>-tis)	Urethrocystitis is a compound word meaning inflammation of the bladder and urethra. "urethr/o" is a combining form meaning urethra. "cyst/o" is a combining form meaning bladder. -*itis* is a suffix meaning inflammation.
9-64	"cyst/o" "urethr/o" -*itis* Urethrocystitis	_____ is a combining form meaning bladder. _____ is a combining form meaning urethra. _____ is a suffix meaning inflammation. _____ is inflammation of the bladder and urethra.

BLOCK	DATA AND ANSWERS	DESCRIPTIONS AND QUESTIONS
9-65		We have finished with the disorders of the organs of the urinary system. Let us turn our attention to the urine and associated clinical conditions.
	dysuria (dis′-u-<u>re</u>-ah)	Dysuria is difficult or painful urination.
		dys- is a prefix meaning painful or difficult.
9-66	prefix, difficult painful	*dys-* is a _____ meaning _____ or _____.
	difficult or painful urination	Dysuria is _____ _____ _____ _____.
9-67	pyuria (pi′-u-<u>re</u>-ah)	Pyuria is pus in the urine.
		"py" is a word root meaning pus.
		"py/o" is the combining form.
	"py/o"	_____ is a combining form meaning pus.
	Pyuria	_____ is pus in the urine.
9-68		There are two word roots referring to urine: "ur" and "urin."
		The corresponding combining forms are "ur/o" and "urin/o."
		-ary is a suffix meaning pertaining to.
	urinary (u-<u>rih</u>-nah′-re)	Select one of the two combining forms and build a medical term meaning pertaining to urine: _____ _____
9-69	uremia (u′-<u>re</u>-me-ah)	Uremia is a disorder in which there is urine in the blood.
		"ur" is a word root meaning urine.
		"ur/o" is the combining form.
		-emia is a suffix meaning condition of the blood.

BLOCK	DATA AND ANSWERS	DESCRIPTIONS AND QUESTIONS
9-70	"ur" *-emia* Uremia	_____ is a word root meaning urine. _____ is a suffix meaning condition of the blood. _____ is a disorder in which there is urine in the blood.
9-71	polyuria (pol'-e-u-<u>re</u>-ah)	Polyuria is a condition of excessive urine. *poly-* is a prefix meaning excessive or much. "ur/o" is a combining form meaning urine. *-ia* is a suffix meaning condition.
9-72	prefix, much excessive combining form urine suffix, condition a condition of excessive urine	*poly-* is a _____ meaning _____ or _____. "ur/o" is a _____ _____ meaning _____. *-ia* is a _____ meaning _____. Polyuria is ___ _____ _____ _____ _____.
9-73	testes (<u>tes</u>-tez) urethra (u-<u>re</u>-thrah), seminal vesicles (<u>sem</u>-ih-nal <u>ves</u>-ik-ulz), scrotum (<u>skro</u>-tum), penis (<u>pe</u>-nis)	Our next topic is the male reproductive system. The anatomy starts with the testes (plural; single, testicle) followed by epididymis, vas deferens, urethra, and seminal vesicles. The accessory (external) organs are the scrotum and penis. The sperm travel the entire path during an ejaculation. The prostate is a gland that elaborates chemical and biochemical substances to facilitate the flow of sperm. See Figure 9.1 for locations and names of specific parts.

BLOCK	DATA AND ANSWERS	DESCRIPTIONS AND QUESTIONS
9-74		"andr" is a word root meaning male.
		"andr/o" is the combining form.
		-pathy is a suffix meaning disease.
		Build a medical term meaning diseases of the male:
	andropathy	_____
	(an-<u>drop</u>-ah-the)	_____
9-75	orchitis (<u>or</u>-ki-tis)	Orchitis is inflammation of the testes.
		"orch," "orchi," and "orchid" are three root words meaning testes.
		"orch/o," "orchi/o," and "orchid/o" are the corresponding combining forms.
		-itis is a suffix meaning inflammation.
9-76	combining form	"orch/o" is a _____ _____ meaning
	testes	_____.
	suffix	*-itis* is a _____ meaning
	inflammation	_____.
	inflammation of the	Orchitis is _____ _____ _____
	testes	_____.
9-77	cryptorchidism (<u>krip</u>-tor-kid'-izm)	Cryptorchidism is a condition in which the testicle (or testes) fails to descend into the scrotum.
		"crypt" is a word root meaning hidden.
		"crypt/o" is the combining form.
		"orchid" is a root word meaning testes.
		"orchid/o" is the combining form.
		-ism is a suffix meaning condition.
		Build a medical term meaning condition of hidden testes:
	cryptorchidism	_____

BLOCK	DATA AND ANSWERS	DESCRIPTIONS AND QUESTIONS
9-78	"crypt/o," combining form	_____ is a _____ _____ meaning hidden.
	testes	"orchid" is a root word meaning _____.
	-ism	_____ is a suffix meaning condition.
9-79	orchidectomy (or′-ki-<u>dek</u>-to-me)	Orchidectomy is excision or surgical removal of one or both testicles.
		"orchid/o" is a combining form meaning testes.
		-ectomy is a suffix meaning excision.
	orchiectomy (or′-ke-<u>ek</u>-to-me)	Orchiectomy is another term meaning excision or surgical removal of one or both testicles.
		"orchi/o" is a combining form meaning testes.
9-80		Name two medical terms that refer to the excision or surgical removal of one or both testicles:
	orchidectomy	1. _____
	orchiectomy	2. _____
	"orchid"	"orchid/o" is the combining form of the root word _____.
	"orchi"	"orchi/o" is a combining form of the root word _____.
	suffix, excision	-ectomy is a _____ meaning _____.
	surgical removal of one or both testes	Orchidectomy or orchiectomy is _____ _____ _____ _____ _____ _____ _____.
9-81		-pexy is a suffix meaning surgical fixation.
		-tomy is a suffix meaning incision.

BLOCK	DATA AND ANSWERS	DESCRIPTIONS AND QUESTIONS
9-82		Give two medical terms that mean surgical fixation of a testicle:
	orchidopexy (or'-kid-o-<u>pek</u>-se)	1. _____ _____
	orchiopexy (or'-ke-<u>o</u>-pek-se)	2. _____ _____
9-83		Give two medical terms that mean incision into a testis:
	orchidotomy (or'-ki-<u>dot</u>-o-me)	1. _____ _____
	orchiotomy (or'-ke-<u>ot</u>-o-me)	2. _____ _____
9-84		From the testes, the sperm travel through ducts to the urethra during an ejaculation. There are two important ducts, the epididymis (a duct looping around the testes) and the vas deferens, which leads into the ejaculatory duct. The seminal vesicles are situated near the location where the vas deferens enters the ejaculatory duct. See Figure 9.1. We will learn the medical terms associated with this path.
9-85	orchiepididymitis (or-ke-ep'-e-did-ih-<u>mi</u>-tis)	Orchiepididymitis is inflammation of the testes and epididymis. "orchi/o" is a combining form meaning testes. "epididym/o" is a combining form meaning epididymis. *-itis* is a suffix meaning inflammation.

BLOCK	DATA AND ANSWERS	DESCRIPTIONS AND QUESTIONS
9-86	combining form testes	"orchi/o" is a _____ _____ meaning _____.
	combining form epididymis	"epididym/o" is a _____ _____ meaning _____.
	suffix inflammation	-itis is a _____ meaning _____.
	inflammation of the testes and epididymis	Orchiepididymitis is _____ _____ _____ _____ _____ _____.
9-87	epididymectomy (ep'-e-did-ih-<u>mek</u>-to-me)	Epididymectomy is excision or surgical removal of the epididymis. -ectomy is a suffix meaning excision.
	"epididym/o"	_____ is a combining form meaning epididymis.
	-ectomy	_____ is a suffix meaning excision.
	Epididymectomy	_____ is excision or surgical removal of the epididymis.
9-88	vasectomy (va-<u>sek</u>-to-me)	Vasectomy is excision or surgical removal of a duct. (In this case, the duct referred to is the vas deferens, which transports sperm from the testes to the ejaculatory duct.) "vas" is a root word meaning duct. "vas/o" is the combining form. -ectomy is a suffix meaning excision.
9-89	Vasectomy	_____ is excision of the vas deferens.
	"vas/o"	_____ is a combining form meaning duct.
	-ectomy	_____ is a suffix meaning excision.

BLOCK	DATA AND ANSWERS	DESCRIPTIONS AND QUESTIONS
9-90		Seminal vesicles are glands that secrete a thick, yellowish fluid, known as seminal fluid, into the vas deferens.
9-91	vesiculectomy (veh'-sik'-u-<u>lek</u>-to-me)	Vesiculectomy is excision or surgical removal of a vesicle (in this case, the seminal vesicles). "vesicul" is a root word meaning a seminal vesicle. "vesicul/o" is the combining form. -*ectomy* is a suffix meaning excision.
9-92	root word seminal vesicles suffix, excision surgical removal surgical removal of the seminal vesicles	"vesicul" is a _____ _____ meaning _____ _____. -*ectomy* is a _____ meaning _____ or _____ _____. Vesiculectomy is _____ _____ ____ _____ _____ _____.
9-93	spermatozoa (sper'-ma-<u>to</u>-zo-ah)	Spermatozoa are mature male germ cells formed in the testes. They are also known as sperm. "spermat/o" is a combining form meaning sperm. -*zoa* (plural) is a suffix meaning lives. -*zoon* (singular) is a suffix meaning life.
9-94	Spermatozoa suffix, lives	_____ are the male sex cells. -*zoa* is a _____ meaning _____.
9-95	spermatolysis (sper'-mah-to-<u>lih</u>-sis)	-*lysis* is a suffix meaning destruction. Build a medical term meaning dissolution (destruction) of sperm: _____ _____

BLOCK	DATA AND ANSWERS	DESCRIPTIONS AND QUESTIONS
9-96	oligospermia (ol'-i-go-sper-me-ah)	Oligospermia is a condition of scanty sperm (in the semen). *oligo-* is a prefix meaning scant or scanty. "sperm/o" is a combining form meaning sperm. *-ia* is a suffix meaning pertaining to.
9-97	*oligo-* "sperm/o" suffix, pertaining to Oligospermia	_____ is a prefix meaning scant or scanty. _____ is a combining form meaning sperm. *-ia* is a _____ meaning _____ ____. _____ is a condition of scanty sperm (in the semen).
9-98	balanoplasty (bah'-lah-no-plas-te)	Our next group of medical terms is related to the penis, the external structure of the male reproductive system. Balanoplasty is surgical or plastic repair of the glans penis. "balan/o" is a combining form meaning glans penis. *-plasty* is a suffix meaning plastic repair.
9-99	surgical repair of the glans penis combining form glans penis suffix, surgical or plastic repair	Balanoplasty is _____ _____ ____ _____ _____ _____. "balan/o" is a _____ _____ meaning _____ _____. *-plasty* is a _____ meaning _____ ____ _____ _____.
9-100	balanorrhea (bah'-lah-no-re-ah)	*-rrhea* is a suffix meaning discharge. Build a medical word that means discharge from the glans penis: _____ _____

BLOCK	DATA AND ANSWERS	DESCRIPTIONS AND QUESTIONS
9-101	balanitis (bal´-ah-<u>ni</u>-tis)	*-itis* is a suffix meaning inflammation. Build a medical term meaning inflammation of the glans penis: _____ _____
9-102	prostatorrhea (pros´-tat-or-<u>re</u>-ah)	The remaining blocks dealing with the male reproductive system discuss medical terms affecting the prostate glands. The prostate glands are structures near the base of the urethra where ejaculation occurs. They manufacture and secrete substances to facilitate sperm flow. Prostatorrhea is discharge from the prostate. "prostat/o" is a combining form meaning prostate. *-rrhea* is a suffix meaning discharge.
9-103	"prostat/o" *-rrhea*	_____ is a combining form meaning prostate gland. _____ is a suffix meaning discharge.
9-104	prostatitis (pros´-tah-<u>ti</u>-tis)	*-itis* is a suffix meaning inflammation. Build a medical term meaning inflammation of the prostate gland: _____ _____
9-105	prostatocystitis (pros´-tah-to-sis-<u>ti</u>-tis)	Prostatocystitis is inflammation of the prostate gland and urinary bladder. "prostat/o" is a combining form meaning prostate gland. "cyst/o" is a combining form meaning urinary bladder. *-itis* is a suffix meaning inflammation.
9-106	Prostatocystitis	_____ is inflammation of the prostate gland and urinary bladder.

BLOCK	DATA AND ANSWERS	DESCRIPTIONS AND QUESTIONS
9-107	prostatovesiculitis (pros'-tah-to-ves-i-ku-<u>li</u>-tis)	Prostatovesiculitis is inflammation of the prostate gland and (seminal) vesicles. "prostat/o" is a combining form meaning prostate gland. "vesicul/o" is a combining form meaning vesicles (seminal). -*itis* is a suffix meaning inflammation.
9-108	"prostat/o," combining form combining form vesicles (seminal) -*itis*	_____ is a _____ _____ meaning prostate gland. "vesicul/o" is a _____ _____ meaning _____ _____. _____ is a suffix meaning inflammation.
9-109	Prostatovesiculitis	_____ is inflammation of the prostate gland and seminal vesicles.
9-110	prostatolithotomy (pros'-tat-o-<u>lith</u>-o-to-me)	Prostatolithotomy is incision in the prostate gland to remove a stone. "prostat/o" is a combining form meaning prostate gland. "lith" is a root word meaning stone. -*tomy* is a suffix meaning incision.
9-111	"prostat/o" "lith" -*tomy*	_____ is a combining form meaning prostate. _____ is a root word meaning stone. _____ is a suffix meaning incision.
9-112	prostatolith (pros'-tat-<u>o</u>-lith)	Build a medical term meaning stone in the prostate: _____ _____

BLOCK	DATA AND ANSWERS	DESCRIPTIONS AND QUESTIONS
9-113	ovaries (o′-<u>vah</u>-rez), fallopian tubes (fah′-lo-pe-an tubz), uterus (<u>u</u>-ter-us), vagina (vah-<u>ji</u>-nah), vulva (<u>vul</u>-vah)	We have completed our discussion of the male reproductive system. We now turn to the female reproductive system. The female reproductive system consists of two ovaries, two fallopian tubes, the uterus, the vagina, the vulva (external genitalia), and two breasts. See Figure 9.2 for location and names of specific parts. The breasts do not play a role in the reproductive process. However, they are part of the reproductive system because they produce milk in direct relationship to the physiological status of other components of the reproductive system.
9-114	gynecologist (gi′-neh-<u>kol</u>-o-jist)	A gynecologist is a physician who specializes in diseases of women. "gynec/o" is a combining form meaning female. *-logist* is a suffix meaning one who specializes in.
9-115	"gynec/o" *-logist*	_____ is a combining form meaning female. _____ is a suffix meaning one (a physician) who specializes in.
9-116	gynecology (gi′-neh-<u>kol</u>-o-ji)	*-logy* is a suffix meaning the study of. Build a medical term meaning the branch of medicine dealing with diseases of the female reproductive system: _____ _____
9-117	cervix (ser′-<u>viks</u>)	We will start with the medical terms associated with the uterus. The cervix is the part of the uterus that protrudes into the cavity of the vagina. "cervic/o" is a combining form meaning cervix and literally refers to the neck (in this case, the neck of the uterus that protrudes into the vaginal cavity).

BLOCK	DATA AND ANSWERS	DESCRIPTIONS AND QUESTIONS
9-118	cervicitis (ser'-vih-<u>si</u>-tis)	Cervicitis is inflammation of the cervix.
		"cervic/o" is a combining form meaning cervix or neck of the uterus.
		-itis is a suffix meaning inflammation.
	Cervicitis	_____ is inflammation of the cervix.
	combining form	"cervic/o" is a _____ _____ meaning
	neck	_____.
	suffix	*-itis* is a _____ meaning
	inflammation	_____.
9-119		*-ectomy* is a suffix meaning excision.
	Cervicectomy	_____ is excision of the cervix.
9-120	endocervicitis (en'-do-ser-vih-<u>si</u>-tis)	Endocervicitis is inflammation of the inner lining of the cervix.
		endo- is a prefix meaning within or inside.
9-121	*endo-*	_____ is a prefix meaning within or inside.
	"cervic"	_____ is a root word meaning cervix.
	-itis	_____ is a suffix meaning inflammation.
	Endocervicitis	_____ is inflammation of the inner lining of the cervix.

BLOCK	DATA AND ANSWERS	DESCRIPTIONS AND QUESTIONS
9-122		We have learned some medical terms associated with the cervix of the uterus. The next stage covers the uterus in general.
	myometritis (my′-o-me-tri-tis)	Myometritis is inflammation of the uterine muscle.
		"my/o" is a combining form meaning muscle.
		"metr" is the root word for uterus. There are three combining forms for "metr:" metr/o", "metr/i," and "metri/o." All three combining forms are used interchangeably. Also, recall that each of the following can be used to indicate a combining form: a, e, i, o, and u.
		-itis is a suffix meaning inflammation.
9-123	Myometritis	_____ is inflammation of the uterine muscle.
	combining form muscle	"my/o" is a _____ _____ meaning _____.
	"metr/i," combining form	_____ is a _____ _____ meaning uterus.
9-124	perimetritis (peh′-re-me-tri-tis)	Perimetritis is inflammation of the tissues around the uterus.
		peri- is a prefix meaning around.
		"metr" is a word root meaning uterus.
		"metr/o" is the combining form.
		-itis is a suffix meaning inflammation.
9-125	*peri-*	_____ is a prefix meaning around.
	"metr"	_____ is a word root meaning uterus.
	-itis	_____ is a suffix meaning inflammation.
	Perimetritis	_____ is inflammation of the tissue around the uterus.

BLOCK	DATA AND ANSWERS	DESCRIPTIONS AND QUESTIONS
9-126	prefix, within root word, uterus suffix inflammation inflammation of the lining of the uterus	*endo-* is a _____ meaning _____. "metr" is a _____ _____ meaning _____. *-itis* is a _____ meaning _____. Endometritis is _____ ____ _____ _____ ____ _____ _____.
9-127	salpingitis (sal'-pin-<u>gi</u>-tis)	Having studied the uterus, we will now learn medical terms related to the two fallopian tubes that form the horns of the uterus. Salpingitis is inflammation of the fallopian tube. "salpinx" (singular) is a word root meaning tube (in this case, the fallopian tube). "salpinge" is the plural form of "salpinx." "salping/o" is the combining form. *-itis* is a suffix meaning inflammation.
9-128	Salpingitis "salpinx" "salpinge"	_____ is inflammation of the fallopian tube. _____ is a root word meaning a fallopian tube. _____ is the root word meaning fallopian tubes.
9-129	salpingectomy (sal'-pin-<u>jek</u>-to-me)	*-ectomy* is a suffix meaning excision. Build a medical term meaning excision of the fallopian tube: _____ _____

BLOCK	DATA AND ANSWERS	DESCRIPTIONS AND QUESTIONS
9-130	salpingostomy (sal'-pin-jos-to-me) combining form fallopian tube suffix, artificial opening creation of an artificial opening in the fallopian tube	Salpingostomy is creation of an artificial opening in the fallopian tube. "salping/o" is a _____ _____ meaning _____ _____. -*stomy* is a _____ meaning _____ _____. Salpingostomy is _____ _____ _____ _____ _____ _____ _____ _____ _____.
9-131	salpingocele (sal'-pin-jo-sel) combining form fallopian tube suffix, herniation herniation of the fallopian tube	Salpingocele is herniation of the fallopian tube. "salping/o" is a _____ _____ meaning _____ _____. -*cele* is a _____ meaning _____. Salpingocele is _____ _____ _____ _____ _____.
9-132	hydrosalpinx (hi-dro-sal'-pinks)	Hydrosalpinx is fluid in the fallopian tube. "hydro" is a root word meaning water. *hydro-* also can be a prefix. "hydr/o" is the combining form.
9-133	combining form water word root fallopian tube	"hydr/o" is a _____ _____ meaning _____. "salpinx" is a _____ _____ meaning _____ _____.

BLOCK	DATA AND ANSWERS	DESCRIPTIONS AND QUESTIONS
9-134	hematosalpinx (he-<u>mat</u>-o-sal'-pinks) "hemat/o" "salpinx"	Hematosalpinx is blood in the fallopian tube. hemat/o is a combining form meaning blood. _____ is a combining form meaning blood. _____ is a root word meaning fallopian tube.
9-135	Hematosalpinx	_____ is blood in the fallopian tube.
9-136	hysterosalpingogram (<u>his</u>-ter-o-sal'-pin-jo-gram)	A hysterosalpingogram is an X-ray film of the uterus and fallopian tube. "hyster/o" is a combining form meaning uterus. "salping/o" is a combining form meaning fallopian tube. -gram is a suffix meaning record (in this case, X-ray film).
9-137	combining form uterus combining form fallopian tube suffix, X-ray film	"hyster/o" is a _____ _____ meaning _____. "salping/o" is a _____ _____ meaning _____ _____. -gram is a _____ meaning _____ _____.
9-138	an X-ray film of the uterus and fallopian tube	A hysterosalpingogram is _____ _____ _____ _____ _____ _____ _____ _____ _____.
9-139	oophorectomy (o-o'-fo-<u>rek</u>-to-me)	We have studied the cervix, uterus, and fallopian tubes. Let us turn our attention to the ovaries. Oophorectomy is excision of the ovary. "oophor/o" is a combining form meaning ovary. -ectomy is a suffix meaning excision.

BLOCK	DATA AND ANSWERS	DESCRIPTIONS AND QUESTIONS
9-140	"oophor/o"	_____ is a combining form meaning ovary.
	-*ectomy*	_____ is a suffix meaning excision.
9-141	Oophorectomy	_____ is excision of the ovary.
9-142	oophorosalpingectomy (o-o-fo′-ro-sal′-pin-<u>jek</u>-to-me)	Oophorosalpingectomy is excision of the ovary and fallopian tube.
9-143	"oophor/o"	_____ is a combining form meaning ovary.
	"salping/o"	_____ is a combining form meaning fallopian tube.
	-*ectomy*	_____ is a suffix meaning excision.

BOX 9.1
Allied Health Professions

Radiologic Technologists and Radiation Therapists

Radiologic technologists take X-rays and administer nonradioactive materials into patients' bloodstreams for diagnostic purposes. They are also referred to as radiographers, and they produce X-ray films (radiographs) of parts of the human body for use in diagnosing medical problems. They prepare patients for radiologic examinations by explaining the procedure, removing jewelry and other articles through which X-rays cannot pass, and positioning patients so that the parts of the body can be appropriately radiographed. To prevent unnecessary exposure to radiation, these workers surround the exposed area with radiation protection devices, such as lead shields, or limit the size of the X-ray beam. Radiographers position radiographic equipment at the correct angle and height over the appropriate area of a patient's body. Using instruments similar to a measuring tape, they may measure the thickness of the section to be radiographed and set controls on the X-ray machine to produce radiographs of the appropriate density, detail, and contrast. They place the X-ray film under the part of the patient's body to be examined and make the exposure. They then remove the film and develop it.

Treating cancer in the human body is the principal use of radiation therapy. As part of a medical radiation oncology team, radiation therapists use machines—called linear accelerators—to administer radiation treatment to patients. Linear accelerators, used in a procedure called external beam therapy, project high-energy X-rays at targeted cancer cells. As the X-rays collide with human tissue, they produce highly energized ions that can shrink and eliminate cancerous tumors. Radiation therapy is sometimes used as the sole treatment for cancer, but it is usually used in conjunction with chemotherapy or surgery.

A great resource is the American Society of Radiologic Technologists at www.asrt.org.

Source: P. S. Stanfield, N. Cross, Y. H . Hui, eds. *Introduction to the Health Professions,* 5th ed. (Sudbury, MA: Jones & Bartlett, 2009).

BLOCK	DATA AND ANSWERS	DESCRIPTIONS AND QUESTIONS
9-144	Oophorosalpingectomy	_____ is excision of the ovary and fallopian tube.
9-145	hysterosalpingo-oophorectomy (his-ter-o-sal-pin-jo-o-o-fo-rek'-to-me)	Hysterosalpingo-oophorectomy is excision of the uterus, ovaries, and fallopian tubes.
9-146	combining form uterus	"hyster/o" is a _____ _____ meaning _____.
	combining form fallopian tubes	"salping/o" is a _____ _____ meaning _____ _____.
	combining form ovaries	"oophor/o" is a _____ _____ meaning _____.
	suffix, excision	-ectomy is a _____ meaning _____.
9-147	hysterosalpingo-oophorectomy	_____ _____ is excision of the uterus, ovaries, and fallopian tubes. (Take your time, this is a long word!)
9-148	colporrhaphy (kol-po-rah'-fe)	Colporrhaphy is suture of the vagina. "colp" is a word root meaning vagina. "colp/o" is the combining form. -rrhaphy is a suffix meaning suture.
	colporrhaphy	_____ is suture of the vagina.
	-rrhaphy	_____ is a suffix meaning suture.
9-149		-scopy is a suffix meaning visual examination. Build a medical term meaning visual examination of the vagina:
	colposcopy (kol-pos-ko'-pe)	_____ _____

BLOCK	DATA AND ANSWERS	DESCRIPTIONS AND QUESTIONS
9-150	vulvovaginal (vul-vo-vah-jin'-al)	Vulvovaginal means pertaining to the vulva and vagina. "vulva" is a root word meaning the external genitalia of the female. "vulv/o" is a combining form meaning vulva. "vagin/o" is a combining form meaning vagina.
9-151	combining form vulva combining form vagina suffix, pertaining to Vulvovaginal	"vulv/o" is a _____ _____ meaning _____. "vagin/o" is a _____ _____ meaning _____. -al is a _____ meaning _____ _____. _____ is pertaining to the vulva and vagina.
9-152	vulvovaginitis (vul'-vo-vaj'-ih-nigh-tis)	Vulvovaginitis is inflammation of the vulva and vagina. -itis is a suffix meaning inflammation.
9-153	Vulvovaginitis "vulv/o" "vagin/o"	_____ is inflammation of the vulva and vagina. _____ is a combining form meaning vulva. _____ is a combining form meaning vagina.
9-154	episiorrhaphy (ep-iz-e-o-rah'-fe)	Episiorrhaphy is suture of a tear in the vulva. "episi" is a root word meaning pubic region or, sometimes, the vulva. "episi/o" is the combining form. -rrhaphy is a suffix meaning suture.

BLOCK	DATA AND ANSWERS	DESCRIPTIONS AND QUESTIONS
9-155	"episi"	_____ is another root word meaning vulva.
	-rrhaphy	_____ is a suffix meaning suture.
	Episiorrhaphy	_____ is suture of a tear of the vulva.
9-156	episioperineoplasty (ep-iz-e-o-peh-rih-ne'-o-plas-te)	Episioperineoplasty is plastic repair of the vulva and perineum. "episi/o" is a combining form meaning vulva.
	perineum (per'-uh-nee-uh-m)	"perineum" is a root word meaning the area between the vagina opening and the anus.
		"perine/o" is the combining form.
		-plasty is a suffix meaning plastic repair.
9-157	combining form vulva	"episi/o" is a _____ _____ meaning _____.
	combining form perineum	"perine/o" is a _____ _____ meaning _____.
	suffix, plastic repair	-plasty is a _____ meaning _____ _____.
	plastic repair of the vulva and perineum	Episioperineoplasty is _____ _____ ____ _____ _____ _____ _____.
9-158	leukorrhea (lu-ko-re'-ah)	Leukorrhea is white discharge from the vagina.
		"leuk/o" is a combining form meaning white.
		-rrhea is a suffix meaning discharge.
9-159	"leuk/o"	_____ is a combining form meaning white.
	-rrhea	_____ is a suffix meaning discharge.
9-160	Leukorrhea	_____ is white vaginal discharge.

BLOCK	DATA AND ANSWERS	DESCRIPTIONS AND QUESTIONS
9-161		The Bartholin's gland is a small, mucus-secreting gland near the vagina.
	Bartholin's adenitis (bar-to-linz ad'-eh-<u>ni</u>-tis)	Bartholin's adenitis is inflammation of a Bartholin gland.
		"aden" is the root word for gland.
		"aden/o" is a combining form meaning gland.
		-itis is a suffix meaning inflammation.
9-162	"aden/o"	_____ is a combining form meaning gland.
	-itis	_____ is a suffix meaning inflammation.
9-163	inflammation of a Bartholin gland	Bartholin's adenitis is _____ _____ __ _____ _____.
9-164		Menstruation is one important physiological feature of a female's reproductive system. It refers to the bloody discharge from the uterus at a regular interval (3–4 weeks) in a female who is not pregnant.
	menometrorrhagia (men'-o-me-<u>tro</u>-ra-je-a)	Menometrorrhagia is excessive menstrual uterine bleeding.
		"men" is a root word meaning to menstruate.
		"men/o" is a combining form meaning to menstruate.
		"metr/o" is a combining form meaning uterus.
		-rrhagia is a suffix meaning excessive bleeding (hemorrhage).
9-165	"men/o"	_____ is a combining form meaning to menstruate.
	"metr/o"	_____ is a combining form meaning uterus.
	-rrhagia	_____ is a suffix meaning excessive bleeding (hemorrhage).
	Menometrorrhagia	_____ is excessive uterine bleeding.

BLOCK	DATA AND ANSWERS	DESCRIPTIONS AND QUESTIONS
9-166	amenorrhea (a´-men-o-<u>re</u>-ah) Amenorrhea	Amenorrhea is absence of menstrual discharge. *a-* is a prefix meaning without or absence. "men/o" is a combining form meaning to menstruate. *-rrhea* is a suffix meaning discharge. _____ is absence of menstrual discharge.
9-167	menarche (men-<u>ar</u>-ke) root word, to menstruate suffix, beginning the beginning of menstruation	Menarche is the beginning of menstruation. "men" is a root word meaning to menstruate. "men/o" is the combining form. *-arche* is a suffix meaning beginning. "men" is a _____ _____ meaning _____ _____. *-arche* is a _____ meaning _____. Menarche is _____ _____ _____ _____..
9-168	 menopause (<u>men</u>-o-pawz)	*-pause* is a suffix meaning stop or stopping of. Build a medical term meaning stopping of menstruation: _____ _____
9-169	oligomenorrhea (ol´-i-go-men-o-<u>re</u>-ah) Oligomenorrhea	Oligomenorrhea is scanty menstrual discharge. "olig/o" is a combining form meaning scant or scanty. *oligo-* also can be a prefix. "men/o" is a combining form meaning to menstruate. *-rrhea* is a suffix meaning discharge. _____ is scanty menstrual flow.

BLOCK	DATA AND ANSWERS	DESCRIPTIONS AND QUESTIONS
9-170	metrorrhea (me-<u>tro</u>-re-ah)	Metrorrhea is excessive uterine discharge.
		"metr" is a word root for uterus.
		"metr/o" is the combining form.
		-rrhea is a suffix meaning excessive discharge.
	Metrorrhea	_____ is excessive uterine discharge.
9-171	dysmenorrhea (dis'-men-o-<u>re</u>-ah)	Dysmenorrhea is difficult or painful menstrual discharge.
		dys- is a prefix meaning difficult or painful.
		"men/o" is a combining form meaning to menstruate.
		-rrhea is a suffix meaning discharge.
	Dysmenorrhea	_____ is difficult or painful menstrual discharge.
	dys-	_____ is a prefix meaning difficult or painful.
9-172		**Table 9.1** summarizes the word components you have learned in this chapter about the genitourinary system.
		The next chapter focuses on the bones, muscles, and joints.

BOX 9.2	
Abbreviations	
AB	abortion
ARF	acute renal failure
BUN	blood urea nitrogen
Cx	cervix
D&C	dilation and curettage
ERT	estrogen replacement therapy
ESRD	end-stage renal disease
GU	genitourinary
HD	hemodialysis
LMP	last menstrual period
PAP	Papanicolaou smear
PID	pelvic inflammatory disease
TAH	total abdominal hysterectomy
TVH	total vaginal hysterectomy
TUR or TURP	transurethral resection of the prostate gland

TABLE 9.1   Word Components in this Chapter

WORD ROOTS	COMBINING FORMS	PREFIXES
aden	aden/o	a-
andr	andr/o	dys-
balan	balan/o	endo-
cervic	cervic/o	hydro-
colp	colp/o	hyper-
crypt	crypt/o	oligo-
cyst	cyst/o	peri-
episi	epididym/o	poly-
hydro	episi/o	SUFFIXES
hyster	gynec/o	-al
leuk	hemat/o	-arche
lith	hydr/o	-ary
men	hyster/o	-cele
metr	leuk/o	-ectomy
my	lith/o	-emia
nephr	men/o	-gram
olig	metr/i	-ia
oophor	metr/o	-iasis
orch	metri/o	-ism

TABLE 9.1   Word Components in this Chapter (continued)

WORD ROOTS	COMBINING FORMS	SUFFIXES
orchi	my/o	-ist
orchid	nephr/o	-itis
pelvis	olig/o	-logist
perineum	oophor/o	-logy
prostat	orch/o	-lysis
py	orchi/o	-megaly
pyel	orchid/o	-oma
ren	perine/o	-osis
salpinge	prostat/o	-pathy
salpinx	py/o	-pause
sperm	pyel/o	-pexy
spermat	ren/o	-plasty
stern	salping/o	-rrhagia
trachel	sperm/o	-rrhaphy
ur	spermat/o	-rrhea
ureter	sten/o	-scopy
urethr	trachel/o	-stomy
urin	ur/o	-tomy
vagin	ureter/o	-tripsy
vas	urethr/o	-trophy
vesic	urin/o	-zoa
vesicul	vagin/o	-zoon
vulva	vas/o	
	vesic/o	
	vesicul/o	
	vulv/o	

Progress Check

A. Multiple Choice

1. A word root meaning glans penis is:
   a. hyster
   b. balan
   c. urin
   d. vas

2. A word root meaning vulva is:
   a. colp
   b. episi
   c. nephr
   d. orch

3. A word root meaning pus is:
   a. ureter
   b. trachel
   c. ur
   d. py

4. A word root meaning neck is:
   a. trachel
   b. metr
   c. cyst
   d. ren

5. A combining form meaning hidden is:
   a. trachel/o
   b. ur/o
   c. crypt/o
   d. men/o

6. A combining form meaning male is:
   a. andr/o
   b. orchid/o

   c. perine/o
   d. cervic/o

7. A combining form meaning uterus or womb is:
   a. gynec/o
   b. hydr/o
   c. aden/o
   d. metr/o

8. A combining form meaning narrow is:
   a. sten/o
   b. leuk/o
   c. lith/o
   d. prostat/o

9. A prefix meaning scanty is:
   a. oligo-
   b. hemi-
   c. tachy-
   d. ultra-

10. A prefix meaning around is:
    a. endo-
    b. peri-
    c. supra-
    d. primi-

11. A suffix meaning condition is:
    a. -ism
    b. -logy
    c. -oma
    d. -cele

12. A suffix meaning hemorrhage is:
   a. -osis
   b. -pexy
   c. -rrhagia
   d. -rrhea

13. A suffix meaning disease is:
   a. -tomy
   b. -pause
   c. -pathy
   d. -zoon

14. A suffix meaning crush is:
   a. -gram
   b. -ia
   c. -lysis
   d. -tripsy

B. Building Medical Terms

Use the following word components to build medical terms matching the definitions given.

crypt	lith/o	py/o
crypt/o	nephr	pyel
cyst	nephr/o	pyel/o
cyst/o	orchi	sten
episi	orchi/o	sten/o
episi/o	orchid	-tomy
hydr	orchid/o	ureter
hydr/o	-osis	ureter/o
hydro-	perine	-uria
-iasis	perine/o	vesic
-ism	-pexy	vesic/o
-itis	-plasty	
lith	py	

1. condition of stone(s) in the kidney

2. surgical fixation of a testicle

3. condition of distention of part of the kidney due to accumulation of urine or water

4. incision of the bladder

5. inflammation of the renal pelvis and the kidney

6. pus in the urine

7. narrowing of the ureter(s)

8. condition where the testicle(s) or testis(es) fails to descend into the scrotum

9. plastic repair of the vulva and perineum

10. plastic repair of the bladder

C.   Definitions and Word Components

	TERM	DEFINITION	PREFIX	WORD ROOT	VOWEL	WORD ROOT	VOWEL	SUFFIX
1.	episiorrhaphy							
2.	cystotrachelotomy							
3.	prostatovesiculitis							
4.	amenorrhea							
5.	urethrocystitis							
6.	orchiepididymitis							
7.	menometrorrhagia							
8.	oligomenorrhea							
9.	trachelocystitis							
10.	nephromegaly							

D. Abbreviations

	ABBREVIATION	MEANINGS
1.	AB	
2.	ARF	
3.	BUN	
4.	Cx	
5.	D&C	
6.	ERT	
7.	ESRD	
8.	GU	
9.	HD	
10.	LMP	
11.	PAP	
12.	PID	
13.	TAH	
14.	TVH	
15.	TUR or TURP	

The Bones, Muscles, and Joints

BLOCK	DATA AND ANSWERS	DESCRIPTIONS AND QUESTIONS
10-1	musculoskeletal (muss-kyoo'-loh-<u>skell</u>-eh-tal)	This chapter presents major medical terms associated with the physiology, anatomy, and disorders of the bones, muscles, and joints of the body. This body system is generally known as the musculoskeletal system. Refer to **Figure 10.1** for the medical names of organs and their parts. Consult this figure throughout this chapter. The chapter studies the bones, followed by the joints.
10-2	musculoskeletal	The bones and muscles of the body are called the _____ system. "muscul" is a root word meaning muscle. "muscul/o" is a combining form meaning muscle. "skelet/o" is a combining form meaning skeleton. -al is a suffix meaning pertaining to.
10-3		We start with terms associated with the skull or head. "crani" is a root word meaning the skull bones or cranium. "crani/o" is a combining form meaning skull bones or cranium.

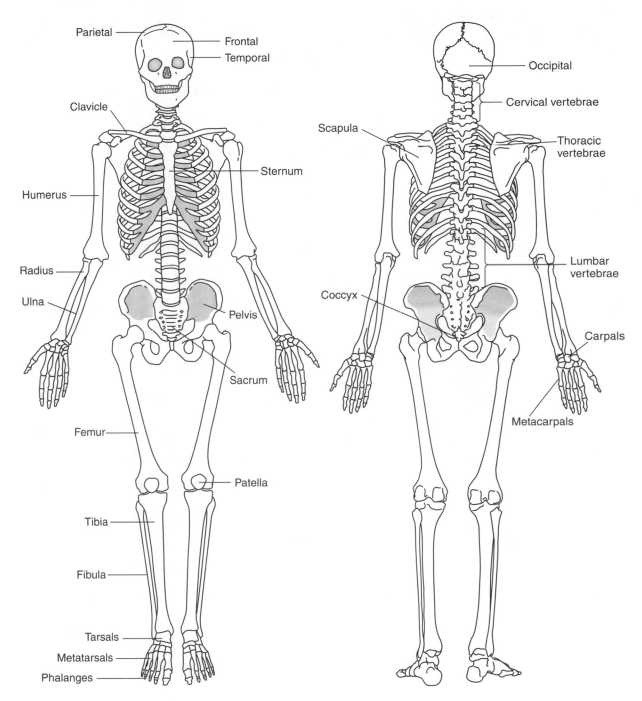

FIGURE 10.1 The human body's musculoskeletal system

BLOCK	DATA AND ANSWERS	DESCRIPTIONS AND QUESTIONS
10-4	cephalad (<u>sef</u>-ah′-lad)	Cephalad means toward the head. "cephal" is a root word meaning head. "cephal/o" is a combining form meaning head. *-ad* is a suffix meaning toward.
10-5	Cephalad	_____ means toward the head.
10-6	craniomalacia (kra′-ne-o-<u>mah</u>-la-se-ah)	Craniomalacia is softening of the skull bones. "crani/o" is a combining form meaning skull bones or cranium. *-malacia* is a suffix meaning softening.
10-7	combining form skull bones or cranium suffix, softening Craniomalacia	"crani/o" is a _____ _____ meaning _____ _____ _____ _____. *-malacia* is a _____ meaning _____. _____ is softening of the skull bones.
10-8	craniectomy (kra′-<u>ne</u>-ek-to-me) craniotomy (kra′-<u>ne</u>-ot-o-me)	*-ectomy* is a suffix meaning excision or removal. *-tomy* is a suffix meaning incision (opening into). Build a medical term (with pronunciation) meaning excision of part of the cranium: _____ _____ Build a medical term meaning incision into the cranium: _____ _____

BLOCK	DATA AND ANSWERS	DESCRIPTIONS AND QUESTIONS
10-9		Our next group of medical terms is related to the bone system from the jaw to the toes.
	maxilla (mak-<u>sih</u>-lah)	The maxilla is the upper jawbone.
		Maxillary means pertaining to the upper jawbone.
	mandible (<u>man</u>-dih-bul)	The mandible is the lower jawbone.
		Mandibular means pertaining to the lower jawbone.
10-10		"maxilla" is the root word meaning the upper jaw.
		"maxill/o" is a combining form meaning the upper jaw.
		-*ary* is a suffix meaning pertaining to.
		"mandibul" is the root word meaning the lower jaw.
		"mandibul/o" is a combining form meaning the lower jaw.
		-*ar* is a suffix meaning pertaining to.
		Note the different suffixes for the two words.
10-11	"maxill/o," combining form	_____ is a _____ _____ meaning the upper jaw.
	combining form the lower jaw	"mandibul/o" is a _____ _____ meaning _____ _____ _____.
		Two suffixes that mean pertaining to are:
	-*ary*	1. _____
	-*ar*	2. _____
10-12	Mandible	_____ is the lower jawbone.
	Maxilla	_____ is the upper jawbone.

BLOCK	DATA AND ANSWERS	DESCRIPTIONS AND QUESTIONS
10-13	submaxillary (sub'-mak-<u>sih</u>-lar-e)	Submaxillary means pertaining to below the upper jawbone
	submandibular (sub'-man-<u>dib</u>-u-lar)	Submandibular means pertaining to below the lower jawbone. *sub-* is a prefix meaning below.
10-14	Submaxillary	_____ means pertaining to below the upper jawbone.
	Submandibular	_____ means pertaining to below the lower jawbone.
	sub-	_____ is a prefix meaning below.
10-15		"maxill/o" is a combining form meaning the upper jawbone. *-itis* is a suffix meaning inflammation. *-ectomy* is a suffix meaning excision or removal. Build a medical term meaning inflammation of the upper jaw
	maxillitis (mak'-sil-<u>li</u>-tis)	bone: _____ _____
		Build a medical term meaning excision of the upper jaw bone:
	maxillectomy (mak'-sil-<u>lek</u>-to-me)	_____ _____
10-16	scapula (<u>skap</u>-u-lah)	"scapula" or "scapul" is a root word referring to one of the pair of large bones forming the shoulder blade.
	subscapular (sub-<u>skap</u>-u-lar)	Subscapular means below the shoulder blade. "scapul/o" is a combining form meaning scapula. *sub-* is a prefix meaning below. *-ar* is a suffix meaning pertaining to.
10-17	Subscapular	_____ is below the shoulder blade.
	pertaining to	*-ar* is a suffix meaning _____ _____.
	below	*sub-* is a preface meaning _____.

BLOCK	DATA AND ANSWERS	DESCRIPTIONS AND QUESTIONS
10-18	suprascapular (su'-prah-<u>skap</u>-u-lar) prefix, above	*supra-* is a prefix meaning above. Build a medical term meaning pertaining to above the shoulder blade: _____ _____ *supra-* is a _____ meaning _____.
10-19	subcostal (sub-<u>kos</u>-tal)	Subcostal means pertaining to below the rib. *sub-* is a prefix meaning below. "cost" is a root word meaning the rib. "cost/o" is a combining form meaning the rib. *-al* is a suffix meaning pertaining to.
10-20	Subcostal "cost/o" pertaining to	_____ means pertaining to below the rib. _____ is a combining form meaning rib. *-al* is a suffix meaning _____ _____.
10-21	sternum (<u>ster</u>-num) sternoid (<u>ster</u>-noyd)	Sternum is the anatomical term meaning breastbone. "stern" is the root word meaning breastbone. Sternoid means resembling the breastbone. "stern/o" is a combining form meaning sternum. *-oid* is a suffix meaning resembling.
10-22	Sternoid "stern/o" *-oid*	_____ means resembling the breastbone. _____ is a combining form meaning breastbone. _____ is a suffix meaning resembling.

BLOCK	DATA AND ANSWERS	DESCRIPTIONS AND QUESTIONS
10-23	intrasternal (in´-trah-<u>stern</u>-al)	Intrasternal means pertaining to within the sternum.
		intra- is a prefix meaning within.
		"stern/o" is a combining form meaning breastbone.
		-al is a suffix meaning pertaining to.
10-24	Intrasternal	_____ is pertaining to within the sternum.
	prefix, within	*intra-* is a _____ meaning _____.
	-al, suffix	_____ is a _____ meaning pertaining to.
10-25	clavicle (<u>klah</u>-vih´-kul)	The clavicle is the collarbone.
10-26	sternoclavicular (ster´-no-<u>klah</u>-vih-ku-lar)	Sternoclavicular refers to the breastbone and collarbone.
		"stern/o" is a combining form meaning breastbone (sternum).
		"clavicul" is a root word meaning clavicle or collarbone.
		"clavicul/o" is a combining form meaning clavicle or collarbone.
		-ar is a suffix meaning pertaining to.
10-27	Sternoclavicular	_____ refers to the breastbone and collarbone.
	combining form	"stern/o" is a _____ _____ meaning _____ _____.
	breastbone (sternum)	
	"clavicul/o"	_____ is a combining form meaning clavicle (collarbone).
	-ar, suffix	_____ is a _____ meaning pertaining to.
10-28	carpals (<u>kar</u>-pals)	Carpals are the wristbones.
	wristbones	Carpals are the _____.

BLOCK	DATA AND ANSWERS	DESCRIPTIONS AND QUESTIONS
10-29	metacarpals (met'-ah-<u>kar</u>-pals)	Metacarpals are the hand bones.
	hand bones	Metacarpals are _____ _____.
10-30	carpoptosis (kar'-pop-<u>to</u>-sis)	Carpoptosis is a drooping or falling wrist.
		"carp" is a root word meaning wrist.
		"carp/o" is a combining form meaning wrist.
		-ptosis is a suffix meaning drooping or falling.
10-31	combining form wrist	"carp/o" is a _____ _____ meaning _____.
	suffix, drooping falling	-ptosis is a _____ meaning _____ or _____.
	a drooping or falling wrist	Carpoptosis is ___ _____ _____ _____ _____.
10-32	femur (<u>fe</u>-mur)	The femur is the large upper leg bone.
	the large upper leg bone	The femur is _____ _____ _____ _____ _____.
10-33	iliofemoral (il'-e-o-<u>fem</u>-or-al)	Iliofemoral means pertaining to the hip bone (pelvic) and large thigh bone (femur).
		The ilium is the medical term for the upper, wing-shaped part of the pelvic bone.
		"ilium" or "ili" is the root word meaning upper, wing-shaped part of the pelvic bone.
		"ili/o" is a combining form meaning ilium.
		"femor/o" is a combining form meaning femur.
		-al is a suffix meaning pertaining to.

BLOCK	DATA AND ANSWERS	DESCRIPTIONS AND QUESTIONS
10-34	combining form ilium	"ili/o" is a _____ _____ meaning _____.
	combining form femur	"femor/o" is a _____ _____ meaning _____.
	suffix, pertaining to	-al is a _____ meaning _____ _____.
	pertaining to the hipbone (pelvic) and large thigh bone (femur)	Iliofemoral is _____ _____ _____ _____ _____ _____ _____ _____ _____ _____.
10-35		Recall that the ilium is the upper, wing-shaped part of the pelvic bone.
	ischium (ish-e-um)	The ischium is the lower rear portion of the pelvic bone.
	the lower rear portion of the pelvic bone	The ischium is _____ _____ _____ _____ _____ _____ _____ _____.
10-36	pubis (pu-bis)	The pubis is the front portion of the pelvic bone.
	the front portion of the pelvic bone	The pubis is _____ _____ _____ _____ _____ _____ _____.
10-37	interpubic (in'-ter-pu-bik)	Interpubic means between the pubic bones.
		inter- is a prefix meaning between.
		"pubic" or "pub" is the root word meaning pubic bones.
		"pub/o" is a combining form referring to the pubic bones.
		-ic is a suffix meaning pertaining to.
10-38	Interpubic	_____ is between the pubic bones.
	between	inter- is a prefix meaning _____.
	combining form pubic bones	"pub/o" is a _____ _____ referring to the _____ _____.

BLOCK	DATA AND ANSWERS	DESCRIPTIONS AND QUESTIONS
10-39	patella (pah-<u>tel</u>-ah) the kneecap	The patella is the kneecap. The patella is _____ _____.
10-40	patellapexy (pah′-tel-ah-<u>pek</u>-se)	Patellapexy is fixation of the patella. "patell" is a root word meaning kneecap. "patell/o" is a combining form meaning kneecap. *-pexy* is a suffix meaning fixation.
10-41	combining form kneecap suffix, fixation fixation of the patella	"patell/o" is a _____ _____ meaning _____. *-pexy* is a _____ meaning _____. Patellapexy is _____ _____ _____ _____.
10-42	tibiofemoral (tib′-e-o-<u>fem</u>-or-al)	Tibiofemoral means pertaining to the large bone of the lower leg (tibia, the shinbone) and the large bone of the thigh (femur). "tibi" is a root word meaning the large inner bone of the lower leg or shinbone. "tibi/o" is a combining form meaning the large inner bone of the lower leg or shinbone. "femor/o" is a combining form meaning thigh bone. "femur" is a root word meaning thigh bone. *-al* is a suffix meaning pertaining to.

BLOCK	DATA AND ANSWERS	DESCRIPTIONS AND QUESTIONS
10-43	combining form the large inner bone of the lower leg or shinbone	"tibi/o" is a _____ _____ meaning _____ _____ _____ _____ ____ _____ _____ ____ ____ _____.
	combining form thigh bone	"femor/o" is a _____ _____ meaning _____ _____.
	suffix, pertaining to	-*al* is a _____ meaning _____ ____.
	pertaining to the large bone of the lower leg (tibia, the shinbone) and the large bone of the thigh (femur)	Tibiofemoral means _____ ____ _____ _____ _____ ____ _____ _____ _____ _____ _____ _____ _____ ____ _____ _____ ____ _____ _____ _____.
10-44	tarsals (<u>tar</u>-salz)	The tarsals are the ankle bones. "tar" is a root word meaning ankle bones. "tar/o" is the combining form meaning ankle bones.
	the ankle bones	The tarsals are _____ _____ _____.
10-45	metatarsals (met'-ah-<u>tar</u>-salz)	The metatarsals are the foot bones.
	the foot bones	The metatarsals are _____ _____ _____.
10-46	tarsectomy (tar'-<u>sek</u>-to-me)	Tarsectomy is excision of one or more ankle bones. "tar/o" is a combining form meaning one or more ankle bones. -*ectomy* is a suffix meaning excision or removal.
10-47	Tarsectomy	_____ is excision of one or more ankle bones.
	"tar/o"	_____ is a combining form meaning one or more ankle bones.
	suffix, excision	-*ectomy* is a _____ meaning _____.

BLOCK	DATA AND ANSWERS	DESCRIPTIONS AND QUESTIONS
10-48	pedialgia (ped'-e-<u>al</u>-je-ah)	Pedialgia is pain in the foot (or feet). "ped" and "pod" are root words meaning foot. "ped/i" and "pod/o" are both combining forms meaning foot. *-algia* is a suffix meaning pain.
10-49	Pedialgia "ped/i," "pod/o" *-algia*	_____ is foot pain. _____ and _____ are both combining forms meaning foot. _____ is a suffix meaning pain.
10-50	phalanges (fa'-<u>lan</u>-jez)	"phalanges" and "phalang" are root words meaning finger or toe bones. "phalang/o" is the combining form.
10-51	phalangectomy (fal'-an-<u>jek</u>-to-me)	Phalangectomy is excision of a finger or toe bone. *-ectomy* is a suffix meaning excision or removal.
10-52	Phalangectomy "phalang/o," combining form *-ectomy*, suffix *-itis*, suffix	_____ is excision of a finger or toe bone. _____ is a _____ _____ meaning finger or toe bone. _____ is a _____ meaning excision or removal. _____ is a _____ meaning inflammation.
10-53	phalangitis (fal'-an-<u>ji</u>-tis)	Phalangitis is an inflammation of the bones of the fingers or toes. *-itis* is a suffix meaning inflammation.

BLOCK	DATA AND ANSWERS	DESCRIPTIONS AND QUESTIONS
10-54	Phalangitis	_____ is an inflammation of the bones of the fingers or toes.
	"phalang/o," combining form	_____ is a _____ _____ meaning finger or toe bone.
	-itis, suffix	_____ is a _____ meaning inflammation.
10-55	dactyl (dak'-<u>til</u>)	Dactyl is a finger or a toe.
		"dactyl" is a root word meaning finger or toe.
		"dactyl/o" is the combining form.
10-56	dactylomegaly (dak'-ti-lo-<u>meg</u>-ah-le)	Dactylomegaly means enlarged digit (a finger or toe)
		"dactyl/o" is a combining form meaning digit (a finger or toe).
		-megaly is a suffix meaning enlarged.
10-57	digit (a finger or toe)	"dactyl/o" is a combining form meaning _____ ____ _____ ____ _____.
	enlarged	*-megaly* is a suffix meaning _____.
	an enlarged digit (a finger or toe)	Dactylomegaly is _____ _____ _____ ___ _____ _____ _____.
10-58	ankylodactylia (ang'-ke-lo-dak-<u>til</u>-e-ah)	Ankylodactylia is the condition of stiffened, crooked, or conjoined fingers or toes.
		"ankyl/o" is a combining form meaning fusion or growing together of parts.
		ankylo- also can be a prefix.
		"dactyl/o" is a combining form meaning digit (a finger or toe).
		-ia is a suffix meaning condition. The condition can be normal or abnormal.

BLOCK	DATA AND ANSWERS	DESCRIPTIONS AND QUESTIONS
10-59	Ankylodactylia	_____ is the condition of stiff, crooked, or fused fingers or toes.
	fusion or growing together of parts	"ankyl/o" is a combining form meaning _____ _____ _____ _____ _____ _____.
	digit (fingers or toes)	"dactyl/o" is a combining form meaning _____ _____ _____ _____.
	condition	-*ia* is a suffix meaning _____.
10-60	calcaneodynia (kal-kah′-ne-o-<u>din</u>-e-ah)	Calcaneodynia is heel bone pain. -*dynia* is a suffix meaning pain. "calcane" is a root word meaning heel bone. "calcane/o" is a combining form meaning heel bone.
10-61	Calcaneodynia	_____ is heel bone pain.
	suffix, pain	-*dynia* is a _____ meaning _____.
	combining form heel bone	"calcane/o" is a _____ _____ meaning _____ _____.
10-62	lumbodynia (lum′-bo-<u>din</u>-e-ah)	Lumbodynia is loin pain. -*dynia* is a suffix meaning pain. "lumb" is a root word meaning loins. "lumb/o" is a combining form meaning loins.
10-63	Lumbodynia	_____ is loin pain.
	suffix, pain	-*dynia* is a _____ meaning _____.
	combining form loins	"lumb/o" is a _____ _____ meaning _____.

BLOCK	DATA AND ANSWERS	DESCRIPTIONS AND QUESTIONS
10-64	cervical vertebrae (ser′-vih-ih-<u>kal</u> <u>ver</u>-teh-bra′)	We will now look at medical terms associated with the vertebra, which starts at the neck and goes to our tail bone and forms five sets of vertebrae bones. The neck bones are called the cervical vertebrae and contain seven bones. They form the first set of vertebrae (of the vertebral column) starting from the neck down. The vertebral column is our backbone.
10-65	neck bones	Cervical vertebrae are _____ _____.
10-66	thoracic vertebrae (tho′-<u>rah</u>-sik <u>ver</u>-teh-bra′)	The 12 vertebrae that connect the cervical vertebrae to the lumbar vertebrae are called the thoracic (at chest level) vertebrae. They form the second set of vertebrae.
10-67	12 vertebrae that connect the cervical vertebrae to the lumbar vertebrae	The thoracic vertebrae are ____ _____ _____ _____ _____ _____ _____ _____ _____ _____ _____.
10-68	lumbar vertebrae (lum-<u>bar</u> <u>ver</u>-teh-bra′)	The lumbar vertebrae are five bones making up the third part of the vertebra.
10-69	five bones making up the third part of the vertebrae	The lumbar vertebrae are _____ _____ _____ _____ _____ _____ _____ _____ _____ _____.
10-70	sacrum (<u>sa</u>-krum)	The sacrum, the fourth part of the vertebrae, consists of four vertebrae fused together.
10-71	four vertebrae fused together to form the fourth part of the vertebrae	The sacrum is made of _____ _____ _____ _____ _____ _____ _____ _____ _____ ____ _____ _____.
10-72	coccyx (<u>kok</u>-siks)	The coccyx, also known as the tailbone, is the last part of the vertebrae.
10-73	the tailbone	The coccyx is _____ _____.

BLOCK	DATA AND ANSWERS	DESCRIPTIONS AND QUESTIONS
10-74	laminectomy (lam′-in-<u>ek</u>-to-me)	Laminectomy is excision of the lamina. "laminas" and "laminae" are root words meaning the flat layers of the vertebrae that form the vertebral arch of the spinal column. "lamin" is another root word meaning the same as above. "lamin/o" is a combining form meaning lamina. *-ectomy* is a suffix meaning excision or removal.
10-75	Laminectomy combining form lamina *-ectomy*, suffix	_____ is excision of the lamina. "lamin/o" is a _____ _____ meaning _____. _____ is a _____ meaning excision or removal.
10-76	spondylodynia (spon′-di-lo-<u>din</u>-e-a)	Spondylodynia is pain in the vertebrae. "spondyl" is a root word meaning vertebrae. "spondyl/o" is a combining form meaning vertebrae. *-dynia* is a suffix meaning pain.
10-77	Spondylodynia combining form vertebrae *-dynia*, suffix	_____ is pain in the vertebrae. "spondyl/o" is a _____ _____ meaning _____. _____ is a _____ meaning pain.

BLOCK	DATA AND ANSWERS	DESCRIPTIONS AND QUESTIONS
10-78	vertebrosternal (ver'-te-bro-<u>stern</u>-al)	Vertebrosternal means pertaining to the vertebra (vertebrae) and breastbone (sternum). "vertebra" and "vertebr" also are root words. "vertebr/o" is a combining form meaning vertebrae. "stern" is a root word meaning sternum or breastbone. "stern/o" is a combining form meaning sternum or breastbone. -*al* is a suffixing meaning pertaining to.
10-79	Vertebrosternal combining form vertebra combining form sternum suffix, pertaining to	_____ means pertaining to the vertebrae and breastbone. "vertebr/o" is a _____ _____ meaning _____. "stern/o" is a _____ _____ meaning _____. -*al* is a _____ meaning _____ _____.
10-80	rachischisis (<u>rak</u>-is-kih'-sis)	Rachischisis is fissure of the vertebral column. "rach" or "rachi" (more common) are root words meaning vertebral column. The corresponding combining forms are "rach/o" and "rachi/o" (more common). -*schisis* is a suffix meaning fissure.
10-81	Rachischisis combining form vertebral column suffix, fissure	_____ is fissure of the vertebral column. "rachi/o" is a _____ _____ meaning _____ _____. -*schisis* is a _____ meaning _____.
10-82	rachicentesis (rak'-ih-<u>sen</u>-te-sis)	Rachicentesis is a puncture into the spinal column. -*centesis* is a suffix meaning puncture.

BLOCK	DATA AND ANSWERS	DESCRIPTIONS AND QUESTIONS
10-83	combining form vertebral column suffix, puncture puncture into the spinal column	"rachi/o" is a _____ _____ meaning _____ _____. -*centesis* is a _____ meaning _____. Rachicentesis is a _____ _____ _____ _____ _____.
10-84	kyphosis (kih'-<u>fo</u>-sis)	Kyphosis is an abnormal hump of the thoracic (chest) spine (also called hunchback). "kyph" is the root word. "kyph/o" is a combining form meaning thoracic hump. -*osis* is a suffix meaning condition. The condition can be normal or abnormal.
10-85	combining form abnormal hump of the thoracic spine suffix, condition Kyphosis	"kyph/o" is a _____ _____ meaning _____ _____ ___ _____ _____ _____. -*osis* is a _____ meaning _____. _____ is an abnormal hump of the thoracic spine (also called hunchback).
10-86	scoliosis (sko'-<u>leo</u>-sis)	Scoliosis is an abnormal (lateral) curve of the spine. "scoli/o" is a combining form meaning lateral curve of the spine. -*osis* is a suffix meaning condition.
10-87	Scoliosis "scoli/o" -*osis*	_____ is an abnormal (lateral) curve of the spine. _____ is a combining form meaning lateral curve of the spine. _____ is a suffix meaning condition.

BLOCK	DATA AND ANSWERS	DESCRIPTIONS AND QUESTIONS
10-88	coccygectomy (kok'-sih-jek-to-me)	Coccygectomy is excision of the tailbone. "coccyx" is a root word meaning the tailbone. "coccyg/o" is the combining form. -ectomy is a suffix meaning excision or removal.
10-89	Coccygectomy "coccyg/o" -ectomy	_____ is excision of the tailbone. _____ is a combining form meaning tailbone. _____ is a suffix meaning excision or removal.
10-90	myeloma (mi-el-o'-mah)	Myeloma is tumor of the bone marrow (its cells) of the spinal cord. "myel/o" is a combining form meaning bone marrow of the spinal cord. -oma is a suffix meaning tumor.
10-91	Myeloma "myel/o" -oma	_____ is tumor of the bone marrow (its cells) of the spinal cord. _____ is a combining form meaning bone marrow of the spinal cord. _____ is a suffix meaning tumor.
10-92		Our next group of medical terms is related to general bone disorders of various parts of the entire skeletal system.
10-93	osteitis (os-te-i'-tis)	Osteitis is inflammation of the bone. "oste" is a root word for bone. "oste/o" is a combining form meaning bone. -itis is a suffix meaning inflammation.
10-94	Osteitis	_____ is inflammation of the bone.

BOX 10.1
Allied Health Professions

Clinical Laboratory (Medical) Technologists and Technicians; Medical, Dental, and Ophthalmic Laboratory Technicians

Changes in body fluids, tissues, and cells are often a sign that something is wrong. Clinical laboratory testing plays a crucial role in the detection and diagnosis of disease. Clinical laboratory and medical technologists perform laboratory testing in conjunction with pathologists (physicians who diagnose the cause and nature of disease) and other physicians or scientists who specialize in clinical chemistry, microbiology, or the other biological sciences. Medical technologists develop data on the blood, tissues, and fluids in the human body by using a variety of precision instruments.

The following are some resources for further information:

- American Medical Technologists, www.amt1.com
- American Society for Clinical Laboratory Science, www.ascls.org

Medical appliance technicians construct, fit, maintain, and repair braces, artificial limbs, joints, arch supports, and other surgical and medical appliances. They follow prescriptions or detailed instructions from podiatrists or orthotists, who request braces, supports, corrective shoes, or other devices. They also follow the instructions of prosthetists in constructing replacement limbs—arms, legs, hands, or feet—for patients who need them due to a birth defect, accident, or amputation. Other health professionals may also order medical appliances to be produced by medical appliance technicians. Medical appliance technicians who work with orthotic and prosthetic devices are called orthotic and prosthetic technicians. Other medical appliance technicians work with medical appliances that help correct other medical problems, such as aids to correct hearing loss.

Dental laboratory technicians fill prescriptions from dentists for crowns, bridges, dentures, and other dental prosthetics. First, dentists send a specification of the item to be manufactured, along with an impression or mold of the patient's mouth or teeth. Then dental laboratory technicians, also called dental technicians, create a model of the patient's mouth by pouring plaster into the impression and allowing it to set. They place the model on an apparatus that mimics the bite and movement of the patient's jaw. The model serves as the basis of the prosthetic device.

Ophthalmic laboratory technicians should not be confused with workers in other vision care occupations. Ophthalmologists are eye doctors who examine eyes, diagnose and treat vision problems, and prescribe corrective lenses. They are physicians who also perform eye surgery. Ophthalmic laboratory technicians read prescription specifications, select standard glass or plastic lens blanks, and then mark them to indicate where the curves specified on the prescription should be ground. They place the lens in the lens grinder, set the dials for the prescribed curvature, and start the machine. After a minute or so, the lens is ready to be finished by a machine that rotates it against a fine abrasive to grind it and smooth out rough edges. The lens is then placed in a polishing machine with an even finer abrasive to polish it to a smooth, bright finish.

The following are some resources for further information:

- American Academy of Orthotists and Prosthetists, www.opcareers.org
- National Association of Dental Laboratories, www.nadl.org
- Commission on Opticianry Accreditation, P.O. Box 4342, Chapel Hill, NC 27515

Source: P. S. Stanfield, N. Cross, Y. H . Hui, eds. *Introduction to the Health Professions,* 5th ed. (Sudbury, MA: Jones & Bartlett, 2009).

BLOCK	DATA AND ANSWERS	DESCRIPTIONS AND QUESTIONS
10-95	osteomyelitis (os′-te-o-mi-<u>eli</u>-tis)	Osteomyelitis is inflammation of the bone and bone marrow. "oste/o" is a combining form meaning bone. "myel/o" is a combining form meaning bone marrow. -*itis* is a suffix meaning inflammation.
10-96	combining form bone combining form bone marrow suffix inflammation	"oste/o" is a _____ _____ meaning _____. "myel/o" is a _____ _____ meaning _____ _____. -*itis* is a _____ meaning _____.
10-97	Osteomyelitis	_____ is inflammation of the bone and bone marrow.
10-98		We will apply the following combining form to general medical terms in the next few blocks: "oste/o."
10-99	osteomalacia (os′-te-o-mah-<u>la</u>-se-ah)	-*malacia* is a suffix meaning softening. Build a medical term meaning softening of the bones: _____ _____
10-100	osteoblast (os-<u>teo</u>-blast′)	"blast" is a root word for a developing or immature cell. -*blast* also can be a suffix. Build a medical term meaning developing bone cell: _____ _____
10-101	osteocyte (os′-<u>teo</u>-sit)	-*cyte* is a suffix meaning cell. Build a medical term meaning bone cell: _____ _____

BLOCK	DATA AND ANSWERS	DESCRIPTIONS AND QUESTIONS
10-102	osteotome (os′-<u>teo</u>-tom)	*-tome* is a suffix meaning an instrument used for cutting. Build a medical term meaning an instrument used for cutting the bone: _____ _____
10-103	osteometry (os′-<u>teo</u>-met-re)	*-metry* is a suffix meaning measurement. Build a medical term meaning measurement of bone: _____ _____
10-104	osteoma (os′-<u>teo</u>-mah)	*-oma* is a suffix meaning tumor. Build a medical term meaning tumor of the bone: _____ _____
10-105	osteolysis (os′-te-o-<u>li</u>-sis)	*-lysis* is a suffix meaning dissolution. Build a medical term meaning dissolution of bone: _____ _____
10-106	osteosclerosis (os′te-o-skleh-<u>ro</u>-sis)	Osteosclerosis is the hardening of bone cells. "oste/o" is a combining form meaning bone. "scler/o" is a combining form meaning hardening. *-osis* is a suffix meaning condition.
10-107	"oste/o" "scler/o" *-osis* Osteosclerosis	_____ is a combining form meaning bone. _____ is a combining form meaning hardening. _____ is a suffix meaning condition. _____ is the hardening of bone cells.

BLOCK	DATA AND ANSWERS	DESCRIPTIONS AND QUESTIONS
10-108	osteoporosis (os′-te-o-po-ro-sis)	Osteoporosis is the condition of bones with cavities or pores (due to a lack of calcium).
		"oste/o" is a combining form meaning bone.
		"pore" or "por" is a root word meaning pores or holes.
		"por/o" is a combining form meaning pores or holes.
		-osis is a suffix meaning condition.
10-109	Osteoporosis	_____ is the condition of bones with cavities or pores (due to a lack of calcium).
	"oste/o"	_____ is a combining form meaning bone.
	-porosis	_____ is a suffix meaning a condition of holes, pores, or cavities.
10-110		You have learned a large number of terms related to the bones. Our next group of medical terms is related to the joints.
		"arthr" is a root word meaning joint.
		"arthr/o" is the combining form. Use this combining form in the next several blocks.
10-111		-clasia is a suffix meaning artificial breaking to provide movement.
		Build a medical term meaning the artificial breaking of a joint to provide movement: _____
	arthroclasia (ar′-thro-kla-ze-ah)	_____
10-112		-centesis is a suffix meaning surgical puncture.
		Build a medical term meaning surgical puncture of a joint:
	arthrocentesis (ar′-thro-sen-te-sis)	_____
		_____

BLOCK	DATA AND ANSWERS	DESCRIPTIONS AND QUESTIONS
10-113	arthrogram (<u>ar</u>-thro-gram)	*-gram* is a suffix meaning record (X-ray). Build a medical term meaning X-ray film of a joint: _____ _____
10-114	arthroscopy (ar'-thro-<u>skop</u>-e)	*-scopy* is a suffix meaning visual examination. Build a medical term meaning visual examination of the inside of a joint: _____ _____
10-115	arthroplasty (ar'-thro-<u>plas</u>-te) arthrotomy (ar'-<u>throt</u>-to-me) arthralgia (ar'-<u>thral</u>-je-ah)	*-plasty* is a suffix meaning surgical (plastic) repair. Build a medical term meaning surgical repair of a joint: _____ _____ *-tomy* is a suffix meaning incision. Build a medical term meaning incision of a joint: _____ _____ *-algia* is a suffix meaning pain. Build a medical term meaning pain in a joint: _____ _____
10-116		Note what happens when "arthr/o" is applied at the beginning of another component that begins with a vowel.
10-117	arthredema (arth'-re-<u>de</u>-mah)	"edema" is a root word meaning abnormal accumulation of fluid in intercellular spaces of the body. Build a medical term meaning accumulation of fluid around a joint: _____ _____

BLOCK	DATA AND ANSWERS	DESCRIPTIONS AND QUESTIONS
10-118	arthritis (ar´-<u>thri</u>-tis)	*-itis* is a suffix meaning inflammation. Build a medical term meaning inflammation of a joint: _____ _____
10-119	polyarthritis (pol´-e-ar-<u>thri</u>-tis)	Polyarthritis is inflammation of many joints. *poly-* is a prefix meaning many. "arthr/o" is a combining form meaning joint. *-itis* is a suffix meaning inflammation.
10-120	Polyarthritis *poly-* "arthr/o" *-itis*	_____ is inflammation of many joints. _____ is a prefix meaning many. _____ is a combining form meaning joint. _____ is a suffix meaning inflammation.
10-121	spondylarthritis (spon´-dil-ar-<u>thri</u>-tis)	Spondylarthritis means inflammation of the vertebral joints. "spondyl" is a root word meaning vertebrae. "spondyl/o" is a combining form meaning vertebrae. "arthr/o" is a combining form meaning joints. *-itis* is a suffix meaning inflammation.
10-122	Spondylarthritis combining form vertebrae combining form joints suffix inflammation	_____ is inflammation of the vertebral joints. "spondyl/o" is a _____ _____ meaning _____. "arthr/o" is a _____ _____ meaning _____. *-itis* is a _____ meaning _____.

BLOCK	DATA AND ANSWERS	DESCRIPTIONS AND QUESTIONS
10-123	tendon (<u>ten</u>-dun)	Our last group of medical terms is related to muscles and tendons. A tendon attaches muscles to bones. Tendons are made of connective tissue. The word tendon has three combining forms: "ten/o," "tendon/o," and "tendin/o." In the next several blocks, select the correct combining forms to build medical terms.
10-124	tendinitis (ten'-di-<u>ni</u>-tis)	*-itis* is a suffix meaning inflammation. Build a medical term meaning inflammation of a tendon: _____ _____
10-125	tenodynia (ten'-o-<u>de</u>-ne-ah)	*-dynia* is a suffix meaning pain. Build a medical term meaning pain in a tendon: _____ _____
10-126	tenotomy (<u>ten</u>-ot-o'-me)	*-tomy* is a suffix meaning incision. Build a medical term meaning incision into a tendon: _____ _____
10-127	tenodesis (ten'-<u>od</u>-e-sis)	*-desis* is a suffix meaning binding or stabilizing. Build a medical term meaning binding or stabilizing (surgical) of a tendon: _____ _____
10-128	tenalgia (ten-al-<u>je</u>-a)	*-algia* is a suffix meaning pain. Build a medical term meaning pain in a tendon: _____ _____
10-129	tenorrhaphy (ten'-o-<u>raf</u>-e)	*-rrhaphy* is a suffix meaning suture. Build a medical term meaning suture of a tendon: _____ _____

BLOCK	DATA AND ANSWERS	DESCRIPTIONS AND QUESTIONS
10-130	tenomyoplasty (ten'-o-mi'-o-<u>plas</u>-te)	Tenomyoplasty is surgical repair of the tendon and muscle.
	combining form tendon	"ten/o" is a _____ _____ meaning _____.
	combining form muscle	"my/o" is a _____ _____ meaning _____.
	suffix, surgical (plastic) repair	*-plasty* is a _____ meaning _____ _____ _____.
	Tenomyoplasty	_____ is surgical repair of the tendon and muscle.
10-131		See **Table 10.1** for a summary of the word components you have learned in this chapter. The next chapter focuses on the sensory organs.

BOX 10.2 Abbreviations	
BKA	below-the-knee amputation
C1, C2, … C7	identifies a specific cervical vertebra starting with the first of the seven for the cervical segment of the entire vertebral column
DIP	distal interphalangeal (joint)
Fx	fracture
L1, L2, … L5	identifies a specific lumbar vertebra starting with the first of the five for the lumbar segment of the entire vertebral column
MCP	metacarpophalangeal (joint)
MTP	metatarsophalangeal (joint)
PIP	posterio interphalangeal (joint)
BMD	bone mineral density, also bone mass measurement
DJD	degenerative joint disease
THR	total hip replacement

TABLE 10.1   Word Components in this Chapter

WORD ROOTS	COMBINING FORMS	PREFIXES
ankyl	ankyl/o	ankylo-
arthr	arthr/o	sub-
blast	calcane/o	supra-
calcane	carp/o	inter-
carp	cephal/o	intra-
cephal	clavicul/o	poly-
clavicul	coccyg/o	**SUFFIXES**
coccyx	cost/o	-ad
cost	crani/o	-al
crani	dactyl/o	-algia
dactyl	femor/o	-ar
edema	ili/o	-ary
femor	kyph/o	-blast
ili	lamin/o	-centesis
kyph	lumb/o	-clasia
lamin	mandibul/o	-cyte
lumb	maxill/o	-desis
mandibul	muscul/o	-dynia
maxill	my/o	-ectomy
muscul	myel/o	-gram
my	oste/o	-ia

TABLE 10.1   Word Components in this Chapter (continued)

WORD ROOTS	COMBINING FORMS	SUFFIXES
myel	patell/o	-ic
oste	ped/i	-itis
patell	phalang/o	-lysis
ped	pod/o	-malacia
phalang	por/o	-megaly
pod	pub/o	-metry
por	rach/i	-oid
pub	scapul/o	-oma
rach	scler/o	-osis
scapul	scoli/o	-pexy
scler	skelet/o	-plasty
scoli	spondyl/o	-porosis
skelet	stern/o	-ptosis
spondyl	tar/o	-rrhaphy
stern	ten/o	-schisis
tar	tendin/o	-scopy
tendon	tendon/o	-tome
tibi	tibi/o	-tomy
vertebr	vertebr/o	

Progress Check

A. Multiple Choice

1. A root word meaning joint is:
   a. ili
   b. kyph
   c. ankyl
   d. lumb

2. A root word meaning wrist is:
   a. clavicul
   b. carp
   c. vertebr
   d. coccyx

3. A root word meaning spinal column or vertebrae is:
   a. myel
   b. oste
   c. por
   d. rach

4. A root word meaning breastbone is:
   a. crani
   b. dactyl
   c. stern
   d. tibi

5. A combining form meaning foot is:
   a. stern/o
   b. tar/o
   c. ten/o
   d. pod/o

6. A combining form meaning loins is:
   a. arthr/o
   b. lumb/o
   c. calcane/o
   d. phalang/o

7. A combining form meaning finger or toe is:
   a. ili/o
   b. dactyl/o
   c. kyph/o
   d. mandibul/o

8. A combining form meaning head is:
   a. crani/o
   b. femor/o
   c. cephal/o
   d. tibi/o

9. A prefix meaning between is:
   a. inter-
   b. intra-
   c. hetero-
   d. para-

10. A suffix meaning drooping or sagging is:
    a. -metry
    b. -ptosis
    c. -scopy
    d. -tome

11. A suffix meaning binding or fusion is:
    a. -desis
    b. -gram
    c. -itis
    d. -malacia

12. A suffix meaning resemble is:
    a.   -porosis
    b.   -rrhaphy
    c.   -schisis
    d.   -oid

13. A suffix meaning dissolution or breakdown is:
    a.   -ary
    b.   -centesis
    c.   -lysis
    d.   -plasty

B.   Building Medical Terms

Use the following word components to build medical terms matching the definitions given.

-al	femor/o	-plasty
-algia	ili	skelet
arthr	ili/o	skelet/o
arthr/o	-itis	spondyl
-ary	-malacia	spondyl/o
calcane	maxill	sub-
calcane/o	maxill/o	tars
crani	muscul/o	tars/o
crani/o	my	ten
-dynia	my/o	ten/o
-ectomy	pedi	tibi
femor	pedi/o	tibi/o

1. surgical repair of the tendon and muscle
2. pertaining to the large bone of the thigh and inner lower leg
3. pain in the heel bone
4. softening of the skull bones
5. pertaining to the hip bone (pelvic) and upper leg bone
6. bones and muscles of the body
7. inflammation of the vertebral joints
8. pertaining to below the upper jawbone
9. painful foot
10. excision of one or more ankle bones

C. Definitions and Word Components

	TERM	DEFINITION	PREFIX	WORD ROOT	VOWEL	WORD ROOT	VOWEL	SUFFIX
1.	ankylodactylia							
2.	carpoptosis							
3.	intrasternal							
4.	osteoporosis							
5.	osteosclerosis							
6.	rachicentesis							
7.	sternoclavicular							
8.	sternoid							
9.	suprascapular							
10.	vertebrosternal							

D. Abbreviations

	ABBREVIATION	MEANING
1.	BKA	
2.	C1, C2, … C7	
3.	DIP	
4.	Fx	
5.	L1, L2, … L5	
6.	MCP	
7.	MTP	
8.	PIP	
9.	BMD	
10.	DJD	
11.	THR	

The Sensory Organs

BLOCK	DATA AND ANSWERS	DESCRIPTIONS AND QUESTIONS
11-1		The first part of this chapter covers terminology related to the eye, its component parts, and medical conditions that affect vision. The eye consists of many parts: the cornea, pupil, retina, and others. It also contains nerves and muscles that control movement and support it. Each eye has two (upper and lower) eyelids lined with a mucous membrane called the conjunctiva. Each eye also contains a lacrimal gland that secretes tears through a series of ducts. The eye is contained in a bony compartment of the skull called the orbit and is surrounded by a cushion of fatty tissue.
	cornea (<u>kor</u>-ne′-a), pupil (<u>pu</u>-pil′), retina (<u>ret</u>-in-ah′) conjunctiva (kon′-junk-tih-<u>vah</u>), lacrimal gland (<u>lak</u>-rih′-mal gland)	For every block of study in this chapter, please refer to **Figure 11.1**, **Figure 11.2**, and **Table 11.1**.
11-2	ophthalmologist (opf′-thal-<u>mol</u>-o-jist)	An ophthalmologist is a physician whose specialty is treatment of the eyes. "ophthalm" is a word root meaning the eye. "ophthalm/o" is a combining form meaning the eye. -*logist* is a suffix meaning one who specializes. An opthalmologist is a physician whose specialty is
	treatment of the eyes	_____ ____ _____ _____.
	"ophthalm/o"	_____ is the combining form meaning eye.

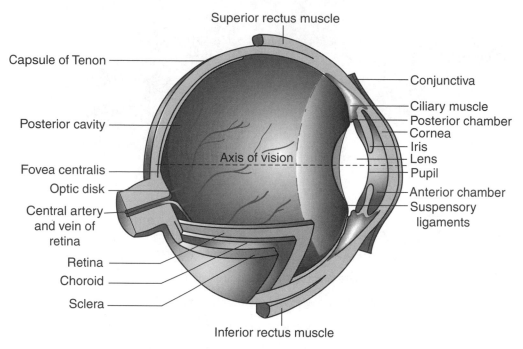

FIGURE 11.1 Parts of the eye

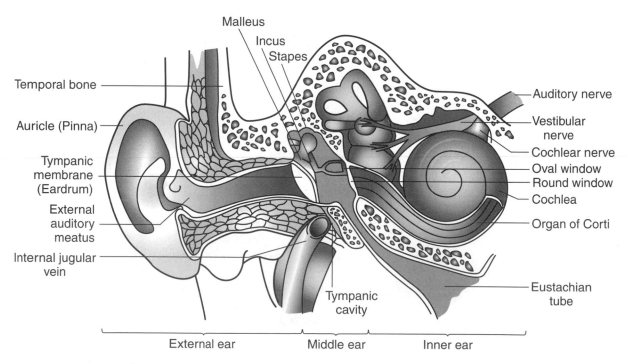

FIGURE 11.2 Parts of the ear

TABLE 11.1 Word Components in this Chapter

WORD ROOTS	COMBINING FORMS	PREFIXES
ambly	acoust/o	an-
antr	an/a	ana-
audi	antr/o	ex-
aur	audi/o	exo-
blephar	aur/o	hemi-
choroid	blephar/o	intra-
chromat	chromat/o	hyper-
cochlea	cochle/o	photo-
conjunctiv	conjunctiv/o	**SUFFIXES**
corne	corne/o	-al
cyst	cyst/o	-algia
dacry	dacry/o	-ar
dipl	dacryoaden/o	-centesis
edema	dacryocyst/o	-cusis
emmetr	dipl/o	-gram
exo	ex/o	-ectomy
heter	heter/o	-ia
kerat	ir/o	-ic
ir	irid/o	-ist
irid	is/o	-itis
iso	kerat/o	-logist
lachrym	lachrym/o	-logy
lacrim	lacrim/o	-malacia
laryng	laryng/o	-meter
leuk	leuk/o	-metry
mastoid	mastoid/o	-opia
ment	ment/o	-osis
meter	meter/o	-pathy
metr	metr/o	-phobia
myc	my/o	-plasty
myo	myc/o	-plegia
myring	myring/o	-ptosis
nas	nas/o	-rrhagia
ocul	ot/o	-rrhaphy
ophthalm	ocul/o	-rrhea
opt	ophthalm/o	-scope
optic	opt/o	-scopy
oto	optic/o	-stenosis

TABLE 11.1   Word Components in this Chapter (continued)

WORD ROOTS	COMBINING FORMS	SUFFIXES
pharyng	ot/o	-stomy
photo	pharyng/o	-tome
presby	phot/o	-tomy
retin	presby/o	-tropia
rhin	pupil/o	
salping	py/o	
sclera	retin/o	
staped	rhin/o	
ton	salping/o	
tympan	scler/o	
	staped/o	
	ton/o	
	tympan/o	

BLOCK	DATA AND ANSWERS	DESCRIPTIONS AND QUESTIONS
11-3	optometrist (op-<u>tom</u>-eh-trist)	An optometrist is a specialist who, after examining and testing the eyes, prescribes and fits lenses.
	optician (op'-<u>tish</u>-an)	An optician is a specialist skilled in filling prescriptions for lenses.
11-4		"optic" or "opt" is another word root meaning the eye.
		"optic/o" is another combining form meaning the eye.
		"opt/o" also is a combining form meaning the eye.
		"metr" is a word root meaning measure.
		"metr/o" is a combining form meaning measure.
		-ist is another suffix meaning a person or specialist.
11-5	optometrist	An _____ is a specialist in testing the eyes and correcting vision.
	optician	An _____ is one who is skilled in filling prescriptions for lenses.

BLOCK	DATA AND ANSWERS	DESCRIPTIONS AND QUESTIONS
11-6	ophthalmic (opf-<u>thal</u>-mik) *-ic*	"ophthalm/o" is a combining form meaning the eye. *-ic* is a suffix meaning pertaining to. Build a medical term (with pronunciation) meaning pertaining to the eye: _____ _____ _____ is a suffix meaning pertaining to.
11-7	intraocular (in'-trah-<u>ok</u>-u-lar)	*intra-* is a prefix meaning within. "ocul" also is a word root meaning the eye. "ocul/o" is another combining form referring to the eye. *-ar* is a suffix meaning pertaining to. "ocular" is a word root meaning pertaining to the eye. Build a medical term meaning pertaining to within the eye: _____ _____
11-8	"ophthalm/o" "optic/o" "opt/o" "ocul/o"	The four combining forms for the eye are: 1. _____ 2. _____ 3. _____ 4. _____
11-9	blepharectomy (blef'-ah-<u>rek</u>-to-me)	Blepharectomy is excision of a lesion of the eyelid. "blephar" is a word root meaning eyelid. "blephar/o" is a combining form meaning eyelid. *-ectomy* is a suffix meaning excision.

BLOCK	DATA AND ANSWERS	DESCRIPTIONS AND QUESTIONS
11-10	"blephar/o" -*ectomy* Blepharectomy	_____ is a combining form meaning eyelid. _____ is a suffix meaning excision. _____ is excision (of a lesion) of the eyelid.
11-11	blepharorrhaphy (blef-<u>ah</u>-ro-r′-fe)	-*rrhaphy* is a suffix meaning suture. Build a medical term meaning suturing of eyelid: _____ _____
11-12	blepharedema (blef′-ar-<u>eh</u>-de-mah	Blepharedema is fluid collection in the eyelid. "edema" is a word root meaning fluid collection.
11-13	combining form eyelid word root, fluid collection fluid collection in the eyelid	"blephar/o" is a _____ _____ meaning _____. "edema" is a _____ _____ meaning _____ _____. Blepharedema is _____ _____ ____ _____ _____.
11-14	"blephar/o"	_____ is a combining form meaning eyelid.
11-15	blepharoptosis (blef′-ah-rop-<u>to</u>-sis) combining form eyelid suffix, falling or drooping the condition of a falling or drooping eyelid	Blepharoptosis is the condition of a falling or drooping eyelid. -*ptosis* is a suffix meaning falling or drooping. "blephar/o" is a _____ _____ meaning _____. -*ptosis* is a _____ meaning _____ ____ _____. Blepharoptosis is _____ _____ ____ __ _____ ____ _____ _____.

BLOCK	DATA AND ANSWERS	DESCRIPTIONS AND QUESTIONS
11-16	ophthalmorrhagia (opf-thal'-mo-<u>rah</u>-je-ah) combining form eye suffix hemorrhage hemorrhage from the eye	Opthalmorrhagia is hemorrhage from the eye. "ophthalm/o" is a _____ _____ meaning _____. -*rrhagia* is a _____ meaning _____. Ophthalmorrhagia is _____ _____ _____ _____.
11-17	ophthalmalgia (opf'-thal-mal-je-<u>ah</u>) -*algia*	"opthalm/o" is a combining form meaning the eye. -*algia* is a suffix meaning pain. Build a medical term meaning pain in the eye: _____ _____ _____ is a suffix meaning pain.
11-18	oculomycosis (ok'-u-lo-mi-<u>ko</u>-sis)	Oculomycosis is a disease of the eye caused by a fungus. "ocul" is a word root meaning eye. "ocul/o" is a combining form meaning eye. "myc" is a word root meaning fungus. "myc/o" is a combining form meaning fungus. -*osis* is a suffix meaning condition. It can be normal or abnormal.
11-19	"ocul/o" "myc/o" -*osis* Oculomycosis	_____ is a combining form meaning eye. _____ is a combining form meaning fungus. _____ is a suffix meaning condition. _____ is a disease of the eye caused by a fungus.

BLOCK	DATA AND ANSWERS	DESCRIPTIONS AND QUESTIONS
11-20	tonometer (to´-<u>nom</u>-eh-ter)	A tonometer is an instrument used to measure pressure within the eye.
		"ton" is a word root meaning pressure.
		"ton/o" is a combining form meaning pressure.
		"meter" is a word root meaning an instrument used to measure.
		-*meter* also is a suffix.
	tonometer	A _____ is an instrument that measures pressure within the eye.
	"ton/o"	_____ is a combining form meaning pressure.
11-21		-*metry* is a suffix meaning measurement.
	tonometry (to´-<u>nom</u>-et-re)	Build a medical term meaning measurement of pressure within the eye: _____ _____
11-22	ophthalmoscope (opf-<u>thal</u>-mo-skop´)	An ophthalmoscope is an instrument that examines the interior of the eye.
	"ophthalm/o"	_____ is a combining form meaning the eye.
	-*scope*	_____ is a suffix meaning an instrument that measures.
	ophthalmoscope	An _____ is an instrument used to examine the interior of the eye.
11-23		-*pathy* is a suffix meaning disease.
	ophthalmopathy (opf-thal´-<u>mop</u>-ah-the)	Build a medical term meaning any disease of the eye: _____ _____

BLOCK	DATA AND ANSWERS	DESCRIPTIONS AND QUESTIONS
11-24	pupil (<u>pu</u>-poh'ol)	Next we will study the medical terms related to the pupil. The pupil is the eye or opening of the iris in the eye. "pupil" is a root word. "pupil/o" is the combining form.
11-25	pupilometer (pu'-pih-<u>lom</u>-e-ter)	A pupilometer is an instrument used to measure the pupil. "pupil/o" is a combining form meaning pupil. "meter" is a root word meaning an instrument used to measure. -*meter* also is a suffix.
11-26	"pupil/o" -*meter* Pupilometer	_____ is a combining form meaning pupil. _____ is a suffix meaning a measuring device. A _____ is an instrument used to measure the pupil.
11-27	leukocoria (loo'-ko-<u>ko</u>-re-ah) Leukocoria	Leukocoria means condition of white pupil. "leuk" is a word root meaning white. "leuk/o" is a combining form meaning white. "cor" is a root word meaning pupil. -*ia* is a suffix meaning condition. _____ is a condition of white pupil.
11-28	iridoplegia (ir'-id-o-<u>ple</u>-je-ah)	Iris is the structure surrounding the pupil. "iris," "ir," and "irid" can be the word root. Iridoplegia is paralysis of the iris. "irid/o" is a combining form meaning iris. -*plegia* is a suffix meaning paralysis.

BLOCK	DATA AND ANSWERS	DESCRIPTIONS AND QUESTIONS
11-29	combining form iris suffix, paralysis paralysis of the iris	"irid/o" is a _____ _____ meaning _____. *-plegia* is a _____ meaning _____. Iridoplegia is _____ ____ _____ _____.
11-30	corneal (<u>kor</u>-ne'-al)	Corneal means pertaining to the cornea of the eye. "corne" is a word root meaning corneal. "corne/o" is the combining form. "kerat/o" also is a combining form meaning the cornea.
11-31	keratocentesis (ker-ah'-to-<u>sen</u>-te-sis)	*-centesis* is a suffix meaning surgical puncture. Build a medical term meaning surgical puncture of the cornea: _____ _____
11-32	keratoplasty (ker'-ah-to-<u>plas</u>-te)	*-plasty* is a suffix meaning plastic repair. Build a medical term meaning plastic repair of the cornea: _____ _____
11-33	corneoiritis (kor'-ne-o-i-<u>ri</u>-tis)	Corneoiritis is inflammation of the cornea and iris. Note the unusual placement of the three adjacent vowels: e, o, and i.
11-34	Corneoiritis	"corne/o" is another combining form meaning cornea. "ir/o" is a combining form meaning iris. *-itis* is a suffix meaning inflammation. _____ is inflammation of the cornea and iris.

BLOCK	DATA AND ANSWERS	DESCRIPTIONS AND QUESTIONS
11-35	combining form cornea	"corne/o" is a _____ _____ meaning _____.
	combining form iris	"ir/o" is a _____ _____ meaning _____.
	suffix inflammation	-itis is a _____ meaning _____.
11-36		"kerat/o" is a combining form for cornea.
		"meter" is a word root meaning an instrument that measures.
	keratometer (keh'-rah-to-meh-ter)	Build a medical term meaning instrument used to measure the cornea: _____ _____ (In this case, the measurement is of the curvature of the cornea.)
11-37	conjunctiva (kon'-junk-tih-vah)	The conjunctiva is a clear mucous membrane that covers the white part of the eye and the lines inside of the eyelids.
		"conjunctiv/o" is a combining form meaning conjunctiva.
		-itis is a suffix meaning inflammation.
	conjunctivitis (kon'-junk-tih-vi-tis)	Build a compound medical term meaning inflammation of the conjunctiva: _____ _____
11-38	aqueous (a-kwe-us) vitreous (vit-re-us)	The eye has two chambers between the cornea and the lens. The front chambers contain a clear, watery fluid called aqueous humor. The back chamber (between the lens and the retina) also contains a clear, jellylike substance called vitreous humor. Aqueous means watery and vitreous means glassy.
11-39	Aqueous humor	_____ _____ is the watery fluid that fills the front two chambers of the eye.
	Vitreous humor	_____ _____ is the jellylike substance that fills the back chamber of the eye.

BLOCK	DATA AND ANSWERS	DESCRIPTIONS AND QUESTIONS
11-40	scleritis (skleh'-<u>ri</u>-tis)	The outermost layer of the eye is a white fibrous tissue (membrane) structure called the sclera (the white of the eye). Scleritis is inflammation of the sclera. "sclera" and "scler" are the word roots meaning sclera. "scler/o" is a combining form meaning the sclera. -*itis* is a suffix meaning inflammation.
11-41	combining form white fibrous tissue of the eye suffix inflammation inflammation of the sclera	"scler/o" is a _____ _____ meaning _____ _____ _____ ____ _____ _____. -*itis* is a _____ meaning _____. Scleritis is _____ _____ _____ _____.
11-42	sclerostomy (skleh'-<u>ros</u>-to-me)	-*stomy* is a suffix meaning the forming of a new opening. Build a medical term meaning surgical formation of an opening in the sclera: _____ _____
11-43	sclerotomy (skleh'-<u>rot</u>-o-me)	-*tomy* is a suffix meaning incision. Build a medical term meaning incision into the sclera: _____ _____
11-44	sclerokeratitis (skleh'-ro-keh-rah-<u>ti</u>-tis)	Sclerokeratitis is inflammation of the sclera and the cornea. "scler/o" is a combining form meaning the sclera. "kerat" is a word root meaning the cornea. "kerat/o" is the combining form. -*itis* is a suffix meaning inflammation.

BLOCK	DATA AND ANSWERS	DESCRIPTIONS AND QUESTIONS
11-45	"scler/o" "kerat/o" -itis Sclerokeratitis	_____ is a combining form meaning the sclera. _____ is a combining form meaning the cornea. _____ is a suffix meaning inflammation. _____ is inflammation of the sclera and the cornea.
11-46	scleromalacia (skleh'-ro-mah-la-se-ah)	Scleromalacia is softening of the sclera. "scler/o" is a combining form meaning the sclera. -malacia is a suffix meaning softening.
11-47	"scler/o" -malacia Scleromalacia	_____ is a combining form meaning the sclera. _____ is a suffix meaning softening. _____ is softening of the sclera.
11-48	retina (ret-ih-nah') retinopathy (ret'-in-op-ath-e)	The next section covers medical terms associated with the retina, which is located at the back of the eye and serves to receive and transmit visual images. "retin" is a word root meaning retina. "retin/o" is a combining form meaning retina. -pathy is a suffix meaning disease. Build a medical term meaning disease of the retina: _____ _____
11-49	retinal (ret-in-al')	-al is a suffix meaning pertaining to. Build a medical term that means pertaining to the retina: _____ _____

BLOCK	DATA AND ANSWERS	DESCRIPTIONS AND QUESTIONS
11-50	photoretinitis (fo′-to-ret-in-i-tis)	Photoretinitis is inflammation of the retina caused by light. "photo" is a word root meaning light. "phot/o" is a combining form meaning light. *photo-* also is a prefix. "retin/o" is a combining form for retina. *-itis* is a suffix meaning inflammation.
11-51	Photoretinitis "phot/o" "retin/o"	_____ is inflammation of the retina caused by light. _____ is a combining form meaning light. _____ is a combining form meaning retina.
11-52	choroiditis (ko′-royd-i-tis)	The choroid is the outside layer of the retina. Choroiditis is inflammation of the choroid. "choroid" is a root word meaning choroid. "choroid/o" is a combining form meaning choroid. *-itis* is a suffix meaning inflammation.
11-53	"choroid" *-itis* Choroiditis	_____ is a a root word meaning choroid. _____ is a suffix meaning inflammation. _____ is inflammation of the choroid.
11-54	amblyopia (am′-ble-o-pe-ah)	The next section discusses medical terms associated with vision. Amblyopia is dull or dim vision. "ambly" is a word root meaning dull or dim. "ambly/o" is a combining form meaning dull or dim. *-opia* is a suffix meaning vision.

BLOCK	DATA AND ANSWERS	DESCRIPTIONS AND QUESTIONS
11-55	"ambly" -*opia* Amblyopia	_____ is a root word meaning dim. _____ is a suffix meaning vision. _____ is dull or dim vision.
11-56	presbyopia (prez'-be-<u>o</u>-pe-ah)	Presbyopia is a defect in vision that occurs normally with age (farsightedness). "presby" is a root word meaning old or aged. "presby/o" is the combining form. -*opia* is a suffix meaning vision.
11-57	root word, old or aged "presby/o" suffix, vision a defect in vision that occurs normally with aging (farsightedness)	"presby" is a _____ _____ meaning _____ _____ _____. _____ is the combining form. -*opia* is a _____ meaning _____. Presbyopia is ___ _____ ____ _____ _____ _____ _____ _____ _____ _____.
11-58	emmetropia (em'-eh-<u>tro</u>-pe-ah)	Emmetropia is ideal vision. "emmetr" is a root word meaning correct measure. "emmetr/o" is the combining form. -*opia* is a suffix meaning vision.
11-59	"emmetr/o" -*opia* Emmetropia	_____ is a combining form meaning correct measure. _____ is a suffix meaning vision. _____ is ideal vision.
11-60	exotropia (ek'-so-<u>tro</u>-pe-ah)	Exotropia means outward-turning and is one of many words to describe the movement of the eye.

BLOCK	DATA AND ANSWERS	DESCRIPTIONS AND QUESTIONS
11-61	Exotropia	"ex/o" is a combining form meaning outward. *exo-* also is a prefix meaning outward. *-tropia* is a suffix meaning turning. _____ means outward-turning.
11-62	heterometropia (het'-eh-ro-met-<u>ro</u>-pe-ah)	Heterometropia is having different vision in the two eyes. "heter" is a root word meaning different. "heter/o" is the combining form. "metr/o" is a combining form meaning measure. *-opia* is a suffix meaning vision.
11-63	combining form different suffix, vision having different vision in the two eyes	"heter/o" is a _____ _____ meaning _____. *-opia* is a _____ meaning _____. Heterometropia is _____ _____ _____ ___ _____ _____ _____.
11-64	anopsia (an-op-se'-ah)	*an-* is a prefix meaning without. *-opsia* is another suffix meaning vision. Build a medical term meaning blindness: _____ _____
11-65	hemianopia (hem-ee-uh'-<u>noh</u>-pee-uh)	Hemianopia is blindness in half of the visual field. *hemi-* is a prefix meaning half. *an-* is a prefix meaning without. *-opia* a suffix meaning vision.

BLOCK	DATA AND ANSWERS	DESCRIPTIONS AND QUESTIONS
11-66	*hemi-*	_____ is a prefix meaning half.
	an-	_____ is a prefix meaning without.
	-opia	_____ is a suffix meaning vision.
	Hemianopia	_____ is blindness in half the visual field.
11-67	anisometropia (an'-i-so-meh-<u>tro</u>-pe-ah)	Anisometropia is the condition of unequal refractive powers in the two eyes.
		an- is a prefix meaning not or without.
		"is/o" is a combining form meaning equal.
		"metr/o" is a combining form meaning measure.
		-opia is a suffix meaning vision.
11-68	*an-*	_____ is a prefix meaning not or without.
	"is/o"	_____ is a combining form meaning equal.
	"metr/o"	_____ is a combining form meaning measure.
	-opia	_____ is a suffix meaning vision.
	Anisometropia	_____ is unequal refractive powers in the two eyes.
11-69	hyperchromatopsia (hi'-per-kro-mah-<u>top</u>-se-ah)	Hyperchromatopsia is a defect of vision in which all objects appear colored.
		hyper- is a prefix meaning excessive.
		"chromat" is a word root meaning color.
		"chromat/o" is a combining form meaning color.
		-opsia is a suffix meaning vision.
11-70	Hyperchromatopsia	_____ is a defect of vision in which all objects appear colored.

BLOCK	DATA AND ANSWERS	DESCRIPTIONS AND QUESTIONS
11-71	diplopia (dip'-lo-<u>pe</u>-ah)	Diplopia is double vision. "dipl" is a word root meaning double. "dipl/o" is the combining form. -*opia* is a suffix meaning vision.
11-72	"dipl/o" -*opia* Diplopia	_____ is a combining form meaning double. _____ is a suffix meaning vision. _____ is double vision.
11-73	photophobia (fo'-to-<u>fo</u>-be-ah)	*photo-* is a prefix meaning light. "phot/o" is a combining form meaning light. -*phobia* is a suffix meaning abnormal fear. Build a medical term meaning abnormal aversion to light: _____ _____
11-74	optomyometer (op'-to-mi-<u>om</u>-eh-ter)	An optomyometer is an instrument used to measure (the power of) the muscles of vision.
11-75	optomyometer	"opt" is a word root meaning eye or vision. "opt/o" is a combining form meaning vision. "my/o" is a combining form meaning muscles. "meter" is a root word meaning an instrument used to measure. -*meter* is also a suffix. An _____ is an instrument that measures (the power of) the muscles of vision.

BLOCK	DATA AND ANSWERS	DESCRIPTIONS AND QUESTIONS
11-76	"opt/o" "my/o" *-meter*	_____ is a combining form meaning vision. _____ is a combining form meaning muscles. _____ is a suffix meaning an instrument used to measure.
11-77	optometry (op'-<u>tom</u>-et-re)	*-metry* is a suffix meaning measurement. Build a medical term meaning measurement of the eye: _____ _____ (Usually this term refers to testing for visual acuity and prescribing corrective lenses.)
11-78	lacrimal (<u>lak</u>-rih'-mal) lachrymal (<u>lak</u>-rih'-mal)	Another group of medical terms is related to tears. Lacrimal means pertaining to tears or tear ducts. "lacrim" is a word root meaning tears or tear ducts. "lacrim/o" is the combining form. *-al* is a suffix meaning pertaining to. Lachrymal is another term meaning pertaining to tears or tear ducts. "lachrymal" or "lachrym" are other root words meaning tears or tear ducts. "lachrym/o" is the combining form.
11-79	Lacrimal Lachrymal	Two medical terms that mean pertaining to tears or tear ducts are: 1. _____ 2. _____

BLOCK	DATA AND ANSWERS	DESCRIPTIONS AND QUESTIONS
11-80	nasolacrimal (na′-zo-<u>lak</u>-rih-mal)	"nas/o" is a combining form meaning nose. "lacrim/o" is a combining form meaning tears or tear ducts. *-al* is a suffix meaning pertaining to. Build a word that means pertaining to the nose and tear ducts: _____ _____
11-81	dacryorrhea (<u>dak</u>-re-o-re′-ah)	Dacryorrhea is the condition of flowing tears. "dacry" is a word root meaning tear. "dacry/o" is another combining form meaning tear. *-rrhea* is a suffix meaning flowing.
11-82	combining form tear suffix, flowing the condition of flowing tears	"dacry/o" is a _____ _____ meaning _____. *-rrhea* is a _____ meaning _____. Dacryorrhea is _____ _____ _____ _____ _____.
11-83	dacryoadenectomy (dak′-re-o-ad-e-<u>nek</u>-to-me)	Dacryoadenectomy is excision of the tear gland. "dacry/o" is a combining form meaning tear. "aden" is a word root meaning gland. "aden/o" is a combining form meaning gland. "dacryoaden/o" is a combining form meaning tear gland. *-ectomy* is a suffix meaning excision.

BLOCK	DATA AND ANSWERS	DESCRIPTIONS AND QUESTIONS
11-84	"dacryoaden/o"	_____ is a combining form meaning tear gland.
	-*ectomy*	_____ is a suffix meaning excision.
	Dacryoadenectomy	_____ is excision of the tear gland.
11-85	dacryostenosis (dak′-re-o-<u>sten</u>-o-sis)	Dacryostenosis is constriction of a tear duct. "dacry/o" is a combining form meaning tear gland or duct. -*stenosis* is a suffix meaning constriction (narrowing).
11-86	Dacryostenosis	_____ is constriction of a tear duct.
	-*stenosis*	_____ is a suffix meaning constriction.
11-87	dacryocystitis (dak′-re-o-sis-<u>ti</u>-tis)	Dacrocystitis is inflammation of the tear cyst or sac. "dacry/o" is a combining form meaning tear. "cyst" is a word root meaning cyst or sac. "cyst/o" is a combining form meaning cyst or sac. "dacryocyst/o" is a combining form meaning tear sac. -*itis* is a suffix meaning inflammation.
11-88	Dacryocystitis	_____ is inflammation of the tear sac.
	"dacry/o"	_____ is a combining form meaning tear.
	"cyst/o"	_____ is a combining form meaning cyst or sac.
	-*itis*	_____ is a suffix meaning inflammation.

BLOCK	DATA AND ANSWERS	DESCRIPTIONS AND QUESTIONS
11-89		The second part of this chapter discusses terms associated with the ears.
		The ear consists of three distinct parts: the external, middle, and inner ear. Each part contains structures that allow it to perform specialized functions.
		Refer to Figure 11.2.
11-90	audiologist (<u>aw</u>-de-<u>ol</u>-o-ji′-st)	An audiologist is a person who specializes in diagnosing hearing disorders.
		"audi" is a word root meaning hearing.
		"audi/o" is a combining form meaning hearing.
		-*logist* is a suffix meaning one who specializes in.
11-91	combining form hearing	"audi/o" is a _____ _____ meaning _____.
	suffix, one who specializes in	-*logist* is a _____ meaning _____ _____ _____ ____.
	a person who specializes in diagnosing hearing disorders	An audiologist is ___ _____ _____ _____ ___ _____ _____ _____.
11-92		-*logy* is a suffix meaning the study of.
		Build a medical term meaning the study of hearing:
	audiology (aw′-de-<u>ol</u>-o-ji)	_____ _____
11-93		"audi/o" is a combining form meaning hearing.
		-*meter* is a suffix meaning an instrument used to measure.
		-*metry* is a suffix meaning measurement.

BOX 11.1

Allied Health Professions

Dispensing Opticians, Pharmacy Technicians, Pharmacy Aides, and Medical Assistants

Dispensing opticians fit eyeglasses and contact lenses, following prescriptions written by ophthalmologists or optometrists. They examine written prescriptions to determine corrective lens specifications. They recommend eyeglass frames, lenses, and lens coatings after considering the prescription and the customer's occupation, habits, and facial features. Dispensing opticians measure clients' eyes, including the distance between the centers of the pupils and the distance between the eye surface and the lens. Dispensing opticians prepare work orders that give ophthalmic laboratory technicians the information needed to grind and insert lenses into a frame.

The following are some resources for further information:

- American Board of Opticianry, www.abo.org
- National Contact Lens Examiners, www.abo-ncle.org

Pharmacy technicians, assistants, and/or aides help licensed pharmacists provide medication and other health care products to patients. Pharmacy technicians usually perform more complex tasks than assistants do, although in some states their duties and job titles overlap. Technicians typically perform routine tasks, such as counting and labeling, to help prepare prescribed medication for patients. A pharmacist must check every prescription before it can be given to a patient, however. Technicians refer any questions regarding prescriptions, drug information, or health matters to the pharmacist. Pharmacy assistants or aides usually have fewer, less complex responsibilities than pharmacy technicians do. Aides and assistants are often clerks or cashiers who primarily answer telephones, handle money, stock shelves, and perform other clerical duties.

The following are some resources for further information:

- Pharmacy Technician Certification Board, www.ptcb.org
- Institute for the Certification of Pharmacy Technicians, www.nationaltechexam.org
- American Society of Health-System Pharmacists, www.ashp.org
- National Pharmacy Technician Association, www.pharmacytechnician.org

Medical assistants perform administrative and clinical tasks to keep the offices of physicians, podiatrists, chiropractors, and other health practitioners running smoothly. They should not be confused with physician's assistants, who examine, diagnose, and treat patients under the direct supervision of a physician. The duties of medical assistants vary from office to office, depending on the location and size of the practice and the practitioner's specialty.

A great resource is the American Association of Medical Assistants at www.aama-ntl.org.

Source: P. S. Stanfield, N. Cross, Y. H . Hui, eds. *Introduction to the Health Professions,* 5th ed. (Sudbury, MA: Jones & Bartlett, 2009).

BLOCK	DATA AND ANSWERS	DESCRIPTIONS AND QUESTIONS
11-94	audiometer (aw'-de-om-eh-ter) audiometry (aw'-di-<u>om</u>-eh-tre)	Build a medical term meaning instrument used to measure hearing: _____ _____ Build a medical term meaning measurement of hearing: _____ _____
11-95	audiogram (aw-de-o-gram)	*-gram* is a suffix meaning a record (in this case, a graphic record of a hearing test). Build a medical term that means graphic record of a hearing test: _____ _____
11-96	otorhinolaryngologist (o'-to-<u>ri</u>-no-lah-rin-<u>joh</u>-lo-jist) otorhinolaryngology (o'-to-<u>ri</u>-no-lah-rin-<u>joh</u>-lo-ge)	An otorhinolaryngologist is a physician who studies and treats diseases of the ear, nose, and throat (commonly referred to as an ENT specialist). Otorhinolaryngology is a medical specialty that deals with diseases of the ear, nose, and throat.
11-97		"oto" is a word root meaning ear. "ot/o" is a combining form meaning ear. "rhin" is a word root meaning nose. "rhin/o" is a combining form meaning nose. "laryngx" is a word root meaning throat. "laryng/o" is a combining form meaning throat. *-logist* is a suffix meaning one who studies. *-logy* is a suffix meaning the study of.

BLOCK	DATA AND ANSWERS	DESCRIPTIONS AND QUESTIONS
11-98	"ot/o"	_____ is a combining form meaning ear.
	"rhin/o"	_____ is a combining form meaning nose.
	"laryng/o"	_____ is a combining form meaning throat.
	-logist	_____ is a suffix meaning one who specializes in.
	-logy	_____ is a suffix meaning the study of.
	otorhinolaryngologist	An _____ is a physician who studies and treats diseases of the ear, nose, and throat.
	Otorhinolaryngology	_____ is a medical specialty that deals with diseases of the ear, nose, and throat.
11-99		We will now turn our attention to medical terms related to the study and disorders of the ear.
	otoscope (o'-to-<u>skop</u>)	An otoscope is an instrument used to examine the ear.
	otoscopy (o'-to-<u>sko</u>-pe)	An otoscopy is an examination of the ear.
11-100		"ot/o" is a combining form meaning the ear.
		"scope" is a word root meaning an instrument used for examination.
		-scope also is a suffix.
		"scopy" is a word root meaning a study or examination.
		-scopy is also a suffix.
11-101	otoscope	An _____ is an instrument used to examine the ear.
	Otoscopy	_____ is an examination of the ear.

BLOCK	DATA AND ANSWERS	DESCRIPTIONS AND QUESTIONS
11-102	otomycosis (o'-to-mi-<u>ko</u>-sis)	Otomycosis is a fungal disease of the ear.
		"ot/o" is a combining form meaning ear.
		"myc" is a word root meaning fungus.
		"myc/o" is a combining form meaning fungus.
		-osis is a suffix meaning condition.
11-103	Otomycosis	_____ is a fungal disease of the ear.
	"ot/o"	_____ is a combining form meaning ear.
	fungus	"myc/o" is a combining form meaning _____.
	-osis	_____ is a suffix meaning condition.
11-104		There are two medical terms related to the ear that do not break down into word components.
	tinnitus (tin'-<u>eye</u>-tus)	Tinnitus is the condition of a ringing sound in the ears.
	vertigo (<u>ver</u>-tih'-goh)	Vertigo refers to the sensation of spinning around or of things in the room spinning around. Vertigo is caused by a loss of equilibrium.
11-105	Tinnitus	_____ is ringing in the ear.
	Vertigo	_____ is a spinning sensation.
11-106		"aur" is a word root meaning ear.
		"aur/o" is another combining form meaning ear.
		-al is a suffix meaning pertaining to.
	aural (<u>aw</u>-ral)	Build a term that means pertaining to the ear: _____ _____
11-107		"ot/o" is a combining form meaning the ear.
		-algia is a suffix meaning pain.
	Otalgia	_____ is pain in the ear.

BLOCK	DATA AND ANSWERS	DESCRIPTIONS AND QUESTIONS
11-108	otoplasty (o′-to-<u>plas</u>-te) combining form ear suffix, plastic repair repair of the ear	An otoplasty is repair of the ear. "ot/o" is a _____ _____ meaning _____. -*plasty* is a _____ meaning _____ _____. Otoplasty is _____ _____ _____ _____.
11-109	otopyorrhea (o′-to-pi′-o-<u>re</u>-ah)	Otopyorrhea is discharge of pus from the ear. "ot/o" is a combining form meaning ear. "py" is a root word meaning pus. "py/o" is a combining form meaning pus. -*rrhea* is a suffix meaning flowing (discharge).
11-110	"ot/o" "py/o" -*rrhea* Otopyorrhea	_____ is a combining form meaning ear. _____ is a combining form meaning pus. _____ is a suffix meaning flowing (discharge). _____ is discharge of pus from the ear.
11-111	auricle (<u>aw</u>-rik-kuh′), pinna (<u>pin</u>-nah) tympanum (tim-<u>pan</u>-num′)	The next group of medical terms is related to the structures and disorders of the ear, beginning with the earlobe. The auricle or pinna is the fleshy ear flap commonly known as the earlobe. As we proceed from the outside of the ear and move inward, we come across the eardrum. We next concentrate on terms related to the eardrum. Tympanum is the medical term for eardrum.

BLOCK	DATA AND ANSWERS	DESCRIPTIONS AND QUESTIONS
11-112	tympan (tim-<u>pan</u>)	"tympan" is a root word meaning eardrum (membrane).
		"tympan/o" is the combining form.
	myring (mi-<u>rin</u>-ji)	"myring" is another root word meaning eardrum.
		"myring/o" is the combining form.
	"tympan," "myring"	_____ and _____ are two root words meaning eardrum.
11-113		"myring/o" is a combining form meaning eardrum.
		-_itis_ is a suffix meaning inflammation.
	Myringitis	_____ is inflammation of the eardrum.
11-114		"tympan/o" is a combining form meaning eardrum.
		-_plasty_ is a suffix meaning plastic repair.
		Build a medical term that means plastic repair of the eardrum:
	tympanoplasty	_____
	(tim′-pan-o-<u>plas</u>-te)	_____
11-115	myringotomy (mir′-in-<u>jot</u>-o-me)	A myringotomy is an incision into the eardrum.
		-_tomy_ is a suffix meaning incision.
	an incision into	A myringotomy is _____ _____ _____
	the eardrum	_____ _____.
11-116	myringotome (mih′-rin-<u>jo</u>-tom)	Myringotome is a knife that is used for surgery on the eardrum.
		"myring/o" is a combining form meaning eardrum.
		-_tome_ is a suffix meaning knife.
11-117	"myring/o"	_____ is a combining form meaning eardrum.
	-_tome_	_____ is a suffix meaning knife.
	myringotome	A _____ is a knife used for surgery on the eardrum.

BLOCK	DATA AND ANSWERS	DESCRIPTIONS AND QUESTIONS
11-118		After the eardrum, we reach the inner ear, which contains several tiny bones that make up the foundation of our hearing system.
11-119	stapedectomy (sta'-peh-<u>dek</u>-to-me)	The stapes, commonly known as the stirrup, is the stirrup-shaped bone in the inner ear. Stapedectomy is excision of the stapes. "staped" is a root word meaning stapes. "staped/o" is a combining form meaning stapes. -*ectomy* is a suffix meaning excision.
11-120	combining form stapes suffix, excision excision of the stapes	"staped/o" is a _____ _____ meaning _____. -*ectomy* is a _____ meaning _____. Stapedectomy is _____ ____ _____ _____.
11-121	otosclerosis (o'-to-<u>skler</u>-o-sis)	Otosclerosis is the hardening of the bones in the inner ear, especially the stapes. "ot/o" is a combining form meaning the ear. "scler/o" is a combining form meaning hardening. -*osis* is a suffix meaning condition.
11-122	Otosclerosis "ot/o" hardening -*osis*	_____ is hardening of the bones of the inner ear, especially the stapes. _____ is a combining form meaning the ear. "scler/o" is a combining form meaning _____. _____ is a suffix meaning condition.

BLOCK	DATA AND ANSWERS	DESCRIPTIONS AND QUESTIONS
11-123	cochlea (<u>kah</u>-klee-ah)	The cochlea, shaped like a snail, is another bone in the inner ear.
		"cochlea" and "cochle" are word roots meaning bone in the inner ear.
		"cochle/o" is the combining form.
11-124	eustachian (u'-<u>sdad</u>-chee-un)	The eustachian tube is a path leading from the ear to the throat area. Refer to Figure 11.2.
	salpingitis (sal'-pin-<u>ji</u>-tis)	Salpingitis is inflammation of the eustachian tube.
		"salpinge" and "salping" are root words meaning tube (here it refers to the eustachian tube).
		"salping/o" is the combining form.
		-*itis* is a suffix meaning inflammation.
11-125	"salpinge"	Two root words for the eustachian tube are _____
	"salping"	and _____.
	"salping/o"	_____ is a combining form meaning tube.
	-*itis*	_____ is a suffix meaning inflammation.
	Salpingitis	_____ is inflammation of the eustachian tube.
11-126	mastoid (<u>mas</u>-toyd)	The mastoid bone, also called the mastoid process, is the bone right behind the earlobe. It has many functions, including protecting the inner ear. Because it has some empty air space, it is easily subject to inflammation and infection.
		"mastoid" is the word root.
		"mastoid/o" is the combining form.

BLOCK	DATA AND ANSWERS	DESCRIPTIONS AND QUESTIONS
11-127		*-itis* is a suffix meaning inflammation.
		Build a word meaning inflammation of the mastoid:
	mastoiditis	_____
	(mas'-toy-<u>di</u>-tis)	_____
11-128	otomastoiditis (o'-to-mas'-toy-<u>di</u>-tis)	Otomastoiditis is inflammation of the ear and the mastoid bone, the bone behind the earlobe.
		"ot/o" is a combining form meaning ear.
		"mastoid/o" is the combining form of mastoid.
		-itis is a suffix meaning inflammation.
11-129	Otomastoiditis	_____ is inflammation of the ear and the mastoid bone.
	"ot/o"	_____ is a combining form meaning ear.
	"mastoid/o"	_____ is a combining form meaning mastoid, or the bone behind the earlobe.
	-itis	_____ is a suffix meaning inflammation.
11-130		*-ectomy* is a suffix meaning excision.
		-tomy is a suffix meaning incision.
		Build a medical term meaning removal of the mastoid:
	mastoidectomy	_____
	(mas'-toy'-<u>dek</u>-to-me)	_____
		Build a medical term meaning incision into the mastoid:
	mastoidotomy	_____
	(mas'-toy-<u>dot</u>-o-me)	_____

BLOCK	DATA AND ANSWERS	DESCRIPTIONS AND QUESTIONS
11-131	labyrinthitis (lab´-ih-rin-<u>thi</u>-tis)	The labyrinth is the inner ear, where the cochlea is located. "labryinth" is a word root. "labyrinth/o" is a combining form. *-itis* is a suffix meaning inflammation. Build a medical term meaning inflammation of the labyrinth (inner ear): _____ _____
11-132	labyrinthectomy (lab´-ih-rin-<u>thek</u>-to-me)	*-ectomy* is a suffix meaning excision. Build a medical term meaning surgical excision of the labyrinth: _____ _____
11-133	acoustic (ah´-<u>coos</u>-tik)	Our last group of medical terms related to the ear covers the clinical aspects of hearing. Acoustic means pertaining to sound or hearing. "acoust" is the word root. "acoust/o" is the combining form.
11-134	Acoustic	_____ means pertaining to sound or hearing.
11-135	acoustometer (ah´-coos-<u>tom</u>-eh-ter)	An acoustometer is an instrument used to measure (acuteness of) hearing. "acoust/o" is a combining form meaning hearing. "meter" is a word root meaning instrument used to measure. *-meter* is also a suffix.

BLOCK	DATA AND ANSWERS	DESCRIPTIONS AND QUESTIONS
11-136	"acoust/o" "meter" -meter acoustometer	_____ is a combining form meaning hearing. _____ is a word root meaning instrument used to measure. _____ is also a suffix. An _____ is an instrument used to measure (acuteness of) hearing.
11-137	anacusis (an'-ah-<u>ku</u>-sis)	Anacusis means without hearing. "an/a" is a combining form meaning without. (Note that this is a rare case in which 'a' is used instead of 'o' in the combining form.) ana- is a prefix meaning without. -cusis is a suffix meaning hearing.
11-138	"an/a" -cusis Anacusis	_____ is a combining form meaning without. _____ is a suffix meaning hearing. _____ means without hearing.
11-139	presbycusis (pres'-be-<u>ku</u>-sis)	Presbycusis is a gradual loss of hearing that occurs with aging. "presby/o" is a combining form meaning aging or old age. -cusis is a suffix meaning hearing.
11-140	combining form old age suffix, hearing a gradual loss of hearing that occurs with aging	"presby/o" is a _____ _____ meaning _____ _____. -cusis is a _____ meaning _____. Presbycusis is ___ _____ _____ ____ _____ _____ _____ _____ _____.

BLOCK	DATA AND ANSWERS	DESCRIPTIONS AND QUESTIONS
11-141	nasal (<u>nayz</u>-al)	The remaining blocks in this chapter discuss medical terms associated with the nose. Nasal means pertaining to the nose (cavity). "nas" is a root word meaning nose. "nas/o" is the combining form. -al is a suffix meaning pertaining to.
11-142	nasitis (nay'-<u>zi</u>-tis)	-itis is a suffix meaning inflammation. Build a medical term meaning inflammation of the nose (cavity): _____ _____
11-143	nasoscope (nayz'-oh-<u>skope</u>)	"scope" is a root word meaning an instrument used to examine. -scope also is a suffix. Build a medical term meaning an instrument used to examine the nose: _____ _____
11-144	nasoantritis (nayz'-oh-an-<u>try</u>-tis)	Nasoantritis is inflammation of the antrum. The antrum includes the nose and its chamber and mucous membranes, the frontal bone and its chamber and mucous membranes, and/or similar structures near the nose bone. "nas/o" is a combining form meaning nose. "antr" is a root word meaning the nose, chamber, and mucous membranes. "antr/o" is a combining form meaning the nose, chamber, and mucous membranes. -itis is a suffix meaning inflammation.

BLOCK	DATA AND ANSWERS	DESCRIPTIONS AND QUESTIONS
11-145	combining form nose root word nose, chamber, mucous membranes combining form the nose, chamber mucous membranes *-itis*	"nas/o" is a _____ _____ meaning _____. "antr" is a _____ _____ meaning _____, _____, and _____ _____. "antr/o" is a _____ _____ meaning _____ _____, _____, and _____ _____. _____ is a suffix meaning inflammation.
11-146	inflammation of the antrum	Nasoantritis is _____ ____ _____ _____.
11-147	nasomental (nayz'-oh-<u>man</u>-toh)	Nasomental means pertaining to the nose and chin. "nas/o" is a combining form meaning the nose. "ment/o" is a combining form meaning the chin. *-al* is a suffix meaning pertaining to.
11-148	combining form chin *-al* pertaining to the nose and chin	"ment/o" is a _____ _____ meaning the _____. _____ is a suffix meaning pertaining to. Nasomental means _____ ____ _____ _____ _____ _____.
11-149	nasolaryngitis (nayz'-oh-lair'-in-gi-tis)	Nasolaryngitis is inflammation of the nose and the voice box. "nas/o" is a combining form meaning nose. "laryng" is a root word meaning voice box. "laryng/o" is the combining form. *-itis* is a suffix meaning inflammation.

BLOCK	DATA AND ANSWERS	DESCRIPTIONS AND QUESTIONS
11-150	combining form voice box *-itis* inflammation of the nose and the voice box	"laryng/o" is a _____ _____ meaning _____ _____. _____ is a suffix meaning inflammation. Nasolaryngitis is _____ _____ _____ _____ _____ _____ _____ _____.
11-151	nasopharyngitis (nayz´-oh-fair-in-gi-tis)	Nasopharyngitis is inflammation of the nose and the throat. "nas/o" is a combining form meaning nose. "pharyng" is a root word meaning throat. "pharyng/o" is the combining form. *-itis* is a suffix meaning inflammation.
11-152	"pharyn/o" Nasopharynitis	_____ is a combining form meaning throat. _____ is inflammation of the nose and the throat.
11-153	rhinorrhea (rye´-noh-<u>ree</u>-ah)	Rhinorrhea is a runny nose (referring to a thin watery discharge from the nose and the mucous membranes). "rhin" is a word root meaning nose and its mucous membranes. "rhin/o" is the combining form. *-rrhea* is a suffix meaning flowing.

BLOCK	DATA AND ANSWERS	DESCRIPTIONS AND QUESTIONS
11-154	word root nose and its mucous membranes combining form rhin *-rrhea* a runny nose (referring to a thin watery discharge from the nose and its mucous membranes)	"rhin" is a _____ _____ meaning _____ _____ _____ _____ _____. "rhin/o" is a _____ _____ meaning _____. _____ is a suffix meaning flowing. Rhinorrhea is ___ _____ _____ _____ _____ __ _____ _____ _____ _____ _____ _____ _____ _____ _____ _____.
11-155	rhinitis (rye'-<u>nye</u>-tis)	*-itis* is a suffix meaning inflammation. Build a medical term meaning inflammation of the nose and its mucous membranes: _____ _____
11-156	dacryocystorhinostomy (dak'-re-o-sis-to'-ri'-<u>nos</u>-to-me)	Dacryocystorhinostomy is creation of an opening into the nose for drainage of tears. (When the path from the tear sac to the eyes is blocked, physicians make an opening into the nose to drain the tears.) "dacry/o" is a combining form meaning tear. "cyst/o" is a combining form meaning cyst or sac. "rhin/o" is a combining form meaning nose. "dacryocyst/o" is a combining form meaning tear sac. *-stomy* is a suffix meaning surgical opening.

BLOCK	DATA AND ANSWERS	DESCRIPTIONS AND QUESTIONS
11-157	combining form tears	"dacry/o" is a _____ _____ meaning _____.
	combining form cyst or sac	"cyst/o" is a _____ _____ meaning _____ ____ _____.
	combining form nose	"rhin/o" is a _____ _____ meaning _____.
	suffix, surgical opening	-*stomy* is a _____ meaning _____ _____.
11-158	creation of a surgical opening into the nose for drainage of tears	Dacryocystorhinostomy is _____ ____ __ _____ _____ _____ _____ _____ _____ _____ ____ _____.
11-159	nasoalacrimal (na'-zo- <u>lak</u>-rim-al)	Nasolacrimal means pertaining to the nose and lacrimal gland or duct. "nas/o" is a combining form meaning nose. "lacrim/o" is a combining form meaning tear gland, duct, and related structure. -*al* is a suffix meaning pertaining to.
11-160	"nas/o" "lacrim/o" -*al* Nasolacrimal	_____ is a combining form meaning nose. _____ is a combining form meaning tear duct, gland, and apparatus. _____ is a suffix meaning pertaining to. _____ is pertaining to the nose and lacrimal gland.

BOX 11.2 Abbreviations	
ABR	auditory brainstem response
AD	right ear (auris sinistra)
AS	left ear (auris dextra)
BOM	bilateral otitis media
dB	decibel
ENT	ears, nose, and throat
EOM	extraocular movement
REM	rapid eye movement
ST	esotropia
TM	tympanic membrane
VA	visual acuity
XT	exotropia

Progress Check

A. Multiple Choice

1. A word root meaning outside layer of the retina is:
   a. choroid
   b. cor
   c. dacryo
   d. dipl

2. A word root meaning correct measure is:
   a. lacrim
   b. leukocoria
   c. emmetr
   d. acoust

3. A root word meaning fungus is:
   a. heter
   b. lacrim
   c. meter
   d. myc

4. A root word meaning dull is:
   a. scler
   b. stapes
   c. ambly
   d. leukocoria

5. A combining form meaning eyelid is:
   a. ton/o
   b. blephar/o
   c. scler/o
   d. stape/o

6. A combining form meaning tear is:
   a. chromat/o
   b. conjunctiv/o
   c. acoust/o
   d. dacry/o

7. A combining form referring to the eustachian tube is:
   a. salping/o
   b. irid/o
   c. kerat/o
   d. lachrym/o

8. A combining form meaning equal is:
   a. chromat/o
   b. cochle/o
   c. is/o
   d. conjunctiv/o

9. A prefix meaning without is:
   a. an-
   b. ab-
   c. super-
   d. hemi-

10. A prefix meaning within is:
    a. hypo-
    b. inter-
    c. peri-
    d. intra-

11. A suffix meaning surgical puncture is:
    a. -al
    b. -algia
    c. -centesis
    d. -ia

12. A suffix meaning pertaining to is:
 a. -ic
 b. -itis
 c. -logist
 d. -malacia

13. A suffix meaning vision is:
 a. -meter
 b. -metry
 c. -logy
 d. -opia

14. A suffix meaning suture is:
 a. -plegia
 b. -ptosis
 c. -rrhaphy
 d. -rrhea

B. Building Medical Terms

Use the following word components to build medical terms matching the definitions given.

an-	is	-opia
chromat/o	-itis	-opsia
-cusis	laryng	opt
cyst	laryng/o	opt/o
cyst/o	-meter	otopy
dacry	metr	otopy/o
dacry/o	metr/o	presby
dipl	my	presby/o
dipl/o	my/o	rhin
heter/o	myring	rhin/o
hetero-	myring/o	-rrhea
hyper-	nas	-stomy
is/o	nas/o	

1. different vision in the two eyes

2. unequal refractive powers in the two eyes

3. defect of vision in which all objects appear colored

4. double vision

5. instrument that measures the power of the muscles of vision

6. pertaining to the nose and tear ducts

7. discharge of pus from the ear

8. inflammation of the eardrum

9. condition where there is a gradual loss of hearing (with aging)

10. creation of an opening into the nose for drainage of tears

11. inflammation of the nose and voice box

C. Definitions and Word Components

	TERM	DEFINITION	PREFIX	WORD ROOT	VOWEL	WORD ROOT	VOWEL	SUFFIX
1.	hemianopia							
2.	opthalmorrhagia							
3.	oculomycosis							
4.	sclerokeratitis							
5.	leukocoria							
6.	otomastoiditis							
7.	myringotome							
8.	anacusis							
9.	nasomental							
10.	rhinorrhea							

D. Abbreviations

	ABBREVIATION	MEANING
1.	ABR	
2.	AD	
3.	AS	
4.	BOM	
5.	dB	
6.	ENT	
7.	EOM	
8.	REM	
9.	ST	
10.	TM	
11.	VA	
12.	XT	

The Endocrine System

BLOCK	DATA AND ANSWERS	DESCRIPTIONS AND QUESTIONS
12-1	endocrine (<u>en</u>-do-krin′)	The word endocrine means secretions. The endocrine system consists of ductless glands that secrete hormones directly into the bloodstream. The endocrine system produces and regulates the hormones that maintain and regulate body balance, metabolism, sensations, and growth. Consult **Figure 12.1** and **Table 12.1** throughout this chapter.
12-2		*endo-* is a prefix meaning within. "crine" is a root word meaning secretions.
12-3	*endo-* "crine" Endocrine	_____ is a prefix meaning within. _____ is a root word meaning secretions. _____ means secretions (from within).

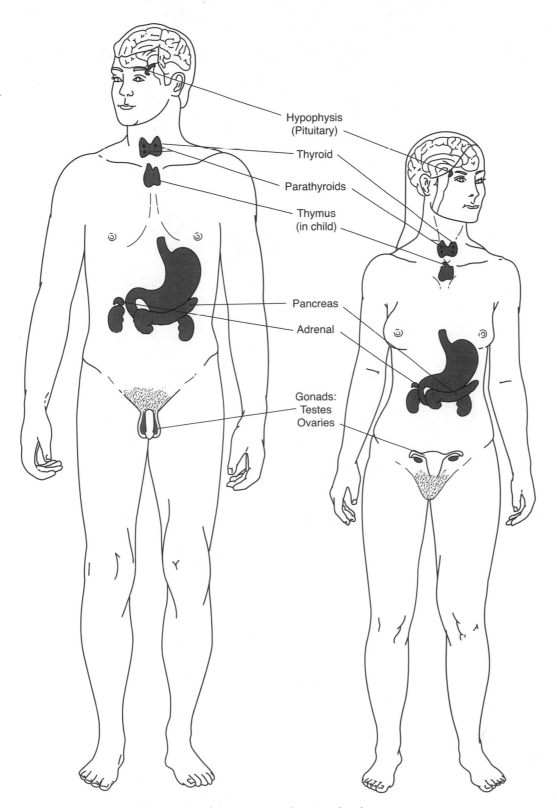

Hypophysis
(Pituitary)

Thyroid

Parathyroids

Thymus
(in child)

Pancreas

Adrenal

Gonads:
Testes
Ovaries

FIGURE 12.1   General locations of the major endocrine glands

TABLE 12.1 Word Components in this Chapter

WORD ROOTS	COMBINING FORMS	PREFIXES
acr	acr/o	adeno-
aden	aden/o	ana-
adip	adip/o	endo-
adipos	adipos/o	epi-
adren	adren/o	eu-
adrenal	adrenal/o	ex-
cyst	cortic/o	hemi-
dips	cyst/o	hyper-
dystrophy	dips/o	hypo-
genital	glyc/o	poly-
gly	gonad/o	syn-
gonad	insulin/o	SUFFIXES
hypophys	lith/o	-al
insulin	oophor/o	-cyte
lith	ophthalm/o	-drome
nephrine	orch/o	-ectomy
oophor	orchi/o	-emia
ophthalm	orchid/o	-ia
orch	pancreat/o	-iasis
orchi	parathyr/o	-ic
orchid	parathyroid/o	-ism
pancreat	pineal/o	-itis
parathyr	test/o	-logy
parathyroid	thym/o	-lysis
pineal	thyr/o	-lytic
pituitar	thyroid/o	-megaly
test		-oid
thym		-oma
thyr		-osis
thyroid		-pathy
toxic		-penia
tropic		-phylaxis
		-physis
		-plasia
		-plasty
		-therapy
		-tomy
		-toxic
		-trophy
		-tropic
		-uria

BLOCK	DATA AND ANSWERS	DESCRIPTIONS AND QUESTIONS
12-4		Locations of the primary endocrine glands:
	pituitary (pi-<u>too</u>-i-ter′-ee), hypophysis (hi′-po-fi-sis), pineal (<u>pi</u>-nee′-al)	brain: pituitary (hypophysis), pineal
	thyroid (thi′-<u>royd</u>), parathyroid (pah′-rah-<u>thi</u>-royd), thymus (<u>thi</u>′-mus)	neck: thyroid, parathyroid, thymus
	pancreas (<u>pan</u>-krc′-uhs), islets of Langerhans (<u>ice</u>-lets of lahng′-er-<u>hahns</u>)	pancreas: islets of Langerhans
	adrenal (ad′-<u>re</u>-no)	kidney: adrenal
		sex glands: ovaries and testes
12-5		Before we proceed to each endocrine gland, let us learn a few key terms applicable to the endocrine system.
	syndrome (<u>sin</u>-drom)	In medicine and psychology, syndrome refers to the association of several clinically recognizable features, signs, and symptoms (observed by a physician) indicative of a specific disease.
		syn- is a prefix meaning together.
		-drome is a suffix meaning a course or set.

BLOCK	DATA AND ANSWERS	DESCRIPTIONS AND QUESTIONS
12-6	prefix, together	*syn-* is a _____ meaning _____.
	suffix, course or set	*-drome* is a _____ meaning _____ _____ _____.
	the association of several clinically recognizable features signs, and symptoms (observed by a physician) indicative of a specific disease	Syndrome is _____ _____ _____ _____ _____ _____ _____, _____, _____ _____ _____ ____ __ _____ _____ ____ __ _____ _____.
12-7		*hypo-* is a prefix meaning under.
		-trophy is a suffix meaning nourishment or development.
	hypotrophy (hi′-po-<u>tro</u>-fe)	Build a medical term (with pronunciation) meaning undernourishment: _____ _____
12-8	anaphylaxis (an′-ah-fil-<u>aks</u>-sis)	Anaphylaxis means without protection.
		ana- is a prefix meaning without.
		-phylaxis is a suffix meaning protection.
12-9	prefix, without	*ana-* is a _____ meaning _____.
	suffix	*-phylaxis* is a _____ meaning _____.
	protection	
	without protection	Anaphylaxis is _____ _____.

BLOCK	DATA AND ANSWERS	DESCRIPTIONS AND QUESTIONS
12-10	adenohypophysis (ad'-en-o-<u>hi</u>-pof-ih-sis)	Adenohypophysis is lack of growth in the glands. "aden" is a word root meaning gland. "aden/o" is a combining form meaning gland. *adeno-* is a prefix meaning gland. *hypo-* is a prefix meaning under. *-physis* is a suffix meaning growth.
12-11	*adeno-* *hypo-* *-physis* Adenohypophysis	_____ is a prefix meaning gland. _____ is a prefix meaning under. _____ is a suffix meaning growth. _____ is lack of growth in the glands.
12-12	endocrinology	"endocrin/o" is a combining form meaning endocrine glands or system. *-logy* is a suffix meaning the study of. Build a medical term meaning the study of the endocrine glands: _____
12-13		Endocrine means secretions within. *endo-* is a prefix meaning within. "crine" is a word root meaning secretions.
12-14	*endo-* "crine" Endocrine	_____ is a prefix meaning within. _____ is a word root meaning secretions. _____ means secretions within.
12-15		We will start with the endocrine glands in the brain. The pituitary gland is the powerful gland responsible for growth. Refer to Figure 12.1.

BLOCK	DATA AND ANSWERS	DESCRIPTIONS AND QUESTIONS
12-16	pituitarism (pi-<u>too</u>-i-ter′-ee-som)	Pituitarism is a condition caused by any disorder of pituitary function. "pituitar" is a root word meaning pituitary gland. -*ism* is a suffix meaning condition. It can be normal or abnormal.
12-17	word root pituitary gland suffix, condition a condition caused by any disorder of pituitary function	"pituitar" is a _____ _____ meaning _____ _____. -*ism* is a _____ meaning _____. Pituitarism is ___ _____ _____ ____ _____ _____ ____ _____ _____
12-18	hypophyseal (<u>hi</u>-poff′-ih-seal)	Hypophysis is another medical term meaning pituitary gland. Hypophyseal means pertaining to the pituitary gland. "hypophys" is a word root meaning pituitary gland and referring to hypophysis. -*al* is a suffix meaning pertaining to.
12-19	"hypophys" -*al* Hypophyseal	_____ is a word root meaning pituitary gland. _____ is a suffix meaning pertaining to. _____ means pertaining to the pituitary gland.
12-20	acromegaly (ak′-ro-<u>meg</u>-ah-le)	Acromegaly occurs when there is excessive growth hormone from the hypophysis after maturity. Enlargement of the extremities and facial bones is called acromegaly. "acr" is a word root meaning extremities (hands and feet). "acr/o" is a combining form meaning extremities (hands and feet). -*megaly* is a suffix meaning enlargement.

BLOCK	DATA AND ANSWERS	DESCRIPTIONS AND QUESTIONS
12-21	"acr/o" *-megaly* Acromegaly	_____ is a combining form meaning extremities (hands and feet). _____ is a suffix meaning enlargement. _____ is enlargement of the extremities and facial bones.
12-22	pineal (<u>pi</u>-nee'-al)	The pineal gland is shaped like a pinecone, which is how it got its name. Look at Figure 12.1 to locate this gland. The exact function of this gland is not known. "pineal" is the root word. "pineal/o" is the combining form. *-ectomy* is a suffix meaning excision.
12-23	pinealectomy (pi'-ne-al-<u>ek</u>-to-me)	Build a medical word that means excision of the pineal gland: _____ _____
12-24	pinealocyte (pi'-ne-al-o-<u>sit</u>)	*-cyte* is a suffix meaning cell. Build a medical word that means a cell of the pineal gland: _____ _____
12-25	piniform (<u>pin</u>-ih-form) pinealoma (pi'-ne-el-<u>o</u>-mah)	Piniform is the shape of the pineal gland. Pinealoma is a tumor of the pineal gland. "pin/o" and "pineal/o" are both combining forms meaning pineal gland. "form" is a word root meaning shape. *-oma* is a suffix meaning tumor.

BLOCK	DATA AND ANSWERS	DESCRIPTIONS AND QUESTIONS
12-26	Piniform	_____ is the shape of the pineal gland.
	Pinealoma	_____ is a tumor of the pineal gland.
12-27		Now, we turn our attention to the neck area. Locate the thymus (a gland) in Figure 12.1. This gland is important in the body's immune system.
	thymus (thi′-<u>mus</u>)	"thymus" and "thym" are word roots for thymus.
		"thym/o" is a combining form meaning thymus.
		-*ectomy* is a suffix meaning excision.
		Build a medical term meaning excision of the thymus gland:
	thymectomy (thi′-<u>mek</u>-to-me)	_____ _____

BOX 12.1
Allied Health Professions

Veterinary Technologists and Technicians: Animal Care and Service Workers

Veterinary technologists and technicians typically conduct clinical work in a private practice under the supervision of a licensed veterinarian. They often perform various medical tests, as well as treat and diagnose medical conditions and diseases in animals. Besides working in private clinics and animal hospitals, veterinary technologists and technicians may work in research facilities.

Many people like animals, but as pet owners can attest, taking care of them is hard work. Animal care and service workers—who include animal caretakers and animal trainers—train, feed, water, groom, bathe, and exercise animals. They also clean, disinfect, and repair their cages. They play with the animals, provide companionship, and observe behavioral changes that could indicate illness or injury. Boarding kennels, pet stores, animal shelters, veterinary hospitals and clinics, stables, laboratories, aquariums, natural aquatic habitats, and zoological parks all house animals and employ animal care and service workers. Job titles and duties vary by employment setting.

A great resource is the American Association for Laboratory Animal Science at www.aalas.org.

Source: P.S. Stanfield, N. Cross, Y. H . Hui, eds. *Introduction to the Health Professions,* 5th ed. (Sudbury, MA: Jones & Bartlett, 2009).

BLOCK	DATA AND ANSWERS	DESCRIPTIONS AND QUESTIONS
12-28	thymolysis (thi′-mo-<u>li</u>-sis)	"thym/o" is a combining form meaning thymus. -*lysis* is a suffix meaning dissolution. Build a medical term meaning dissolution of the thymus: _____ _____
12-29	thyrotoxicosis (thi′-ro-tok′-sih-<u>ko</u>-sis)	Most of us have heard of the thyroid gland, especially those of us with a weight problem. The thyroid gland can secrete a substance to increase our metabolism. Thyrotoxicosis is a toxic condition of the thyroid gland, or thyroid crisis. "thyroid" and "thy" are root words meaning thyroid. "thyroid/o" is a combining form meaning thyroid. "thyr/o" is a combining form meaning thyroid. "toxic" is a root word meaning poison. -*osis* is a suffix meaning condition. It can be normal or abnormal.
12-30	Thyrotoxicosis	_____ is a toxic condition of the thyroid gland or thyroid crisis.
12-31	euthyroid (u′-<u>thi</u>-royd)	*eu*- is a prefix meaning normal or good. Build a medical term meaning normal thyroid: _____ _____
12-32	thyroidotomy (thi′-roy-<u>dot</u>-o-me)	"thyroid/o" is another combining form meaning the thyroid gland. -*tomy* is a suffix meaning incision. Build a medical term meaning surgical incision of the thyroid gland: _____ _____

BLOCK	DATA AND ANSWERS	DESCRIPTIONS AND QUESTIONS
12-33	combining form thyroid gland suffix, surgical incision	"thyroid/o" is a _____ _____ meaning _____ _____. -*tomy* is a _____ meaning _____ _____.
12-34	incision into the thyroid gland	Thyroidotomy is _____ _____ _____ _____ _____.
12-35	hemithyroidectomy (hem'-ih-thi'-roy-<u>dek</u>-to-me)	A hemithyroidectomy is a surgical excision of half (part) of the thyroid gland. *hemi-* is a prefix meaning half. "thyroid/o" is a combining form meaning thyroid gland. -*ectomy* is a suffix meaning excision.
12-36	*hemi-* "thyroid/o" -*ectomy*	_____ is a prefix meaning half. _____ is a combining form meaning thyroid gland. _____ is a suffix meaning excision.
12-37	surgical excision of part (half) of the thyroid gland	Hemithyroidectomy is _____ _____ _____ _____ ____ _____ _____ _____ _____.
12-38	hypothyroidism (hi'-po-<u>thi</u>-roy-dizm)	Hypothyroidism is deficient thyroid gland activity. *hypo-* is a prefix meaning deficient. "thyroid/o" is a combining form meaning thyroid gland. -*ism* is a suffix meaning condition.
12-39	prefix, deficient combining form thyroid gland suffix, condition	*hypo-* is a _____ meaning _____. "thyroid/o" is a _____ _____ meaning _____ _____. -*ism* is a _____ meaning _____.

BLOCK	DATA AND ANSWERS	DESCRIPTIONS AND QUESTIONS
12-40	deficient thyroid gland activity	Hypothyroidism is _____ _____ _____ _____.
12-41	prefix, excess combining form thyroid gland suffix, condition a condition of too much thyroid hormone	*hyper-* is a _____ meaning _____. "thyroid/o" is a _____ _____ meaning _____ _____. *-ism* is a _____ meaning _____. Hyperthyroidism is ___ _____ _____ _____ _____ _____ _____.
12-42	Hypothyroidism Hyperthyroidism	_____ is deficient thyroid gland activity. ' _____ is excessive thyroid gland activity.
12-43	thyrolytic (thi'-ro-<u>lih</u>-tik)	*-lytic* is a suffix meaning destruction. Build a medical term meaning destructive to thyroid tissue: _____ _____
12-44	exophthalmic (eks'-opf-<u>thal</u>-mik)	Exophthalmic means pertaining to eyes bulging outward. One cause of this is a malfunction of the thyroid gland. *ex-* is a prefix meaning outward. "ophthalm/o" is a combining form meaning eyes. *-ic* is a suffix meaning pertaining to.
12-45	pertaining to eyes bulging outward	Exophthalmic means _____ _____ _____ _____ _____.

BLOCK	DATA AND ANSWERS	DESCRIPTIONS AND QUESTIONS
12-46	thyroparathyroidectomy (thi'-ro-pah-rah-thi'-roy-<u>dek</u>-to-me)	Thyroparathyroidectomy is a compound word meaning excision of the thyroid and parathyroid glands. Refer to Figure 12-1 to locate the parathyroid gland. "thyr/o" is a combining form meaning thyroid gland. "parathyroid" is a word root meaning parathyroid. "parathyroid/o" is a combining form meaning parathyroid. -*ectomy* is a suffix meaning excision.
12-47	"thyr/o" "parathyroid/o" -*ectomy* Thyroparathyroidectomy	_____ is a combining form meaning thyroid. _____ is a combining form meaning parathyroid. _____ is a suffix meaning excision. _____ is excision of the thyroid and parathyroid glands.
12-48	parathyroidectomy (pah'-rah-thi-roy-<u>dek</u>-to-me)	Parathyroidectomy is excision of the parathyroid gland.
12-49	combining form parathyroid gland suffix, excision excision of the parathyroid gland	"parathyroid/o" is a _____ _____ meaning _____ _____. -*ectomy* is a _____ meaning _____. Parathyroidectomy is _____ ____ ____ _____ _____.
12-50	parathyroidoma (pah-rah-thi'-roy-<u>do</u>-mah)	Parathyroidoma is a tumor of the parathyroid gland. -*oma* is a suffix meaning tumor.
12-51	Parathyroidoma	_____ is a tumor of the parathyroid gland.

BLOCK	DATA AND ANSWERS	DESCRIPTIONS AND QUESTIONS
12-52	hyperthyroidism (hi′-per-thi-roy-dizm)	Hyperthyroidism is excessive production of thyroid hormone. *hyper-* is a prefix meaning excessive. "thyroid/o" is a combining form meaning thyroid gland. *-ism* is a suffix meaning production.
12-53	prefix, excessive combining form thyroid gland suffix, production	*hyper-* is a _____ meaning _____. "thyroid/o" is a _____ _____ meaning _____ _____. *-ism* is a _____ meaning _____.
12-54	excess production of thyroid hormones	Hyperthyroidism is _____ _____ _____ _____ _____.
12-55	parathyrotropic (pah′-rah-thi-roy-tro-pic)	Parathyrotropic means influencing (stimulating) the activity of the parathyroid gland. "parathyr/o" is a combining form meaning parathyroid gland. "tropic" is a root word meaning influencing (stimulating). *-tropic* also is a suffix meaning influencing (stimulating).
12-56	combining form parathyroid gland suffix, influencing (stimulating) influencing (stimulating) the activity of the parathyroid gland	"parathyr/o" is a _____ _____ meaning _____ _____. *-tropic* is a _____ meaning _____ _____. Parathyrotropic means _____ _____ _____ _____ _____ _____ _____ _____.

BLOCK	DATA AND ANSWERS	DESCRIPTIONS AND QUESTIONS
12-57	thyrotherapy (thi-roy′-theo′-<u>raph</u>-pee)	Thyrotherapy is treatment of the thyroid. "thyr/o" is a combining form meaning thyroid. "therapy" is a root word meaning treatment. -*therapy* also is a suffix meaning treatment.
	combining form thyroid	"thyr/o" is a _____ _____ meaning _____.
	suffix, treatment	-*therapy* is a _____ meaning _____.
12-58	treatment of the thyroid	Thyrotherapy is _____ _____ _____ _____.
12-59		Next we will study medical terms related to the endocrine glands in the abdomen, beginning with the pancreas. Refer to Figure 12.1.
	pancreatolithiasis (pan′-kre-ah-to-<u>lith</u>-i-ah-sis)	Pancreatolithiasis is the presence of stone or calculi in the pancreas. "pancreas" and "pancreat" are word roots meaning pancreas. "pancreat/o" is a combining form meaning pancreas. "lith" is a root word meaning stone (calculi).
		"lith/o" is the combining form. -*iasis* is a suffix meaning the presence of.
12-60	"pancreat/o"	_____ is a combining form meaning pancreas.
	"lith/o"	_____ is a combining form meaning stone (calculi).
	-*iasis*	_____ is a suffix meaning the presence of.
12-61	Pancreatolithiasis	_____ is the presence of calculi in the pancreas.

BLOCK	DATA AND ANSWERS	DESCRIPTIONS AND QUESTIONS
12-62	insulin (in'-<u>soo</u>-lin)	Insulin is a hormone secreted by the islet of Langerhans cells of the pancreas. It lowers blood sugar (glucose) to maintain its normal level in the blood. Because insulin is manufactured by the islets of Langerhans, a structure within the pancreas, insulin is usually synonymous with islets of Langerhans.
12-63	insulinoma (in'-soo-lih-<u>no</u>-mah)	Insulinoma is a tumor of the islets of Langerhans, the source of insulin. "insulin" is a word root meaning insulin. "insulin/o" is a combining form meaning insulin. *-oma* is a suffix meaning tumor.
12-64	"insulin/o" *-oma*	_____ is a combining form meaning insulin. _____ is a suffix meaning tumor.
12-65	a tumor of the islets of Langerhans	Insulinoma is ___ _____ _____ _____ _____ _____ _____.
12-66	insulitis (in'-soo-<u>li</u>-tis)	*-itis* is a suffix meaning inflammation. Build a medical term meaning inflammation of the islets of Langerhans: _____ _____
12-67	insulinopenia (in'-soo-lih-no-<u>pe</u>-ne-ah)	Insulinopenia is a condition of decreased levels of circulating insulin.
12-68	Insulinopenia	"insulin/o" is a combining form meaning insulin. *-penia* is a suffix meaning decreased. _____ is a condition of decreased levels of circulating insulin.
12-69	hyperglycemia (hi'-per-gli-<u>se</u>-me-ah)	Hyperglycemia is a condition of deficient insulin in the blood. This means there is excessive sugar in the blood, one of the major symptoms of diabetes.

BLOCK	DATA AND ANSWERS	DESCRIPTIONS AND QUESTIONS
12-70		*hyper-* is a prefix meaning excessive.
		"glyc" is a word root meaning sugar.
		"glyc/o" is a combining form meaning sugar.
		-emia is a suffix meaning blood.
12-71	prefix, excessive	*hyper-* is a _____ meaning _____.
	combining form	"glyc/o" is a _____ _____ meaning
	sugar	_____.
	suffix, blood	*-emia* is a _____ meaning _____.
12-72	excessive sugar in the blood	Hyperglycemia is _____ _____ ____ _____ _____.
12-73	hypoglycemia (hi'-po-gli-<u>se</u>-me-ah)	Hypoglycemia occurs when there is a deficient level of sugar in the blood. Usually, it is caused by too much insulin in the blood.
		"glyc/o" is a combining form meaning sugar.
		-emia is a suffix meaning blood.
12-74	prefix, deficient	*hypo-* is a _____ meaning _____.
	combining form	"glyc/o" is a _____ _____ meaning
	sugar	_____.
	suffix, blood	*-emia* is a _____ meaning _____.
12-75	a deficient level of sugar in the blood	Hypoglycemia is ___ _____ _____ _____ _____ ____ _____ _____.
12-76	polyglycourea (pol'-e-gli-ko-<u>u</u>-re-ah)	Apart from high blood sugar, one symptom of diabetes is polyglycouria.
		poly- is a prefix meaning much or many.
		"glyc/o" is a combining form meaning sugar.
		-uria is a suffix meaning urine.

BLOCK	DATA AND ANSWERS	DESCRIPTIONS AND QUESTIONS
12-77	*poly-* combining form sugar *-uria* Polyglycourea	_____ is a prefix meaning much or many. "glyc/o" is a _____ _____ meaning _____. _____ is a suffix meaning urine. _____ is too much sugar in the urine.
12-78	polydipsia (poh'-le-<u>dip</u>-se-ah)	One of the cardinal signs of the onset of diabetes is polydipsia, which is an abnormal state of thirst. *poly-* is a prefix meaning much. "dips" is a word root meaning thirst. "dips/o" is a combining form meaning thirst. *-ia* is a suffix meaning state.
12-79	"dips/o" *-ia* Polydipsia	_____ is a combining form meaning thirst. _____ is a suffix meaning state. _____ is a state of much thirst.
12-80		The adrenal glands are located on the top of each kidney. Refer to Figure 12.1. These structures make many hormones for the body, including those related to sexual and nervous functions. "adrenal" and "adren" are two word roots meaning the adrenal glands. "adrenal/o" and "adren/o" are the two combining forms.
12-81	adrenomegaly (ad-re'-no-<u>meg</u>-ah-le)	"adren/o" is a combining form meaning adrenal gland. *-megaly* is a suffix meaning enlargement. Build a medical word meaning enlargement of the adrenal gland: _____ _____

BLOCK	DATA AND ANSWERS	DESCRIPTIONS AND QUESTIONS
12-82	"adren/o"	_____ is a combining form meaning adrenal gland.
	-*megaly*	_____ is a suffix meaning enlargement.
	Adrenomegaly	_____ is enlargement of the adrenal gland.
12-83	epinephrine (ep'-ih-<u>nef</u>-rin)	Epinephrine is a hormone produced by one specific part of the adrenal gland.
		epi- is a prefix meaning above.
		"nephrine" is a root word meaning kidney.
12-84	prefix, above	*epi-* is a _____ meaning _____.
	word root	"nephrine" is a _____ _____ meaning
	kidney	_____.
	hormone produced by one specific part of the adrenal gland	Epinephrine is a _____ _____ ____ _____ _____ _____ ____ _____ _____ _____.
12-85	adrenalopathy (ad-re'-nal-<u>op</u>-ath-e)	Adrenalopathy is any disease of the adrenal glands.
		"adrenal/o" is a combining form meaning adrenal glands.
		-pathy is a suffix meaning disease.
12-86	"adrenal/o"	_____ is a combining form meaning adrenal glands.
	-*pathy*	_____ is a suffix meaning disease.
12-87	adrenal hyperplasia (ad-re'-nal hi'-per-pla-<u>se</u>-ah)	Adrenal hyperplasia is overdevelopment of the adrenal glands or enlarged adrenals.

BLOCK	DATA AND ANSWERS	DESCRIPTIONS AND QUESTIONS
12-88		"adrenal/o" is a combining form meaning adrenal gland.
		hyper- is a prefix meaning excessive.
		-plasia is a suffix meaning growth or development.
12-89	"adrenal/o"	_____ is a combining form meaning adrenal gland.
	hyper-	_____ is a prefix meaning excessive.
	-plasia	_____ is a suffix meaning growth or development.
	Adrenal hyperplasia	_____ _____ refers to enlarged adrenals.
12-90	adrenocortical hyperplasia (ad-re'-no-<u>cor</u>-tih-ko hi'-per-<u>pla</u>-se-ah)	Adrenocortical hyperplasia is excessive development of the adrenal cortex. Cortex refers to a specific part of the adrenal gland. Cortical is the adjective for cortex.
		"cortical" and "cortic" are the word roots.
		"adren/o" is a combining form meaning adrenal gland.
		"cortic/o" is a combining form meaning cortex.
		-al is a suffix meaning pertaining to.
		hyper- is a prefix meaning excessive.
		-plasia is a suffix meaning development.
12-91	"adren/o"	_____ is a combining form meaning adrenal.
	"cortic/o"	_____ is a combining form meaning cortex.
	hyper-	_____ is a prefix meaning excessive.
	-plasia	_____ is a suffix meaning development.
12-92	Adrenocortical hyperplasia	_____
		_____ is excessive development of the adrenal cortex.

BLOCK	DATA AND ANSWERS	DESCRIPTIONS AND QUESTIONS
12-93	hypoadrenocorticism (hi′-po-ad-re-no-<u>kor</u>-ti-sizm)	Hypoadrenocorticism is the condition of underfunctioning of the adrenal cortex. *hypo-* is a prefix meaning under or less. "adren/o" is a combining form meaning adrenal. "cortic/o" is a combining form meaning cortex. *-ism* is a suffix meaning state or condition.
12-94	*hypo-* "adren/o" "cortic/o" *-ism*	_____ is a prefix meaning under or less. _____ is a combining form meaning adrenal. _____ is a combining form meaning cortex. _____ is a suffix meaning state or condition.
12-95	Hypoadrenocorticism	_____ is underfunctioning of the adrenal cortex.
12-96	corticoid (<u>kor</u>-tih′-koyd)	Corticoid means resembling the cortex. "cortic/o" is a combining form meaning cortex. *-oid* is a suffix meaning resembling.
12-97	"cortic/o" *-oid* Corticoid	_____ is a combining form meaning cortex. _____ is a suffix meaning resembling. _____ means resembling the cortex.
12-98	cortical (<u>kor</u>-tih′-kal) adrenocortical (ad-re′-no-<u>kor</u>-tih-kal)	Build a medical term meaning pertaining to the cortex: _____ _____ Build a medical term meaning pertaining to the adrenal cortex: _____ _____

BLOCK	DATA AND ANSWERS	DESCRIPTIONS AND QUESTIONS
12-99	adrenalitis (ad′-re-nal-i̱-tis)	*-itis* is a suffix meaning inflammation. "adrenal/o" is a combining form meaning the adrenal glands. Build a medical term meaning inflammation of an adrenal gland: _____ _____
12-100	Adrenotoxic	*-toxic* is a suffix meaning toxic. "adren/o" is a combining form meaning adrenal gland. _____ is a substance that would be poisonous to the adrenal glands.
12-101		Note that in the above two blocks, two combining forms meaning adrenal glands are used: "adren/o" and "adrenal/o."
12-102	adrenalectomy (ad-re′-nal-e̱k-to-me)	"adrenal/o" is a combining form meaning adrenal gland. *-ectomy* is a suffix meaning excision. Build a medical term meaning excision of the adrenal gland: _____ _____
12-103	combining form adrenal gland suffix, excision excision of the adrenal gland	"adrenal/o" is a _____ _____ meaning _____ _____. *-ectomy* is a _____ meaning _____. Adrenalectomy is _____ _____ _____ _____ _____.
12-104	adrenogenital (ad-re′-nal-je̱n-ih-tal)	Adrenogenital means pertaining to the adrenal glands and genitals. "adren/o" is a combining form meaning adrenal gland. "genital" is a root word meaning genitals.

BLOCK	DATA AND ANSWERS	DESCRIPTIONS AND QUESTIONS
12-105	"adren/o"	_____ is a combining form meaning adrenal gland.
	"genital"	_____ is a root word meaning genitals.
	Adrenogenital	_____ means pertaining to the adrenal glands and genitals.
12-106	adrenitis (ad-re′-<u>ni</u>-tis)	Adrenitis is inflammation of an adrenal gland.
		"adren/o" is a combining form meaning adrenal gland.
		-*itis* is a suffix meaning inflammation.
12-107	"adren/o"	_____ is a combining form meaning adrenal gland.
	-*itis*	_____ is a suffix meaning inflammation.
	inflammation of an adrenal gland	Adrenitis is _____ _____ _____ _____ _____.
12-108		Our final group of medical terms for the endocrine system is related to the sex organs.
	oophorocystectomy (o′-o-fo′-ro-sis-<u>tek</u>-to-me)	An oophorocystectomy is the excision of an ovarian cyst.
		"oophor" is a word root meaning ovary.
		"oophor/o" is a combining form meaning ovary.
		"cyst" is a root word meaning sac.
		"cyst/o" is a combining form meaning sac.
		-*ectomy* is a suffix meaning excision.

BLOCK	DATA AND ANSWERS	DESCRIPTIONS AND QUESTIONS
12-109	"oophor/o," combining form root word, sac *-ectomy* Oophorocystectomy	_____ is a _____ _____ meaning ovary. "cyst" is a _____ _____ meaning _____. _____ is a suffix meaning excision. _____ is excision of an ovarian cyst.
12-110	oophoroplasty (o'-o-fo-ro-<u>plas</u>-te)	"oophor/o" is a combining form meaning ovary. *-plasty* is a suffix meaning plastic repair. Build a medical term meaning plastic repair of an ovary: _____ _____
12-111	oophoritis (o'-o-fo-<u>ri</u>-tis)	"oophor/o" is a combining form meaning ovary. *-itis* is a suffix meaning inflammation. Build a medical term meaning an inflamed ovary: _____ _____
12-112		Testis (testes) means testicle and has four root words and four combining forms. The four root words are "test," "orch," "orchi," and "orchid." The four combining forms are, respectively, "test/o," "orch/o," "orchi/o," and "orchid/o."
12-113	testitis (<u>tes</u>-ti'-tis) orchitis (or'-<u>ki</u>-tis)	*-itis* is a suffix meaning inflammation. Recall that the two combining forms meaning testis (testes) are "test/o" and "orch/o." Build a medical term meaning an inflamed testis: _____ _____ Build another medical term meaning inflammation of a testis: _____ _____

BLOCK	DATA AND ANSWERS	DESCRIPTIONS AND QUESTIONS
12-114		*-ectomy* is a suffix meaning excision. Recall that the two combining forms for testis (testes) are "test/o" and "orchi/o."
		Build two medical terms meaning incision into a testis:
	testectomy (tes-<u>tek</u>-to′-me)	1. _____ _____
	orchiectomy (ord′-ke-<u>ek</u>-to-me)	2. _____ _____
12-115	hypogonadism (hi′-po-go-<u>nad</u>-izm)	Hypogonadism is the condition of decreased function of the gonads.
		hypo- is a prefix meaning decreased.
		"gonad" is a word root meaning gonads.
		"gonad/o" is a combining form meaning gonads.
		-ism is a suffix meaning condition.
12-116	prefix, decreased	*hypo-* is a _____ meaning _____.
	"gonad/o"	_____ is a combining form meaning gonads.
	-ism, suffix	_____ is a _____ meaning condition or function.
	Hypogonadism	_____ is a condition of decreased function of the gonads.
12-117	adiposogenital dystrophy (ad-dih-po′-so-<u>jen</u>-ih-tal <u>dis</u>′-tro-fe)	Adiposogenital dystrophy is abnormal development of the fat tissues in the genitals resulting in decreased sexual development. Adipose tissues are fatty tissues.
		Adipose has two combining forms, "adip/o" and "adipos/o."
		"genital" is a root word meaning the genitals.
		"dystrophy" is a root word meaning disordered (difficult or bad) growth or development.
		dys- is a prefix meaning disordered (difficult or bad).
		-trophy is a suffix meaning growth or development.

BLOCK	DATA AND ANSWERS	DESCRIPTIONS AND QUESTIONS
12-118	combining form fat "genital" root word disordered, difficult, bad Adiposogenital dystrophy	"adipos/o" is a _____ _____ meaning _____. _____ is a root word meaning the genitals. "dystrophy" is a _____ _____ meaning _____, _____, or _____. _____ _____ is abnormal development of the fat tissues in the genitals resulting in decreased sexual development.

BOX 12.2
Abbreviations

ACTH	adrenocorticortropic hormone
ADH	antidiuretic hormone
DM	diabetes mellitus
FBS	fasting blood sugar
GH	growth hormone
GTT	glucose tolerance test
NIDDM	non–insulin-dependent diabetes mellitus
PTH	parathyroid hormone
RAI	radioactive iodine
TFT	thyroid function test

Progress Check

A. Multiple Choice

1. A word root meaning eye(s) is:
   a. insul
   b. nephr
   c. ophthalm
   d. pineal

2. A word root meaning a stone is:
   a. glyc
   b. lith
   c. orch
   d. testes

3. A combining form meaning blood sugar is:
   a. adrenal/o
   b. glyc/o
   c. parathry/o
   d. thyroid/o

4. A combining form meaning fat is:
   a. adipos/o
   b. cortic/o
   c. orchid/o
   d. thym/o

5. A prefix meaning above is:
   a. ana-
   b. endo-
   c. epi-
   d. hemi-

6. A suffix meaning cell is:
   a. -al
   b. -cyte
   c. -drome
   d. -ectomy

7. A suffix meaning normal or abnormal condition is:
   a. -emia
   b. -ism
   c. -ic
   d. -iasis

8. A suffix meaning dissolution is:
   a. -ine
   b. -ia
   c. -itis
   d. -lysis

9. A suffix meaning resembling is:
   a. -lytic
   b. -megaly
   c. -oid
   d. -oma

B. Building Medical Terms

Use the following word components to build medical terms matching the definitions given.

acr/o	hypo-	ophthalm/o
aden	-iasis	pancreat/o
aden/o	-ic	parathyroid
adren	insulin	parathyroid/o
adren/o	insulin/o	-penia
cortic	-ism	-physis
cortic/o	lith	poly-
cyst/o	lith/o	thyr/o
-ectomy	-megaly	thyroid/o
ex-	oophor	uria
glyc	oophor/o	-uria
glyc/o	ophthalm	

1. lack of growth in the glands

2. enlargement of the extremities and facial bones

3. pertaining to eyes bulging outward

4. excision of the thyroid and parathyroid glands

5. stone or calculi in the pancreas

6. condition of decreased levels of circulating insulin

7. excess sugar in the urine

8. pituitary gland

9. underfunctioning of the adrenal cortex

10. excision of an ovarian cyst

C.   Definitions and Word Components

	TERM	DEFINITION	PREFIX	WORD ROOT	VOWEL	WORD ROOT	VOWEL	SUFFIX
1.	hypotrophy							
2.	supradrenals							
3.	endocrinology							
4.	thyrotoxicosis							
5.	hemithyroidectomy							
6.	hyperglycemia							
7.	adrenalopathy							
8.	hyperplasia							
9.	adrenogenital							

D. Abbreviations

	ABBREVIATION	MEANING
1.	ACTH	
2.	ADH	
3.	DM	
4.	FBS	
5.	GH	
6.	GTT	
7.	NIDDM	
8.	PTH	
9.	RAI	
10.	TFT	

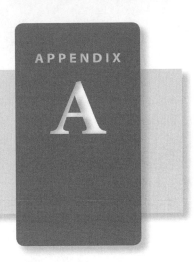

Bibliography

Chabner DE. *The Language of Medicine*, 8th ed. New York: Elsevier; 2007.

Dorland's Illustrated Medical Dictionary, 31st ed. New York: Saunders; 2007.

Jones BD. *Comprehensive Medical Terminology*, 2nd ed. Florence, KY: Delmar Cengage Learning; 2006.

Merriam-Webster's Medical Dictionary. Springfield, MA: Merriam-Webster; 2006.

Mosby's Dictionary of Medicine, Nursing, and Health Professions. New York: Elsevier/ Mosby; 2008.

Stedman's Medical Dictionary for the Health Professions and Nursing, 6th ed (illustrated). Philadelphia: Lippincott Williams & Wilkins; 2007.

Venes D (ed.). *Taber's Cyclopedic Medical Dictionary*. Philadelphia: F. A. Davis; 2009.

WebMD. *Webster's New World Medical Dictionary*, 3rd ed. Hoboken, NJ: Wiley; 2008.

Answers to Chapter Progress Checks

Chapter 2   Eight Keys to Building Medical Terms

A. Multiple Choice

1. a	**3.** d	**5.** a	**7.** c
2. c	**4.** b	**6.** a	**8.** b

B. Definitions and Word Components

	TERM	DEFINITION	PREFIX	WORD ROOT	VOWEL	WORD ROOT	VOWEL	SUFFIX
1.	antitoxin	against a toxic substance	anti-	toxin				
2.	biliary	pertaining to the bile		bil	i			-ary
3.	disinfect	free of infection	dis-	infect				
4.	endometritis	inflammation of the lining of the uterus	endo-	metr	o			-itis
5.	mucous	pertaining to mucus		mu				-ous
6.	quadriplegia	paralysis of all four extremities	quadri-					-plegia
7.	zoophobia	fear of animals		zoo				-phobia
8.	hemophobia	fear of blood		hem	o			-phobia
9.	cerebrospinal	(space flowing) through the brain and spinal cord		cerebr	o	spin	o	-al
10.	natal	pertaining to birth		nat	a			-al

C. Medical Terms and Their Definitions

	TERM	DEFINITION
1.	onychomycosis	condition of fungal infection of the nails
2.	corectasis	dilation of the pupil
3.	rachiotomy	incision into the spine
4.	pelvimetry	process of measuring the pelvis
5.	psychotherapy	treatment of the mind or soul
6.	tracheostenosis	narrowing or constriction of the windpipe
7.	melanoderma	discoloration of the skin
8.	nephropathy	disease of the kidney
9.	laparoscopy	use of a scope to penetrate the abdomen wall to study the abdominal cavity
10.	albumin	specific protein substances in the blood
11.	exophthalmia	condition of protrusion of the eyeballs due to a hormonal disorder
12.	dyspareunia	condition of difficult, painful mating or sexual intercourse
13.	hemigastrectomy	removal of half of the stomach
14.	presbycusis	hearing problems due to old age
15.	panencephalitis	inflammation of the entire brain
16.	hemolysis	breaking down of blood components, cells, or pigments; in biology or medicine it means breaking down of red blood cells
17.	bradypnea	slow breathing
18.	euphoria	state of well-being
19.	dystocia	difficult labor
20.	cholecystitis	inflammation of the gallbladder

D. Abbreviations

See Box 2.2.

Chapter 3   Whole-Body Terminology

A. Multiple Choice

1. c	**4.** a	**7.** a	**10.** a
2. d	**5.** c	**8.** d	**11.** b
3. b	**6.** b	**9.** a	**12.** d

B. Matching

1. i	**4.** g	**7.** d	**9.** f
2. h	**5.** j	**8.** e	**10.** b
3. a	**6.** c		

C. Medical Terms and Their Definitions

	TERM	DEFINITION
1.	connective tissue	one of the fibrous tissues of the body, serving a binding function for special parts of the body (e.g., bones, tendons)
2.	diaphragm	dome-shaped muscle separating the abdominal and thoracic cavities
3.	epigastric region	located between the right and left hypochondriac regions, beneath the cartilage of the lower ribs; usually covers parts of the right and left lobes of the liver and a major portion of the stomach
4.	integumentary system	consists of the skin and accessory organs, such as nail, hair, and oil and sweat glands; in Latin, integument means covering
5.	mediastinum	mass of tissues and organs separating the two lobes of the lungs and separating the sternum in front and the vertebral column behind; includes the heart, its large and small vessels, and all respiratory branches leading to the lungs from the nose
6.	peritoneal cavity	space containing the stomach, intestines, liver, gallbladder, pancreas, spleen, reproductive organs, and urinary bladder
7.	sagittal plane	divides the body into right and left portions that may or may not be equal
8.	tissue	group of cells combined to form a structure that has a special responsibility or function in the body
9.	transverse plane	divides the body into superior and inferior sections (top and bottom)
10.	umbilicus	root word meaning navel

D. Abbreviations

See Box 3.2.

Chapter 4   The Integumentary System

A. Multiple Choice

1. b	**5.** a	**8.** b	**11.** c
2. a	**6.** c	**9.** a	**12.** a
3. d	**7.** d	**10.** c	**13.** d
4. c			

B. Building Medical Terms

1. electrodesiccation	**4.** onychocryptosis	**7.** rhytidoplasty	**9.** tenea pedis
2. dermatofibroma	**5.** escharotomy	**8.** cutis hyperelastica	**10.** epidermis
3. dermatoconiosis	**6.** dermabrasion		

C. Definitions and Word Components

	TERM	DEFINITION	PREFIX	WORD ROOT	VOWEL	WORD ROOT	VOWEL	SUFFIX
1.	dyskeratosis	faulty development of the epidermis in which it has abnormal, premature, or imperfect keratin formation (keratinization)	dys-	kerat	o			-osis
2.	onychophagia	biting of fingernails		onych	o			-phagia
3.	subcutaneous	under the skin	sub-	cutane	o			-ous
4.	autodermato-plasty	plastic repair using a patient's own skin for the skin graft		aut	o	dermat	o	-plasty
5.	heterodermato-plasty	plastic repair using skin from a donor for the skin graft		heter	o	dermat	o	-plasty
6.	keratosis	a horny skin growth		kerat	o			-osis

	TERM	DEFINITION	PREFIX	WORD ROOT	VOWEL	WORD ROOT	VOWEL	SUFFIX
7.	intraepidermal	within the epidermis	intra-	epiderm	o			-al
8.	hyperelastica	excess elasticity	hyper-	elastica				
9.	dermatoplasty	plastic repair of the skin		dermat	o			-plasty
10.	melanocytes	cells that form color pigments (black or dark) in the skin		melan	o			-cytes

D. Abbreviations

See Box 4.2.

Chapter 5   The Gastrointestinal System

A. Multiple Choice

1. c   **3.** d   **5.** d   **7.** d

2. a   **4.** c   **6.** b

B. Building Medical Terms

1. sigmoidoscope   **4.** pancreatolith   **6.** esophagogastric or gastroesophageal   **8.** esophagogastro-duodenocopy

2. enterorrphagia   **5.** colorectal

3. hepatitis   **7.** cheilopathy

C. Definitions and Word Components

	TERM	DEFINITION	PREFIX	WORD ROOT	VOWEL	WORD ROOT	VOWEL	SUFFIX
1.	cheilostomato-plasty	plastic surgery of the lips and mouth		cheil	o	stomat	o	-plasty
2.	gastrorrhagia	hemorrhage of the stomach		gastr	o			-rrhagia
3.	esophageal	pertaining to the esophagus		esophag	o			-eal
4.	colopexy	to fix the colon surgically		col	o			-pexy

	TERM	DEFINITION	PREFIX	WORD ROOT	VOWEL	WORD ROOT	VOWEL	SUFFIX
5.	proctologist	physician who specializes in the diseases of the rectum and anus		proct	o			-logist
6.	hepatomegaly	enlargement of the liver		hepat	o			-megaly
7.	odontalgia	toothache		odont	o			-algia
8.	oligodontia	having less than the normal amount of teeth		olig	o	odont	o	-ia
9.	gingivectomy	surgical removal of gum tissue		gingiv	o			-ectomy
10.	glossosis	pertaining to the tongue		gloss	o			-osis
11.	sialolith	salivary stone		sial	o			-lith
12.	esophagos-tenosis	narrowing of the esophagus		esophag	o			-stenosis

D. Abbreviations

See Box 5.2.

Chapter 6   The Respiratory System

A. Multiple Choice

1. b   5. d   9. a   12. a
2. a   6. b   10. c   13. b
3. c   7. b   11. b   14. d
4. c   8. b

B. Building Medical Terms

1. rhinostenosis
2. nasopharyngitis
3. pleuritis
4. thoracocentesis
5. tracheo-pharyngotomy
6. coccidioido-mycosis
7. orthopnea
8. nasogastric
9. endotracheal
10. bronchospasm

C. Definitions and Word Components

	TERM	DEFINITION	PREFIX	WORD ROOT	VOWEL	WORD ROOT	VOWEL	SUFFIX
1.	tracheopharyngotomy	incision into the trachea and the larynx		trache	o	pharyng	o	-tomy
2.	pneumoconiosis	disease of the lungs caused by breathing dust particles		pneum	o	coni	o	-osis
3.	histoplasmosis	fungal infection of the lungs resembling tuberculosis		hist	o	plasm	o	-osis
4.	nasopharyngeal	pertaining to the nose and pharynx		nas	o	pharynge	o	-al
5.	hemoptysis	spitting of blood or of blood-stained sputum (from the lungs)	hemo-					-ptysis
6.	atelectasis	incomplete expansion of the lungs at birth, or collapse of the adult lung		atel	o			-ectasis
7.	sinusitis	inflammation of the hollow spaces within the nasal cavity (sinus)		sinus	o			-itis
8.	pertussis	whooping cough	per-	tussis				
9.	tuberculosis	infectious disease of the lung, caused by mycobacterium tuberculosis and marked by small swellings (abscesses) in tissues of the lung		tubercul	o			-osis

	TERM	DEFINITION	PREFIX	WORD ROOT	VOWEL	WORD ROOT	VOWEL	SUFFIX
10.	bronchiectasis	chronic dilatation (or expansion) of one or more bronchi or a branch of the respiratory tract		bronchi	o			-ectasis

D. Abbreviations

See Box 6.2.

Chapter 7   The Cardiovascular System

A. Multiple Choice

1. b	**5.** b	**9.** a	**12.** d
2. d	**6.** a	**10.** c	**13.** b
3. a	**7.** d	**11.** b	**14.** a
4. c	**8.** a		

B. Building Medical Terms

1. phlebolithiasis	**3.** sphygmo-manometer	**5.** cardiomyopathy	**8.** thrombocytopenia
2. varicoid	**4.** pericardectomy	**6.** erythroblastosis	**9.** hemosiderosis
		7. agranulocytes	**10.** cardiogenic

C. Definitions and Word Components

	TERM	DEFINITION	PREFIX	WORD ROOT	VOWEL	WORD ROOT	VOWEL	SUFFIX
1.	aortostenosis	narrowing of the aorta		aort	o	sten	o	-osis
2.	lymphadeno-tomy	incision of a lymph node		lymph	o	aden	o	-tomy
3.	pericardec-tomy	removal of the membrane around the heart	peri-	card	o			-ectomy
4.	arterioscle-rosis	hardening of an artery		arteri	o	scler	o	-osis
5.	intracardiac	within or inside the heart	intra-	cardi	o			-ac

	TERM	DEFINITION	PREFIX	WORD ROOT	VOWEL	WORD ROOT	VOWEL	SUFFIX
6.	supravalvular	above a valve	supra-	valvul	o			-ar
7.	thrombocy-tolysis	destruction of blood platelets		thromb	o	cyt	o	-lysis
8.	endocarditis	inflammation of the lining of the heart	endo-	card	o			-itis
9.	venorrhaphy	suturing of a vein		ven	o			-rrhapy
10.	hemangioma	tumor of blood vessels		hem	o	angi	o	-oma

D. Abbreviations

See Box 7.2.

Chapter 8   The Nervous System

A. Multiple Choice

1. b   **5.** c   **8.** b   **11.** b

2. d   **6.** a   **9.** a   **12.** c

3. a   **7.** d   **10.** d   **13.** a

4. c

B. Building Medical Terms

1. dysphasia   **3.** encephalomalacia   **6.** ventriculogram   **9.** myeloschisis

2. meningo-cephalocele   **4.** anencephalia   **7.** dipsomania   **10.** narcolepsy

5. hydromyelocele   **8.** anesthesia

C. Definitions and Word Components

	TERM	DEFINITION	PREFIX	WORD ROOT	VOWEL	WORD ROOT	VOWEL	SUFFIX
1.	encephalo-sclerosis	hardening of the brain		encephal	o	scler	o	-osis
2.	cephalalgia	pain in the head (headache)		cephal	o			-algia
3.	electroen-cephalogram	a record (graphic chart) of the electrical impulses of the brain		electr	o	encephal	o	-gram

	TERM	DEFINITION	PREFIX	WORD ROOT	VOWEL	WORD ROOT	VOWEL	SUFFIX
4.	rachiomyelitis	inflammation of the spinal canal and cord		rachi	o	myel	o	-itis
5.	oligophrenia	little (defective) mental development		olig	o	phren	o	-ia
6.	myelomeningocele	herniation of spinal cord and its membranes		myel	o	mening	o	-cele
7.	hyperesthesia	excessive sensitivity	hyper-	esthes	o			-ia
8.	schizophrenia	major psychosis or mental disorder		schiz	o	phren	o	-ia
9.	poliomyelitis	viral disease causing inflammation of the nerve cells (gray matter) of the spinal cord		poli	o	myel	o	-itis
10.	psychosomatic	pertaining to the body and mind		psych	o	somat	o	-ic

D. Abbreviations

See Box 8.2.

Chapter 9: The Genitourinary System

A. Multiple Choice

1. b	**5.** c	**9.** a	**12.** c
2. b	**6.** a	**10.** b	**13.** c
3. d	**7.** d	**11.** a	**14.** d
4. a	**8.** a		

B. Building Medical Terms

1. nephrolithiasis
2. orchiopexy
3. hydronephrosis
4. vesicotomy
5. pyelonephritis
6. pyuria
7. ureterostenosis
8. cryptorchidism
9. episioperineoplasty
10. cystoplasty

C.   Definitions and Word Components

	TERM	DEFINITION	PREFIX	WORD ROOT	VOWEL	WORD ROOT	VOWEL	SUFFIX
1.	episiorrhaphy	suture of (a tear in the) vulva		episi	o			-rrhaphy
2.	cystotrachelotomy	incision of the neck of the urinary bladder		cyst	o	trachel	o	-tomy
3.	prostatovesiculitis	inflammation of the prostate gland and (seminal) vesicles		prostat	o	vesicul	o	-itis
4.	amenorrhea	no menstrual discharge	a-	men	o			-rrhea
5.	urethrocystitis	inflammation of the bladder and urethra		urethr	o	cyst	o	-itis
6.	orchiepididymitis	inflammation of the testes and epididymis		orchi	o	epididym	o	-itis
7.	menometrorrhagia	excessive uterine bleeding		men	o	metr	o	-rrhagia
8.	oligomenorrhea	scanty menstrual discharge		olig	o	men	o	-rrhea
9.	trachelocystitis	inflammation of the neck of the urinary bladder		trachel	o	cyst	o	-itis
10.	nephromegaly	enlargement of a kidney		nephr	o			-megaly

D.   Abbreviations

See Box 9.2.

Chapter 10   The Bones, Muscles, and Joints

A. Multiple Choice

1. c	5. d	8. c	11. a
2. b	6. b	9. a	12. d
3. d	7. b	10. b	13. c
4. c			

B. Building Medical Terms

1. tenomyoplasty	4. craniomalacia	7. spondylarthritis	9. pedialgia
2. tibiofemoral	5. iliofemoral	8. submaxillary	10. tarsectomy
3. calcaneodynia	6. musculoskeletal		

C. Definitions and Word Components

	TERM	DEFINITION	PREFIX	WORD ROOT	VOWEL	WORD ROOT	VOWEL	SUFFIX
1.	ankylodactylia	stiffened, crooked, or fusion of the fingers or toes		ankyl	o	dactyl	o	-ia
2.	carpoptosis	drop or falling wrist		carp	o			-ptosis
3.	intrasternal	pertaining to within the sternum	intra-	stern	o			-al
4.	osteoporosis	condition of bones with cavities or pores (due to a lack of calcium)		oste	o			-porosis
5.	osteosclerosis	the condition of hardening of bone cells		oste	o	scler	o	-osis
6.	rachicentesis	puncture into the spinal column		rachi	o			-centesis
7.	sternoclavicular	breast bone and collar bone		stern	o	clavicul	o	-ar
8.	sternoid	resembling the breastbone		stern	o			-oid

	TERM	DEFINITION	PREFIX	WORD ROOT	VOWEL	WORD ROOT	VOWEL	SUFFIX
9.	suprascapu-lar	pertaining to above the shoulder blade	supra-	scapul	o			-ar
10.	vertebroster-nal	pertaining to the vertebrae and breastbone		vertebr	o	stern	o	-al

D. Abbreviations

See Box 10.2.

Chapter 11   The Sensory Organs

A. Multiple Choice

1. a	**5.** b	**9.** a	**12.** a
2. c	**6.** d	**10.** d	**13.** d
3. d	**7.** a	**11.** c	**14.** c
4. c	**8.** c		

B. Building Medical Terms

1. heterometropia	**4.** diplopia	**8.** myringitis	**11.** nasolaryngitis
2. anisometropia	**5.** optomyometer	**9.** presbycusis	
3. hyperchro-matopsia	**6.** nasolacrimal	**10.** dacryo-cystorhinostomy	
	7. otopyorrhea		

C. Definitions and Word Components

	TERM	DEFINITION	PREFIX	WORD ROOT	VOWEL	WORD ROOT	VOWEL	SUFFIX
1.	hemianopia	blindness in half of the visual field	hemi-	an	o			-opia
2.	opthalmor-rhagia	hemorrhage from the eye		opthalm	o			-rrhagia
3.	oculomycosis	disease of the eye caused by a fungus		ocul	o	myc	o	-osis
4.	sclerokeratitis	inflammation of the sclera and the cornea		scler	o	kerat	o	-itis
5.	leukocoria	condition of white pupil		leuk	o	cor	o	-ia

	TERM	DEFINITION	PREFIX	WORD ROOT	VOWEL	WORD ROOT	VOWEL	SUFFIX
6.	otomastoiditis	inflammation of the ear and the mastoid bone		ot	o	mastoid	o	-itis
7.	myringotome	knife used for surgery on the eardrum		myring	o			-tome
8.	anacusis	without hearing		an	a			-cusis
9.	nasomental	pertaining to the nose and chin		nas	o	ment	o	-al
10.	rhinorrhea	thin watery discharge from the nose (a runny nose)		rhin	o			-rrhea

D. Abbreviations

See Box 11.2.

Chapter 12 The Endocrine System

A. Multiple Choice

1. c **4.** a **6.** b **8.** d

2. b **5.** c **7.** b **9.** c

3. b

B. Building Medical Terms

1. adenohypophysis **4.** thyroparathyro-idectomy **6.** insulinopenia **9.** hypoadreno-corticism

2. acromegaly **5.** pancreatolithiasis **7.** polyglycouria **10.** oophoro-cystectomy

3. exophthalmic **8.** hypophysis

C. Definitions and Word Components

	TERM	DEFINITION	PREFIX	WORD ROOT	VOWEL	WORD ROOT	VOWEL	SUFFIX
1.	hypotrophy	underdevelopment	hypo-					-trophy
2.	suprarenals	above the kidneys	supra-	renals				
3.	endocrinol-ogy	study of endocrine glands	endo-	crin	o			-logy
4.	thyrotoxicosis	toxic condition of the thyroid		thyr	o	toxic	o	-osis

	TERM	DEFINITION	PREFIX	WORD ROOT	VOWEL	WORD ROOT	VOWEL	SUFFIX
5.	hemithyroi-dectomy	surgical removal of half of the thyroid	hemi-	thyroid	o			-ectomy
6.	hyperglyce-mia	excessive sugar in the blood	hyper-	glyc	o			-emia
7.	adrenalopa-thy	disease of the adrenals		adrenal	o			-pathy
8.	hyperplasia	overdevelopment	hyper-					-plasia
9.	adrenogenital	pertaining to the adrenals and genitals		adren	o	genit	o	-al

D. Abbreviations

See Box 12.2.

Index

All index entries refer to the block where the item can be found. For example, 9-166 refers to Chapter 9, block 166.